S0-DZH-150

An Investigative Approach to Industrial Hygiene

An INVESTIGATIVE APPROACH to INDUSTRIAL HYGIENE

Sleuth at Work

LESTER LEVIN

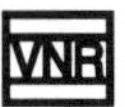

VAN NOSTRAND REINHOLD

I(T)P® A Division of International Thomson Publishing Inc.

New York • Albany • Bonn • Boston • Detroit • London • Madrid • Melbourne
Mexico City • Paris • San Francisco • Singapore • Tokyo • Toronto

I(T)P® A division of International Thomson Publishing, Inc.
The ITP logo is a registered trademark.

Printed in the United States of America

For more information, contact:

Van Nostrand Reinhold
115 Fifth Avenue
New York, NY 10003

Chapman & Hall GmbH
Pappelallee 3
69469 Weinheim
Germany

Chapman & Hall
2-6 Boundary Row
London SEI 8HN
United Kingdom

International Thomson Publishing Asia
221 Henderson Road #05-10
Henderson Building
Singapore 0315

Thomas Nelson Australia
102 Dodds Street
South Melbourne, 3205
Victoria, Australia

International Thomson Publishing Japan
Hirakawacho Kyowa Building, 3F
2-2-1 Hirakawacho
Chiyoda-ku, 102 Tokyo
Japan

Nelson Canada
1120 Birchmount Road
Scarborough, Ontario
Canada M1K 5G4

International Thomson Editores
Campos Eliseos 385, Piso 7
Col. Polanco
11560 Mexico D.F. Mexico

1 2 3 4 5 6 7 8 9 10 BBR 01 00 99 98 97 96

Contents

Preface

This book deals with the recognition and control of health problems associated with working and does so in large part by recounting actual case studies; perhaps, more accurately, *case stories*. Professionally, the field is called occupational health and its practitioners include doctors, nurses, engineers, scientists, and technicians; its clients include just about everybody who goes to work. In particular, it focuses on the role of the occupational health professional who is arguably most directly responsible for protecting our health on the job and solving those problems but who is largely unknown to the general public and therefore needs an introduction; namely, the *industrial hygienist*.

The industrial hygienist can be exasperated trying to explain to an unknowing audience that his or her professional title is not a euphemism for a sanitary worker at an industrial plant, nor does it bear any analogy to a dental hygienist. Failing to convey to the general public by their job title just what they do, industrial hygienists have been trying for years—albeit unsuccessfully—to settle upon a more revealing name. Compounding the problem with their identity, they do not even agree on whether "hygienist" has four syllables (hy-gi-*en*-est) or three (hy-*gien*-ist) with the second, subjectively pronounced either as in "gene" or to rhyme with "ken." They do, however, agree on what they do. Succinctly, they are professionals scientifically trained to protect the health of workers.

Part 1 of the book provides the historical and scientific background which led to the evolution of the profession. Most students—we are told by their professors—flinch at the prospect of reading the history of their subject as if it were a boring irrelevancy. The bias toward history persists among other prospective audiences outside of the classroom. Undismayed, the author believes that the story in this history is neither boring nor irrelevant.

The account is not represented as or intended to be a comprehensive history of the field, citing all the major events and naming all the major contributors and their accomplishments; rather, it explains how the profession evolved as a logical and necessary development in man's progress. It first traces why addressing the health problems from working did not merit a high priority in our social progress. Man initially had to have an understanding of what caused him to get sick outside of work and how to prevent or control illness, particularly epidemic diseases, so that he could survive to work. Other practical considerations—economic, sociological, technological, and legal—which impeded development are also discussed with contemporary references.

Part 2, which constitutes the major portion and focus of the book, is comprised of twelve case studies grouped under four general categories involving mysterious or less than obvious causes of illness at work investigated by an industrial hygienist. This case study/story approach to the subject has a lot to do with the experiences of the author who has spent his career practicing industrial hygiene in industry and as a consultant, and by teaching—and learning from—graduate students in industrial hygiene and the environmental sciences. As Scheherezade and most good teachers have learned, you keep your audiences awake and challenged by telling an intriguing tale in which they can play an informed and reactive role. Many years after my former students have forgotten the formulas or the historical names of the lectures, they can recall why the vat cleaner overexposed earlier to solvent vapors at work flunked a mandated test for drunk driving after causing a highway accident, why the discontented map reproduction workers in a large office building inexplicably complained of getting headaches only at work, why the residents thought they might lose their hearing or their minds from the combined noises from a dog kennel and the new automatic car wash in the neighborhood, and what went on at a college job that caused the normally placid part-time student to become argumentative and show signs of paranoia.

Most industrial hygiene investigations of workplace health complaints and illnesses identify obvious or fairly predictable causes or contributing conditions, but every so often the expert is stumped at the outset. Without being able to identify the likely suspect, it is impossible to establish whether the complaint is work related. Barring a harmless remission of the complaint, the hygienist is further frustrated in achieving the ultimate goal of the profession: to prevent or control the problem. Those few cases in which the hygienist is challenged to act as a "sleuth at work" to solve the mystery provide the most appealing and informative case selections. The what, why, and how of industrial hygiene practice are conveyed and retained more effectively thereby in the mind of the reader by the graphic story.

Attempting to write about nonfiction science in a narrative style invites the same kind of criticisms and concerns that historians might raise about historical novels. Can science, which uniquely employs a methodology to determine truth, be represented in the form used by fiction? Surely liberties have to be taken in the storytelling to represent dialogues and events not personally heard or seen by the writer but which are paradoxically introduced for verisimilitude and drama. The essential elements of the cases described are, indeed, true; whatever the author learned from the case resulted from the experience, which we are reminded has no substitute. Where records are missing and memory is strained, the most reasonable account of the vacuity is introduced consistent with the related facts and professional experience. All names and characters in these stories are fictitious and any resemblance to actual people, however unavoidable, is unintended.

Part 3 deals at length with two vocations with distinctive and unusually high safety and health hazards. Before workmen's compensation laws were enacted, common law held that a worker assumed the risks commonly associated with the job and, therefore, could not be compensated for any incapacitating injury or illness; hence, the term of assumption of risk. In the classic Studs Terkel book *Working*, workers of all stripes report in their own words how they feel about their jobs. A great many workers—though certainly not all—express their discontent and boredom, having little sense of fulfillment or personal satisfaction from their work, and only work because they must. Then, there are the happy dedicated few who love what they do and continue to have inordinate pride in their work. The odd couple of beauticians and firefighters are the essay subjects in Part 3 who represent, in contemporary version, "The Risk Assumers."

It is the author's hope that the book will have appeal to a diverse audience. It can serve as an introductory or supplementary textbook for students in occupational health and the environmental, biological, and physical sciences. Insofar as it introduces a relatively little known field ancillary to our burgeoning focus on human health and the environment, it may well serve in career guidance for science and engineering undergraduates, and for scientifically oriented high school seniors. It provides useful information to medical and health practitioners, plant and office managers, lawyers, claims and insurance adjustors, plant supervisors, business people, employers, and workers; in short, anyone whose responsibilities involve keeping themselves and their workers healthy and safe on the job. Since most people work, or live with, or depend on people who do, and have concern and interest in health matters, the book is aimed at a general-interest audience. Finally, although it may seem like preaching to the converted, even industrial hygienists may find the book informative and useful. The varieties of our individual professional experiences are such that they may overlap but they rarely coincide, so that we may learn by sharing our experiences or enjoy the reinforcement from a common experience.

Acknowledgments

Many friends, colleagues, my Drexel University graduate students—who now span both of the prior categories—and even relatives, who warrant their own category, have offered helpful suggestions with portions of the manuscript. I have also depended on the kindness of strangers who have graciously served as valuable sources of information, or for corroboration and corrections. I have personally thanked each of these literary accessories but without intending any slight or lesser degree of appreciation, there are those who merit special recognition and thanks for their contributions.

My polymath good friend, Nat Matlin, has generously shared with me his technical library and been an unfailing source for information and confirmation in matters of medical history, science and technology, literary references, and the cinema. My wife's sister, Harriet Eisenberg, who as a medical secretary and translator honed her editing skills on the research submissions of her distinguished physician bosses, applied similar surgical and restorative service to my early efforts. Dr. Alex Liddie, Professor of English at Trenton State College, spent an academician's holiday generously reviewing most of the manuscript with judicious editorial suggestions and comments, belying the poet Philip Larkin's warning of the difficulty in communicating ". . . to find words at once true and kind. . ."

Dr. John P. Barry, Adjunct Professor at Drexel University, and former student Dr. Chrysoula J. Komis, CIH, both with OSHA, and Dr. Melvin A. Benarde, Professor and Director of the Asbestos and Lead Abatement Center at Temple University provided technical corrections with valuable suggestions in their reviews of selected case stories and essays. Although the case stories of industrial hygiene investigations deal with technical and scientific subjects in a book intended for classroom application, the book is also intended for a general, albeit reasonably well-read, audience. Consequently, several *relatively* representative readers with diverse backgrounds kindly offered their responses with helpful comments from a nontechnical perspective including: my cousin Henry K. Davis, a retired travel industry executive, who as autobiographer in his own "write," critically blue-penciled drafts of my early case stories; my sister Jean Lauren, a visiting nurse and animal rights advocate; my son Dr. Andrew Levin, an international agricultural development specialist; my daughter-in-law Carole G. Levin, an agricultural resource administrator and apiarist; my daughter Judith Gail Lindenberger, a corporate communication and training manager; and my daughter Laura Ellen Fried, a nurse and a hand clinic administrator.

The background information for the essay dealing with cosmetologists in Part 3 was largely developed from the doctoral research project of my student, Dr. Geraldine K. Stovall, CIH, which entailed the cooperation of over four hundred hairdressers in providing detailed work health histories and interviews. Graduate student Mohamed Basal was the source of the current underground use of *kohl*, or lead-based eye makeup, in the United States. The updated information on the beauty shop health problems and industry practices has been gratefully provided in interviews with veteran cosmetologists, Arnold Tarr and Mitchell Z. Cohen of Philadelphia, and Glenn Culley of Yardley, Pennsylvania.

Background information for the essay on the fire fighters was initially developed from a master's degree research project undertaken by Drexel University graduate student, Gregory L. Siwinski, CIH, who lived at a Philadelphia Fire Department station in order to be available for collecting exposure data during fire calls. Captain Henry Dollberry of the Philadelphia Fire Department freely shared his experiences and knowledge in interviews and kindly provided me with official department reports and photographs for use in the book. M. Armour Floyd and James Henry generously recounted their personal histories and retrospectives as former Philadelphia fire fighters.

Captain John Turner with almost twenty-two years at the Louisville, Kentucky Fire Department similarly provided me with an informative and personal account of the career fire-fighters' lot in another municipal department.

Orville M. Slye, Fire Protection Specialist and President of Loss Control Associates, Incorporated helped clarify for me some of the technical aspects of fire and fire fighting. He kindly assigned his associate employee, Stephan W. Haines, an intensely dedicated professional fire protection engineer and volunteer fire fighter, to provide a comprehensive technical review of the fire fighter essay. In this reversal of roles, I served as the graduate student submitting the term paper to the professor.

Otto Michael Falk, an artist friend living in Israel, whimsically captured the essence of the case stories with his cartoon drawings which I trust will equally delight the readers.

I am, indeed, very appreciative of the above-named contributors and the many more unnamed individuals with whom I have connected in my practice as an industrial hygienist and who have contributed to my professional experiences and, hence, the material for this book; my teachers, my students, my fellow employees and bosses, colleagues and, especially, the workers whose experiences with workplace illnesses and stresses are the genesis for it all.

My foremost critic and supporter, whose judgment, good sense, and love I cherish above all else is my wife Ruth, to whom this book is dedicated.

PART 1 *The Evolution of a Profession*

Chapter 1

Working and Illness

Suffering from illness has always been part of human existence, and early man must have wondered what made him sick; however, any concerns about getting sick or injured from working were late in developing on several counts. That primitive man did not work in the sense we have in "working for a living" explains an obvious delay. The poor fellow spent most of his time trying to survive by feeding, clothing, sheltering, and protecting himself and his family, whereas the communal advantages of specializing in work only later became one of the markers of a civilized society.

The first specialists at work probably continued to toil alone in their fields or in a shop at home with little awareness of how their work might affect their health. The farmer clearing a field under a hot sun probably experienced acute physical hazards which caused him immediate pain and suffering, such as from heat exhaustion or accidentally breaking a bone. However, it was not obvious to the first artisan—the potter—or a tool worker that inhaling the mineral dusts and metal fumes raised by working at home, day after day, could gradually lead to difficulty in breathing and physical deterioration.

In the fourth century B.C., Plato anticipated modern industry by arguing in *The Republic* that as a matter of necessity and efficiency, the ideal state could not develop and succeed without organized group efforts in working and the production of goods. With communal workplaces, we became more aware of work-associated health problems where the exposures were exacerbated by the increased level of production in more crowded and largely unventilated, noisy, and dangerous atmospheres.

Despite awareness since antiquity of the workplace health and safety hazards of enclosed workplaces like mines, there was little action taken to improve the health and safety of miners or, indeed, of any other workers, until well after the Industrial Revolution, almost 2000 years later. In ancient civilizations, the explanation may have a lot to do with an almost disdainful value placed on physical labor and the worker. Arduous physical work was performed by slaves—men, women, and children—and as long as there was a cheap and adequate supply of this work force, there was little economic, let alone humanitarian, incentive to protect the workers' health. Lest one think that all the ancients were totally lacking in social responsibility, Hammurabi (1792–1750 B.C.), a king of Babylon most renowned for the issuance of the first recorded code of laws, decreed: any builder whose structure collapses causing human loss shall be put to death. Presumably, the crime applied to the loss of laborers as well as building residents or passersby.

In a contemporary reminder that *plus ça change, plus c'est la même chose* (the more things change, the more they remain the same), during a recent industrial hygiene survey of an industrial operation of an international corporation in Nigeria, an industrial hygienist from the parent company was shocked to see the native dock loaders in their bare feet precariously carrying drums weighing well over a hundred pounds on their shoulders.

"Can't we provide them with steel toe safety shoes? It might save a lost time injury," the hygienist suggested to the plant manager.

"Why spend the money?" was the slightly puzzled reply. "We only hire them by the day so it's cheaper to get a replacement."

How then did we come to recognize a moral responsibility to protect the health and safety of all workers? There are some who would argue that society does not willingly or naturally pursue altruism and that laws and regulations are necessary to effect the changes. Resistance to this approach is embodied in the latin maxim *leges sine moribus vanae*, which, freely translated, means "laws without tradition don't work."

Consider the hidebound attitudes of employers and the government about compensating workers for injuries from accidents on the job that persisted in the United States until the twentieth century. There were three principles embodied in the common law that effectively excluded any compensation and exculpated the employer of any financial responsibility.

- The Assumption of Risk. Simply stated, the worker assumed the consequences of the well-known risks of his job as a condition of employment and waived any claims in consequence. Because coal miners might be expected to suffocate or die in mine explosions and a falling circus trapeze artist might miss the net, the incapacitated worker or their widows were ineligible for any compensation.
- Causation by Fellow Servants. If it were your misfortune to be hurt on the job by the untoward and unexpected action of a fellow worker, you also had no recourse for compensation from your employer. Thus, if a co-

worker failed to clean up a grease spill in a dark corner which caused you to fall and break your neck, you were financially on your own until such time as you might get back on the job.

- Contributory Negligence. If neither of the two preceding disclaimers applied, no compensation would be allowed it if could be shown that your actions or inactions *in any way* contributed to your workplace injury or accident. With the burden of proof on the worker and considering the traditional bias against workplace awards, it would be virtually impossible to close this loophole designed to shield the employer from liability.

Compensation for contracting an occupational disease was also difficult to obtain but for different reasons. Whereas physical injury from an accident at work is usually prompt and fairly evident, a disease resulting from chronic exposure at work often takes many years before the onset of confirmatory symptoms. Silicosis, the debilitating dust disease of miners, may not produce significant breathing difficulties for ten years at lower levels of exposure, and mesothelioma, a highly malignant cancer seen in asbestos workers, may show up as much as forty years after the initial exposure. For proof of causation, courts require a precise time and location for the disease, which was clearly untenable. Furthermore, many physicians unfamiliar with the occupational diseases would either misdiagnose their working patients or attribute the symptoms to a nonoccupational cause. The net effect of these positions was to render moot any compensation for worker injury and illness by the employer or society and, consequently, there was no financial incentive for an employer to pay much attention to work health problems or institute workplace safety.

Before the end of the nineteenth century, England had enacted compensation for occupational injuries and illnesses; but as an indication of even the judicial resistance to change in the United States, it was not until 1911 that Wisconsin was successful in enacting the first compulsory workmen's compensation, following attempts by other states which were struck down by the Supreme Court as being *unconstitutional.*

There is an overriding practical consideration having nothing to do with social attitudes and values and the absence of laws and compensation which explains why we have been late in recognizing and doing something to control workplace health and safety problems.

Although many workers have died from their injuries and illnesses, the numbers pale by comparison with the massive toll from deadly diseases in the community. The sudden outbreak and uncontrolled spread of communicable diseases, brought about worldwide by the travels of merchants, sailors, and armies, have been so devastating to life, that at times in our history, it was the history of our times. The epidemic of bubonic plague, aptly called the Black Death, erupted in Europe in 1348 and was estimated to have affected two-thirds of the population, most of whom died, representing an astounding twenty-five million people.

Understandably, just surviving and dying left little time for anything else, including working. As rats were common and fecund residents around the garbage piles and homes of the medieval villages, there was little suspicion that they and the tiny fleas they carried were instrumental in spreading the sudden disease. Apart from fleeing from the scene, there were no effective means of limiting the disease, which meant man was powerless until the disease ran its course. Fortunately, each successive cycle of plague produced lower attack and fatality rates, implying that some degree of immunity to the disease was imparted to the survivors and their progeny, or perhaps whatever was causing the illness was losing its potency.

There were many other communicable diseases making frequent appearances throughout history with undulating death and disability rates, including, in part, typhus, smallpox, dysentery, anthrax, malaria, typhoid fever, syphilis, measles, diphtheria, yellow fever, brucellosis, tuberculosis, and leprosy. Those that are always present in a community and cause a more or less predictable number of cases annually are called endemic; if the number of cases rises dramatically and often, without control, it officially becomes an epidemic; and if it erupts within the same period in many countries of the world, it qualifies as pandemic. The massive suffering and death brought on a community by an epidemic disease, in particular, were immediately evident to all, whereas the health problems of the workers were often slower to develop and were largely familiar only to the affected workers and their families. Only when the major epidemic and communicable diseases had been brought under manageable control and we had achieved economic viability could we begin to pay attention to the toll on our health and safety in the workplace. This is evident in the developing "third world" nations where the struggle to survive precludes any practical attention to the problems of the emerging workplaces.

Whether we find our work ennobling or degrading, that is where we still spend more of our time, including getting there, than any other conscious activity in our lives. The profession dedicated to protecting our health in that uniquely dominating environment evolved from a need to identify and control what causes us to get sick in the first place.

Chapter 2

Early Thoughts on Causes and Cures for Illness

The idea that illness was caused by supernatural forces or evil spirits which invaded the body rather than representatives from the natural world was fairly common among many primitive societies. Among people believing the troublemaker was a nonhuman creature like a demon, it was perfectly reasonable to accept that when man started to work in underground mines and shafts that the resident demons were responsible for sucking out the miners' breath and blowing out their lamps on entering dead air spaces. Later, ominous phenomena from the real world, like foul weather and rancid food, were associated with illness. Strange or fetid odors, in particular, have always been taken as bad news, and workers even to this day, whether in an office, a manufacturing plant, or a classroom, are often convinced that their workplace ills are caused by what they can smell. Early man probably did not regard any of these natural candidates as more "real" than the supernatural ones; more likely, he felt more comfortable dealing with the devils he knew. He could merge conflicting views by believing that the real venomous snake that made him ill by a bite was itself invaded by the evil spirit that was after the man. However untenable any of these explanations for disease causation may appear today, the treatment and control logically followed.

Supernatural Invaders and Lost Souls

It was perfectly reasonable to believe that the cure for an illness caused by an invasive spirit required removal. Phlebotomy, or bloodletting by puncture, the enlistment of leeches, suction caps, and even trepination (i.e., crudely drilling a hole in the skull) were all popularly practiced until recent history as a means of purification and release of the invaders and body poisons. In *A History of Medicine*, Douglas Guthrie wryly observes that among primitive tribes in Borneo, the symbolic removal of a victim's pain by sucking on a straw during a trance resembles early psychotherapy.

Although we tend to look down on many of these primitive practices as naive and ineffectual, they sometimes emerge as empirical antecedents for contemporary treatment. For example, physical massage, which did not require the special training of a medicine man, was originally used to indicate the exit route for the disease-causing invader. Manual workers who suffered from muscular aches and strains were soon to recognize that the massage gave them prompt and sometimes more lasting relief than swallowing any noxious potion from the medicine man; more recently, specialized massaging techniques have been applied in relaxation therapy to relieve the psychological and emotional stresses of the upscale workplace.

Natural Causes

The inevitable failures of the shamans, priests, and other nonmedical practitioners must have raised doubts about the effectiveness of their treatments and the diagnoses. Even in the period dominated by belief in the supernatural causes, there were intimations of a more direct and noetic basis for what causes disease; namely, chemical, biological, and physical agents from man's natural environment. The experience of a direct contact during work that caused a rapid response leading to an irritation or illness (e.g., a farmer in the field brushing against a nettle or a poison ivy leaf or getting stung by a bee) might have suggested something more than a spiritual cause. In support of this direct causation, many primitive farmers have learned empirically without benefit of their local shaman or priest that these same irritations could be assuaged by the application of a sorrel leaf or a mud pack.

Efficacious herbs and drugs of the materia medica of this earlier period have been found to have an actual pharmacological basis, such as the willow bark and leaves and other plants chewed for headaches supplying a related natural form of the active ingredient in aspirin. The prescription was based on treating the symptom rather than the cause of the illness, which may still be the case with headaches.

There were other enlightening associations revealed in some of the early beliefs and actions. The conventional wisdom that these nonhuman creatures bearing disease resided in filthy, dank, and smelly atmospheres, such as privies, suggested that sanitation may have had something to do with the etiology of the disease. The ancients' sometime fear that the healthy could be contaminated by close contact with a diseased victim such as drinking from a common cup also implied the concept of person-to-person communicability. Although not much in the way of medical treatment apart from the spiritual is mentioned in the Bible, there are many references to the importance of personal hygiene and environmental sanitation in preventing disease, such as dietary laws based on food protection and purity ("kosher" means ritual cleaning) and possibly the first identification of the rat as a transmitter of bubonic plague. In terms of preventing communicable disease, the sanitary engineering practices and accomplishments of the Roman Empire were exemplary and have formed the cornerstone of public health ever since. Early in the Etruscan period, the swamps adjoining Rome were drained, a malaria-preventive measure that was also practiced in many ancient societies. Unquestionably, the greatest Roman public health achievements were the building of (1) a sanitary sewer system in the sixth century B.C., (2) public baths, and (3) the later construction of a network of aqueducts to carry fresh uncontaminated water to the metropolis. The Roman water system provided a per capita volume of potable water equal to that supplied to our cities today.

Subtly and cumulatively, these peripheral developments led to a more scientific and rational basis—as we now see it—for explaining disease causation and, consequently, for prescribing more effective treatment and control.

Chapter 3

An Emerging Occupational Health Profession

Most historians regard Hippocrates as the progenitor in the fourth century B.C. of the thinking man's medical practitioner. His school of medicine regarded illness to be the human response to the changing forces of man's environment, the importance of which he spelled out to the physician in his treatise "Airs, Waters and Places." He generally does not not cite a specific agent in the environment which causes disease; rather, he focuses on the attributes or qualities of the environmental factors: heat and cold, wetness and dryness, and personal behavior, which we call "life-style" (that is, moderation or excess in eating, drinking and sex, other indulgences, and physical activity or indolence). However, he did cite the importance of the work environment on health, noting that a metal digger exposed to dusty atmospheres developed breathing difficulties, and he seemed to attribute the colic suffered by a lead worker to his high lead exposure in what might be the earliest report of an occupational disease.

About the first century A.D., Pliny the Elder reported that lead and mercury workers, aware of the toxic health hazard from inhaling the dusts, used crude protective face masks. Considering what the civilized world of this time believed made up matter, it was understandable why most observers focused on the work milieu and did not zero in on a specific causative agent there for the occupational disease. One of the earliest philosophers, Thales of Miletus (circa 585 B.C.) propounded that water is the basis of all matter, which was a starting point for subsequent theories suggesting variously fire, air, and earth as the primal stuff. A century later, Leucippus and Democritus explained matter as being made up of indivisible and indestructible atoms; but not until 1808 did John Dalton, the English chemist and physicist, lay the foundations for modern atomic theory which led to the elemental identification of matter and the development of modern chemistry.

The Roman physician, Galen, born circa 131 A.D., had a dominant and stultifying effect on medical theory and practice for over a thousand years. To his credit, he was probably the first physician to undertake experimentation to explain human physiology, describing how the lungs draw in vital air mixed with blood pumped by the heart, pointing out the diagnostic significance of the pulse. He did comment on the dangerous exposures of miners to acid mists and underground gaseous hazards but offered no suggestions; in fact, no other physician made any substantive contributions to occupational safety and health until the era of Galen's unfrocking by Paracelsus in the Renaissance of the sixteenth century.

The distinctive contributions of three disparate medical practitioners of this era were fundamental to the development of occupational health and warrant special recognition.

Paracelsus (c. 1493–1541)

Philippus Aureolus Theophrastus Bombastus von Hohenheim, whom we know as Paracelsus, was born in Einsiedeln near Zurich a year or so after Columbus discovered the New World, the son of a mining town doctor and a matron at a local hospital. A great deal has been written about this iconoclastic and charismatic figure in the history of medicine, variably called a genius and a fraud, a revealer of the truth, and self-serving egotist and liar. However he and his contributions may be judged, no one contends that the concepts and practice of medicine remained the same after his arrival on the scene.

As a boy and young man, he learned about metallurgy, rudimentary chemistry, and botanical medicine from his father. According to his own testimony, he received a medical degree at the University of Ferrara, but there were no confirmatory records from the university. With or without the degree, it is believed he practiced medicine in Strasbourg and left there around 1527 to accept an appointment as the town physician in Basel. It was alleged that he successfully contained an outbreak of plague in Basel caused by the inadequacies of the Latin-speaking medical establishment, whom he called ignoramuses, fools, and frauds. Four hundred years later, the German film director G.W. Pabst reconstructed the event, portraying Paracelsus as a Nazi Fuhrer symbol in an eponymous 1943 propaganda film which extols his battle against "foreigners" (ironically, Paracelsus was Swiss), intellectuals, and pestilence. Paracelsus' medical tenure in Basel, however, lasted barely a year when he faced arrest on charges of fighting with other doctors and at least one patient.

Because he affirmed that experience and experimentation rather than blind acceptance of groundless and erroneous concepts dating back to Galen would lead to truth in medicine, he set out to acquire this knowledge through extensive travels and discussions with people of all stations throughout Europe. Just when he took off on this quest of twelve or thirteen years is in question, but there is some agreement of his itinerary and activities. He traveled in Italy, Spain, and the Netherlands, where he was reported to have been involved in some military operations, and he later ranged as far west as Cornwall in England and as far east as western Russia and Turkey. Perhaps with successes in his diagnoses and practice of medicine en route, he acquired a following. He became a noted and popular lecturer and writer who scorned the use of scholarly Latin in favor of the vernacular German. Much that is recorded about Paracelsus comes from either his admirers or detractors, but he did leave a body of writing expressing his innovative ideas, which are variably insightful and brilliant, provocative and outlandish, and, often, elusive. Most accounts agree, however, that he shared the social graces, dress, drinking habits, and company of roughnecks, but nobody can be certain whether his death in Salzburg in 1541 was actually the result of a tavern brawl.

Surely, one might expect considerable malarkey from a man who in his pivotal work (the "Paramirium") states that medicine is based on the four pillars of philosophy, astronomy, alchemy, and virtue. On closer inspection and understanding of what he really meant, his approach seems only partly half-cocked. Philosophy is his noble catchall for the application of knowledge obtained by observation from nature and the outer world (the "macrocosm") to that in man (the "microcosm"), reflecting the Hippocratic concept. Astronomy (i.e., astrology) as an indicator of man's fate actually was given short shrift by Paracelsus, but because the heavens are part of the microcosm, he would reason that their effects on nature and man's health could not be ignored. The alchemy he referred to was an explanation for the chemical basis of the body, disease, and toxins. Some latter-day commentators have taken too literal a view of his belief that the basic properties of matter are represented by mercury (that which evaporates), sulfur (that which burns), and salt (that which resists heat). In speaking of the existence of different *kinds* of these same elements, Paracelsus implies a more comprehensive view of the nature of matter. Finally, as an essential believer, Paracelsus felt that the fourth and most important factor of virtue resided in faith in God, which was required to effect healing. This would appear to be more of a reinforcement of the Hippocratic requirement for ethical medical practice than a reliance on divine intervention.

Paracelsus may be likened to a blindfolded dart thrower who, given enough shots, is bound to hit some bull's-eyes, but the overall number of hits on his score card suggests elements of substance and intellectual creativity, if not genius. Indeed, some very significant contributions to toxicology, chemistry, biochemistry, medicine, and occupational health emerge from the pile.

He expressed innovative ideas on the inspection of urine as a diagnostic tool, homeopathic and chemical treatments of disease, the antisepsis of wounds, the use of ether as an anesthetic and morphine (as laudanum or tincture of opium) as a pain killer, and the curative value of mineral baths. Some have even claimed he was an early psychiatrist and forerunner of Freud.

However, his greatest contribution to occupational health might well be the science of toxicology, which some admirers claim entitles him to a claim of paternity. He proposed the concept and identification of a specific chemical entity or "toxicon" of the real world that produces an effect in the body, either good or bad, which is embodied in his oft-quoted definition of a poison.

> All substances are poisons: there is none which is not a poison. The right dose differentiates a poison from a remedy.

Even primitive societies had recognized that toxic extracts from certain plants smeared on an arrow tip or spear enhanced the killing power of the weapon in a way that presaged chemical warfare. The further discovery of all sorts of toxic substances in nature led to applications for poisons in lethal sentencing, as in Socrates' downing of the hemlock and political, domestic, and power-play murders perfected earlier by the Borgias in Italy and later by Catherine de Medici in France during the Renaissance. In the minds of these dispensers, a poison is a poison is a poison. They had no awareness that at the other end of the scale, very small doses of their poison might be beneficial as a remedy or, conversely, that even essentials in our diet like common table salt in huge though admittedly less efficient doses could kill. There are, of course, exceptions and confirmations to Paracelsus' suggestion, adopted by present-day advocates of "hormetics," that a little bit of poison can be curative. His prescription of mercury—a well-known toxin—as a treatment for syphilis was ineffectual, whereas the first somewhat successful drug treatment for the same disease three hundred years later in Paul Ehrlich's "magic bullet" was an arsenic compound.

Industrial toxicologists and hygienists following Paracelsus' dictum have come to regard toxicity as a continuum in which very low levels of most known toxins are, if not therapeutic, at least without demonstrable adverse human health effect to normal healthy workers over a lifetime of exposure. This led to the concept of an acceptable safe level of workplace exposure, or **Threshold Limit Value**, which is basic to industrial hygiene practice and the control of chemical exposures for which we are indebted to the eternally elusive Paracelsus.

Georgius Agricola (1494–1555)

Of necessity, man's earliest vocation and industry was agriculture, which absent mechanization and pesticides was less of a hazardous occupation than today, notwithstanding the greater earlier demands on manual labor. In 1550, a German physician who had started his medical career as the doctor for the mining town of Joachimsthal wrote in the preface to his twelve-volume study of mining and metals, " . . . none of the arts is older than agriculture, but that of the metals (viz, mining) is no less ancient . . . for no mortal man ever tilled a field without implements . . . which are made from metals."

He shrewdly adds that as all useful arts of man depend on metal, very many men became rich and kings became richer from the mines. He was not, of course, referring to the lesser fortunes of the laborers working the mines who got sick, suffered, and died early as a result of their work. He specifically describes a rapidly fatal "consumption" developing from the dust-laden lungs of the Carpathian miners, and without citing the diminishing odds for matrimony, he relates that *some* of the miners' widows successively survived seven husbands.

The author who assumed the more illustrious sounding Latin name of Georgius Agricola was born in 1493 in Saxony (present-day Germany) as Georg Bauer, which surname loses status in the English translation as "peasant." He first received a classical education in Leipzig, served as teacher and principal at a school in Zwickau, and in 1524 went to the Italian universities in Bologna, Venice and, probably, Pisa where he studied medicine and natural sciences for almost three years. On his return, he served as town physician in Joachimsthal for three years during which time he learned all he could about mining and smelting practices from actual work-site trips and extensive reading and discussions with the experienced and most knowledgeable miners and smelters. He took a two- or three-year sabbatical, traveling and studying further into the subject of mining; in 1533, he was appointed as the Chemnitz town physician in Saxony, where he remained until his death in 1555.

In contrast to his rambunctious and antiestablishment contemporary, Paracelsus, Agricola was, with the possible exception of his strong Catholicism during the Lutheran Reformation, main-stream Saxony. He quietly continued his scholarly mining studies for about nine years, often serving as a consultant, was married probably for the second time at age 49 in 1543, had several children, and began writing a series of technical books related to mining and metallurgy in 1544. Although he continued to work as a physician and had many wide intellectual pursuits and civic duties, his chief interests and accomplishments were clearly in mining technology and the natural sciences. The early books which included the first treatments of physical geology and systematic mineralogy and works dealing with underground waters and gases, a history of metals and a glossary of Latin and German terms in mineralogy and metallurgy are prelude to his magnum opus, *De Re Metallica*, completed in 1550 and published posthumously in 1556.

By reporting virtually all that was known or needed to be known about mining and metallurgy in sixteenth-century Europe with illustrative drawings commissioned by the author, this scholarly work was what we indiscriminately call "state of the art." For almost two hundred years, it was the foremost reference and how-to-do-it guide to the industry, although the technology has long since been supplanted. Many of his scientific observations were faulty and the conclusions unwarranted, but to his credit, he is fairly circumspect in his extensive discussion of the controversial use of forked twigs as divining rods for prospecting and the dubious claims of wizards using rings and mirrors. He subtly suggests in a reasoned conclusion that for a serious miner there are more reliable natural indicators.

The historical and technical value of the work was greatly enhanced for the modern reader by its translation into English from the original Latin edition with extensive references and authoritative annotation by Herbert Clark Hoover, the thirty-first president of the United States, and his wife, Lou Henry Hoover. Mr. Hoover had a distinguished and highly successful career as a mining engineer before entering public life.

Although the sections in the two books dealing with the health and safety hazards comprise a relatively small portion of the entire twelve-volume text, Agricola underscores the importance he places on the subject by listing Medicine, meaning the protection of miners against their particular occupational diseases, among the seven needs of information for those engaged in the industry. In that Agricola was as much of an engineer and business man in his thinking as a physician, he also includes Arithmetical Sciences so the entrepreneur can calculate his operating costs and Law so he does not get into trouble over mining rights and jurisdictional claims. What he has to say about the mining health and safety hazards, the source of the problem, and the controls is clear, on target, and fundamental to industrial hygiene practice.

In Book V, which deals with excavation and the digging of shafts and tunnels to access the underground ores, he identifies the specific hazards of flooding, particularly from previously worked nearby sections and the need to drain or pump the water out through the shafts and tunnels. Similarly, in this quotation from the Hoover translation, he cautions miners of breathing hazards working in air depleted atmospheres.

> Air, indeed, becomes stagnant both in tunnels and in shafts; . . . This suffices to prevent miners from continuing their work for long in these places even if the mine is full of silver and gold, or if they continue, they cannot breath freely and they have headaches. This more often happens if they work in these places in great numbers, and bring many lamps, which then supply them with a feeble light because the foul air from both lamps and men make the vapors still more heavy.

Agricola's interest in mechanics and engineering is illustrated when he discusses in considerable detail in Book VI the equipment for pumping out the water and ventilating the mine atmospheres. The mechanical equipment employs wooden block and pulley, the windlass, gear wheels and shafts, rods, and pistons in Rube Goldberg configurations which are variably powered by hand-cranking, horse power, and water buckets and wheels. One nonmechanical device proposed simply takes advantage of prevailing wind currents using a large barrel with a square opening on the windward side connected to pipes to direct the air flow into the shafts. Presumably, there was a contingency for calm days.

The last section of Book VI specifically addresses the miners' health and safety problems. With the caveat that Agricola used sixteenth-century terminology to describe certain exposures and alludes to diseases that we cannot precisely identify, he gave a fairly comprehensive account of many of the mining and metal exposure hazards that we still face today, as shown in Table 3.1.

For completeness sake, Agricola mentions "demons of ferocious aspect," in the penultimate paragraph, which we are told are "expelled and put to flight by prayer and fasting." In common with most pioneers, Agricola's great contribu-

Table 3.1. Health Effects Attributed by Agricola to Exposures in Mining (Sixteenth Century)

Mining Exposures/Conditions	Health Effects
1. Cold, dampness	Injures limbs (trench foot), much ill health, especially in advanced years
2. Extreme dryness, low humidity	Aggravates dust exposures, leading to breathing difficulties (called "asthma" by Greeks)
3. Corrosive, toxic dusts	Consumption (silicosis)
Quartz	
Arsenic and cobalt compounds	Skin ulceration, lung and bone cancer, eye damage
Mercury and compounds	"Fatal"
Lead and compounds	
4. Poisonous vapors, mists, atmospheres	Asphyxiation, breathing difficulties, death
Hydrogen sulfide, sulfur dioxide	
Sulfuric acid	
Carbon monoxide, arsine	
Methane, carbon dioxide	
Oxygen deficiency	
5. Accidents	Traumatic injury, fractures, death
Falls	
Slips	
Burial	
Drowning	
6. Insects	Extreme irritation, itching, death
Ants	
Scorpions	

tion to occupational health rests on his novel and pragmatic approach to the field—which we should emulate today—rather than the historical value of his description of an outdated technology and faulty scientific conclusions.

De Re Metallica was written as a treatise for the practicing miner and shelterer, but, for Agricola, protecting the life and health of the worker is considered more important than the profits, so that work protection is integrated into the text wherever it is applicable. As noted, the technical section dealing with digging shafts and tunnels pointedly warns of the operational hazards to the worker from possible mine collapses and flooding and the health hazards and recommended controls in entering oxygen-depleted and toxic atmospheres. Thus, the mine operator and worker actually facing the problems on the job are directly informed on a practical need-to-know basis. Agricola's unique identification of health and safety considerations in the performance of the job is his legacy to all workers.

Bernardino Ramazzini (1633–1714): The Father of Occupational Medicine

Like his two predecessors of the previous century, the Italian-born Ramazzini studied medicine and, after receiving his degree at the University of Parma in 1659, began practicing in Rome and then Carpi until 1671. He accepted an appointment as a professor of medicine at the University of Modena, which he held for eighteen years and continued to practice there, gaining fame throughout Europe for his investigative studies of epidemic disease first in the community and then in the workplace. In 1700 at the age of sixty-seven, he received a prestigious academic appointment at the University of Padua, where, despite blindness, he remained an active lecturer up until his death on his eighty-first birthday. His career path, as often happens, followed interests sparked by random observation and circumstance rather than planning.

In 1690, there was an epidemic in Modena of lathyrism, a noncommunicable and somewhat rare disease which results in irreversible muscle weakness and paralysis of the legs and lower trunk of the body. Apparently, Ramazzini was successful in identifying the consumption of meal made from a toxic bean (genus *Lathyrus*) commonly known as chickling peas—not to be confused with the tastier chickpea or garbanzo popular in Mediterranean cuisines—as the source of the problem. That is less of a coup for the well-read professor than it appears because Hippocrates had described lathyrism and its causes in his book *On Epidemic* and it was also later reported by other physicians including Pliny the Elder and Galen. Contemporaneously, the year Ramazzini moved to Modena, the Duke of Wurttemburg in Germany banned the eating of foods made from the lathyrus flour, notwithstanding that the chickling pea has to constitute the major portion of the diet to cause the disease. Most peasants knew enough to avoid eating chickling peas as a staple, but in modern times, during periods of crop failures in very poor countries, lathyrism will appear and it has also occurred among the inmates whose diet was mainly chickling peas at a Nazi forced-labor camp in the Ukraine early in World War II.

Ramazzini went on to study the etiology of other community-disease outbreaks, notably malaria, and in his careful and thoughtful approach, he helped contribute to the development of the epidemiological method of disease study without formally applying it; that is, the study of the interrelationship of the three components which together produce the illness: namely, the affected human or animal **host**; the specific chemical, biological, or physical **agent**, which uniquely causes the disease; and, finally, the **environment**, or the place and circumstances under which all three meet. Hippocrates and his followers emphasized the contribution of the external environment, Paracelsus identified and highlighted the concept of a specific and natural, as opposed to a supernatural, agent, and all physicians addressed the internal environment of the host. In some cases, the communicable disease requires animal intermediates called vectors to carry the agent to the host or another agent (e.g., infected rats carrying fleas which, in turn, bite man and thereby transmit the causative microorganism). Misled by the prevailing dogmas and limited by their lack of scientific knowledge, Ramazzini and other investigators of that period were severely handicapped in making real progress toward the conquest of disease.

Fortuitously, at home one day, Ramazzini was shocked to watch a laborer cleaning out the sanitary cesspool at fever pitch, driven by the intolerable agony of the work and the stench of the pit. He concluded that the physician had a moral obligation to attend to the health and suffering of the heretofore ignored workers and thereupon practiced his preaching by starting a systematic study of their workplaces and diseases. He did not limit his attention to the obviously hazardous industrial trades of potters, miners, stone cutters, and the like; rather, anticipating our contemporary view that the health of all workers is affected to varying degrees by their work, his population was a motley mix including midwives, voice teachers, athletes, sailors, and learned men. His findings and recommendations were published in 1700 as *De Morbis Artificum* (*On the Diseases of Trades*), which remained the most comprehensive treatment of occupational health until the scientific and industrial revolutions of the next century.

As an astute and tireless observer, he gave reasonably accurate descriptions of the occupational diseases and provided a lot of commonsense recommendations for reducing exposures and their effects by emphasizing the importance of ventilation, personal hygiene, exercise, protective clothing, and rest periods. His ideas on disease causation were handicapped, once again, by his limited scientific knowledge. His accounts are informative, interesting, and sometimes fanciful, as illustrated in this representative section from *De Morbis Artificum* dealing with painters.

Diseases of Painters

> Painters are attacked by various ailments such as palsy of the limbs, cachexy (general ill health), blackened teeth, unhealthy complexions, melancholia, and the loss of smell. It very seldom happens that painters look florid or healthy, though they usually paint the portraits of other people to look handsomer and more florid than they really are, . . . and if one reads the Lives of painters it will be seen that they are by no means long-lived, especially those that were most distinguished. . . . Their sedentary life and melancholic temperament may be partly to blame for they are almost entirely cut off from intercourse with other men and constantly absorbed in the creations of their own immediate cause. But for their liability to disease there is more immediate cause. I mean the materials of the colors that they handle and smell constantly, such as red lead, cinnabar, white lead, varnish, nut-oil and linseed oil which they use for mixing colors; and the numerous pigments made of various mineral substances. The odors of varnish and the above-mentioned oils make their workrooms smell like a latrine; this is very bad for the head and perhaps accounts for the loss of the sense of smell. Moreover, painters when at work wear dirty clothes smeared with paint, so that their mouths and noses inevitably breathe tainted air; this penetrates to the seat of their animal spirits, enters by the breathing passages the abode of the blood, disturbs the economy of the natural functions and excites the disorders mentioned above. We all know that cinnabar is a product of mercury, that cerussa is made from lead, verdigris from copper, and ultramarine from silver; for colors derived from metals are far more durable than those from vegetables and hence are in greater demand by painters. In fact, the mineral world supplies the materials of almost every color in use and this accounts for really serious ailments that ensue. Painters, then, are inevitably attacked by the same disorders as others who work with metals, although in a milder form.

Ramazzini's contribution to a holistic approach to medical diagnosis and practice is capsuled in his advice to physicians to ask their patients, "What's your occupation?"

The question might help with the diagnosis if the physician knew as much about the particular occupation and workplace exposures there as Ramazzini did. It is unlikely that a general practitioner either from his or her medical school training and experiences has such knowledge, particularly with unfamiliar job titles. Would present-day doctors have the foggiest idea what a roustabout, a gaffer, a busheler, or even the more mundanely titled pipe fitter do without asking some specific follow-up questions? To his credit, Ramazzini made physicians and the rest of us start to think about the workplace contribution to health, which explains why he deserves to be dubbed the Father of Occupational Medicine.

The Industrial Revolution and the Workplace

During the period of Paracelsus, Agricola, and Ramazzini, covering roughly 1500–1700, the modern scientific method of inquiry was being developed and applied brilliantly by Copernicus, Kepler, Galileo, Boyle, Robert Hooke, and Newton, among others, in mathematics, astronomy, physics, chemistry, and biology. Our trio was not, however, in the same league as their contemporary seminal scientists about whose methods and work they were probably unaware. Nevertheless, their contributions symbolically and even in some practical measures helped prepare us to recognize the gradual escalation of workplace hazards in consequence of the Industrial Revolution.

In the eighteenth century, population increases in western Europe expanded the market demands for goods, which could not be satisfied by the limited production capabilities and economic insecurities of home tradesmen and cottage industry. The increased production of goods, which characterizes the Industrial Revolution, began slowly in England around 1760. It was made possible by the introduction of mechanical inventions and machinery driven by water and steam power and ultimately optimized by the division and efficient organization of labor. Concomitantly, industrialization brought about changes for the worker and working conditions that were revolutionary. The individual worker's purchasing power, as well as the national wealth from the new productivity, more than kept pace with the needs created by the rise in population, but the effects on the workers' health and safety were far less beneficial.

Although the mass production of goods and the development of the modern assembly line did not emerge until the early twentieth century, the introduction of steam power and boilers and machinery with rotating equipment without safety guards created hazards of serious physical injury. Metal smelting operations and the manufacture of metal tools and pottery kilns created hot atmospheres with the release of toxic metal fumes and lung-damaging dusts. The textile mills where the cotton and wool fibers were spun and woven were noisy, crowded, dirty, and poorly lit. Mining, which had always been hazardous, was made more so by the ability to dig deeper into the earth with mechanized equipment and the discovery of metal ores and minerals with greater health risks. In all work milieus, these exposures were exacerbated by enclosure and congestion, the lack of adequate ventilation, poor sanitation, darkness, dampness, cold and heat, and the excessively long work hours—particularly for children.

The French and American Revolutions of the late eighteenth century may have paved the way for more representative and democratic governments and processes, but the workers' rights to a healthful and safe workplace were not recognized or appreciably acted upon until well after the industrialization had become an integral part of the economy in the twentieth century. The development of a multiscientific discipline dedicated to reducing workplace hazards certainly received its impetus from that industrial "revolution," but no real progress was possible without the equally revolutionary improvements in public health and the later scientific, political, and social achievements.

Chapter **4**

The Chimney Sweeps: Early Success in Controlling an Occupational Disease

What may be the first successful conquest of an occupational disease was begun early in the new industrial age in England over two hundred years ago and impressively so without benefit of sophisticated science and a heavy infusion of capital. Lacking central heating, the homestead in the damp English climate was kept cozy and the residents fed by an open fireplace which continually and not too efficiently burned coal. The chimneys accumulated heavy deposits of soot which required frequent and periodic cleaning, generally performed by young boys who were small and agile enough to enter and sweep out the narrow chimneys. However young, as soon as a child was able to assist in the eighteenth-century English workplace, he or she was considered part of the work force; thus, nobody mistook the chimney sweeps working from dawn to dusk and barely recognizable through their blackened faces and clothing for little men.

Sir Percivall Pott, a noted surgeon who is probably better known to medical students and physicians today for having named a fracture of the lower fibula and a disease of the vertebrae, first described in 1775 a relatively rare cancer of the scrotum that these young male chimney sweeps developed by the time of their puberty. He correctly surmised that the disease resulted from the chimney sweeps' excessive skin contact with the soot and, therefore, could be controlled with the implementation of personal hygienic measures—daily and thorough washing of the contacted skin and the removal and frequent laundering of protective clothing. In a first-ever action by Parliament in the recognition and control of an occupational disease, the Chimney Sweeps' Act was passed in 1788, the year of Potts' death, requiring these simple preventive measures. The practical vindication of Potts' hypothesis came slowly in the succeeding generations, abetted by the use of mechanical means of cleaning, with the virtual elimination of the dreaded cancer among the chimney sweeps. The more radical measures of establishing a minimum age and hourly limits for child labor and, specifically, the apprenticeship of children as chimney sweeps would not receive any consideration and enforcement until late in the next century.

We now know from chemical analysis that a family of organic chemicals called polycyclic aromatic hydrocarbons (PAHs) constituting as much as 40 percent of the chimney soot will promote the formation of cancer when it is painted on the skin of laboratory test animals. The positive animal test results strengthen the human association with cancer promotion. However, without confirming the results on human subjects—for which there are ethical restrictions—we cannot unequivocally say we proved the causation in people, but we cannot deny Potts his success. Because these PAHs are constituents in high-boiling petroleum-derived products like heavy oils, asphalts, and waxes, in coal tar products, and in the combustion products of coal burning power plants, trash incinerators, oil furnaces, wood-burning stoves, and tobacco, their implication in human cancer causation is evident and strong.

Chapter 5

The Conquest of Communicable Diseases

THE SANITARY REVOLUTION

We tend to believe today that the control and the conquest of human disease requires sophisticated scientific knowledge and methods, when, in fact, a great deal of progress had been made in blissful ignorance of science. From the time of Hippocrates through the nineteenth century, malaria (Italian *mal'aria* for bad air) was believed to be caused by the fetid orders arising from swamps and filth. Without the benefit of identifying the causative disease agents, many early civilizations had figured out that draining the marshes and maintaining environmental and personal sanitation helped prevent the outbreak and spread of malaria and other diseases. The ancient Romans, it was noted, had constructed a magnificent aqueduct system for supplying clean water and a separate sewer system for disposing of the sanitary wastes into the Tiber river for natural purification.

In an early and influential advocacy for the healthful effects of sanitation, Jean Jacques Rosseau in the eighteenth century proselytized his belief that man had enjoyed a healthy and happy life in his natural and "pure" state until civilization befouled him and his environment. The wide-scale promotion of environmental sanitation and personal hygiene in the industrialized world of the nineteenth century led to a Sanitary Revolution, which proved to be the greatest single factor in reducing the incidence of communicable diseases and improving the health and longevity of the population.

Although the healthful advantages of sanitation in the community were generally recognized, the workplace did not seem to warrant the same attention.

Factories, mines, shops, and manufacturing plants at the peak of the industrial expansion remained almost unabashedly dirty, poorly lit, noisy, and unventilated with few on-site provisions for personal washing or change of work clothes to remove the workplace contaminants. Until recently, some workers almost pridefully accepted this double standard as if the squalor was a distinguishing mark of their busy machine shop or office.

By the nineteenth century, the greatest potential for the spread of water-borne enteric diseases such as typhoid fever and cholera arose from the contamination of a community water supply with diseased human wastes. In England, as well as in Europe, there probably were periodic but contained outbreaks of enteric disease from contaminated water supplies in the villages and perhaps even occasionally in the rural areas, but the potential for mass epidemics resulted from the large population increases and densities in the cities created by the Industrial Revolution. It is estimated that in the first twenty years of the nineteenth century in England, which had, by far, the highest industrial rate of growth in Europe and the world, many small villages were converted into manufacturing towns with a near doubling of the population in which most of the people lived without water pipes, drainage, and waste collection. The sewer systems were designed primarily for the drainage of swamps and runoff from rain, whereas the human wastes and leachates from open refuse piles were collected in odorous and leaking cesspools throughout the city. Around 1834, the cesspools in London were allowed to drain into the central sewer emptying into the overloaded Thames River, which, in turn, became an open sewer.

There had been a cholera epidemic in London in 1832 and by 1838, Sir Edwin Chadwick, a sanitarian and lawyer, began a lifetime public health campaign to provide clean water supplies, separate sewers, waste collection, and burial sites to the metropolitan areas. Laws passed by the Parliament in 1848 to make the cities clean up their acts were emasculated by the provision that the sanitation measures could not interfere with the mercantile pursuit of profit.

Chadwick's campaign for separate sanitary waste sewers and clean water supply got a major boost in 1854 resulting from the outbreak of cholera in an undrained slum area in London. Dr. John Snow traced the cholera victims there specifically to users of water from the Broad Street water pump, operated by a water company which obtained its supply from a contaminated section of the Thames. Their neighbors who used water provided by a rival company which tapped into the uncontaminated Thames head waters far above the city were unaffected. By locking up the Broad Street pump and reducing the local cholera outbreak, Snow dramatically demonstrated that cholera was transmitted by the contaminated drinking water.

To this day, during civil wars and natural catastrophes in which there are breakdowns in the water supply and sanitation, the major casualties are often the victims of dysentery, cholera, typhoid fever, and related water-borne diseases.

We are periodically reminded of our vulnerability when our modern water-treating systems are compromised. In the spring of 1993, as many as two hundred and eighty thousand people in the Milwaukee area developed diarrhea with perhaps a half-dozen deaths attributed to water contamination from cryptosporida, a tiny protozoan that is resistant to normal chlorination levels and probably got through the filtration system of one of the city water-treatment plants. Nonetheless, the mass epidemic water-borne diseases had effectively been eliminated in the developed world by the sanitary measures initiated during the nineteenth century in England before the great scientific discoveries of disease etiology and control.

The benefits of these life-saving public health measures were crucial, although less obvious, to the promotion of the workers' health and safety. First, as members of the greater community, workers must be able to survive the epidemic diseases and remain healthy to continue working. Second, in the order of priorities, not until a community was largely free of epidemic diseases could resources and attention be directed to the less visible and pressing health problems of the working poor.

Although occupational diseases and illnesses are generally not considered to be communicable or even epidemic in nature, some of the most important advances in the prevention of infectious and chemically induced diseases arose from health problems in the workplace.

Immunization: A Public Health Dividend from the Workplace

When Edward Jenner as a young English doctor learned from the conventional wisdom that dairymaids who developed the mild cowpox disease from their occupational exposures on the milking stool never got smallpox, he conceived the idea of purposely infecting people with cowpox as a preventive measure against the deadly and feared smallpox. In 1796, without knowing that either disease was caused by a microscopic organism, Jenner inoculated, or vaccinated (Latin *Vaccinus*, pertaining to cows), a young boy with some of the oozing material from an active cowpox sore. Two weeks later, he effectively proved that his "volunteer" did not develop smallpox by being injected with material from an active smallpox sore. The ultimate triumph of Jenner's discovery came when the World Health Organization officially declared in 1979 that smallpox had been eradicated worldwide as the result of a massive vaccination program.

The archetypal work of Pasteur and Koch which led to the first unequivocal identification of a specific microbiological pathogen and the scientific development of a vaccine to prevent its infection was based on anthrax, a highly contagious and virulent animal disease which man largely contracts occupationally. The disease is caused by a bacillus bacterium which can revert to a highly resistant dormant spore until it finds favorable conditions inside a host to start growing and releasing its deadly toxins. The dermal form of the disease in man starts with an itch, followed by a pustule and swelling, although rarely with pain, and in a few days the black scab characteristic of anthrax (L. *anthrax* fr. Greek coal) is formed, by which time deadly toxins have been released throughout the body. Workers handing diseased animals and animal products are infected principally through the skin and occasionally by inhalation from the hair and hide of goats, sheep, cattle, horses, and pigs; hence, it has been called Woolsorters' disease and Ragpickers' disease. More recently, the list of occupation-associated cases of anthrax has been bizarrely extended. In 1979, there was a report of an epidemic in the then Soviet industrial city of Sverdlovsk (Ekaterinburg in prerevolutionary days) causing at least sixty-eight deaths that was blamed on eating infected meat or skin contact with diseased animals. More than a dozen years later, a joint investigation by a western scientist and Russian scientists found evidence that suggested that the deaths were caused by the accidental inhalation by military and civilian personnel of an anthrax aerosol that had escaped from a military microbiology facility that was probably engaged in biological warfare.

In 1876, Koch clinched the germ theory of disease by positively identifying the anthrax bacillus from diseased animals, infecting healthy animals with the diseased animal tissue, and isolating and identifying the same organisms from the final victims. In 1881, Pasteur demonstrated the success of his heat-attenuated anthrax vaccine with sheep before the world press and a prestigious group of scientists in a dramatic made-for-movies scene—which it was in the *The Story of Louis Pasteur* starring Paul Muni. The crowd burst into applause as a barking dog startled a seemingly moribund group of anthrax-exposed but inoculated sheep who rose, as if on cue, and started bleating next to a group of their dead and dying uninoculated brethren.

Workers at particular risk of contracting anthrax such as sheepherders, furriers, veterinarians, insulators, and animal husbandry workers, among others, can be effectively protected from contracting the disease by immunization. Even in the developing countries, the animals at risk have largely been inoculated. Sterilization of animal hides and hair, and burning of diseased animals have greatly reduced the occupational incidence of disease, but once in a while, a case occurs in the United States, usually involving the shipment of some unsterilized animal hair or hide from a less vigilant country. If infection does occur, antibiotics must be given promptly to both animals and man, as they are highly effective in killing the organism but ineffectual against the toxins produced by the invaders.

More recently, health care and dental workers, dentists and surgeons who may be exposed at work to blood and other body fluids contaminated with viral hepatitis B are strongly recommended to receive the vaccine which provides almost 100 percent protection for at least seven years. The incubation period averages fifty to ninety days so that the victims may not suspect infection with a nonspecific feeling of nausea, loss of appetite, abdominal pains, and vomiting, but some victims may develop a fatal liver condition. The Center for Disease Control has estimated that twelve thousand health care workers get infected annually and about 10 percent of these become active carriers of the disease. These workers are at similar risk from all blood-borne pathogens including the HIV (human immunodeficiency virus) associated with AIDS.

Pasteur successfully demonstrated in 1885 with human beings infected with rabies that a vaccine may be used *therapeutically*, which, to this day, is standard treatment for the rabies victim. Although no equally successful therapeutic vaccine for other diseases has been developed for over a hundred years following Pasteur's great triumph, more recently there have been attempts to develop such vaccines for other infectious agents, most promisingly with the herpes simplex virus and, less so, with victims of tuberculosis, AIDS, leprosy, and hepatitis B, among others, and there is even interest in a vaccine to reduce blood cholesterol levels.

Protection by vaccination is theoretically applicable to all infectious diseases, and specific vaccines have been successfully developed for many diseases, including the common childhood diseases of diphtheria, pertussis (whooping cough), and as a prophylactic treatment for tetanus. Consequently, the development of a successful vaccine is virtually at the top of the list in strategies for the ultimate prevention of most uncontrolled infectious diseases. In the 1980s, the Institute of Medicine surveyed the world's top vaccine researchers for their priority nominations for the most needed and reasonably achievable vaccines for the developed and developing nations. The top-ranked candidate for both the developed and developing countries was for the human immunosuppressive virus (HIV) associated with AIDS, which by the early 1990s was believed to be responsible for over half a million deaths annually, with projections for greatly increasing numbers. For the developing world, malaria which causes up to an astounding half-*billion* cases and over two and a half million deaths annually was second, followed by tuberculosis, which is responsible for about two million deaths annually.

Ten years later there had been some notable successes in vaccine development, but despite massive efforts by government and industry, none of the major ranked killers was toppled, There are scientific, financial, and organizational reasons proffered for these humbling failures and, eventually, the vaccine researchers may be successful, but the hopes for immunization as the ultimate disease weapon have been somewhat undermined.

Chemical Control of Disease

The most important scientific developments of the twentieth century with probably the greatest impact in advancing public health in both preventing and treating infectious diseases involved a benevolent kind of chemical warfare.

Chemical Disinfection of Drinking Water

Up until the middle of the nineteenth century, a city discharged its raw sewage into a river or large body of flowing water in which the naturally present bacteria, with sufficient dissolved oxygen, would decompose the organic wastes and the human pathogenic organisms would die off. The cities and towns downstream of the discharge could then obtain reasonably clean and safe, (i.e., pathogen-free water), after simple filtration or primary treatment. If no waterways for disposal were available, the human wastes containing disease pathogens were discharged into underground septic systems or collected in cesspools where the same purification processes occurred but more slowly. With more towns springing up and population density increasing in the cities, resulting from the great industrial expansion, the increased waste discharges overloaded the waterway's natural purifying capacity and contaminated ground and surface water supplies from overflows of cesspools and ground seepage. The water-borne diseases which had killed millions before the sanitary revolution similarly resurfaced, so that by the 1880s in the United States, typhoid fever accounted for up to 100 deaths per 100,000 population and cholera outbreaks were once again common with high death tolls.

By the end of the century, it became evident that drinking-water supplies required disinfection treatment to prevent the return of water-borne epidemic diseases. The answer came with inexpensive and simple chemical treatment of the water with chlorine, which even at low concentrations in solution is a powerful oxidizing and germicidal agent. Chlorination has proven to be tremendously effective in knocking out the most common human pathogens in a relatively short time, with a residual concentration remaining in solution to maintain the biological purity by the time the water is used for drinking, eating, and washing. The chlorine may impart a somewhat objectionable odor and impairment of the taste of the water, which sounds carping considering that it has probably been more responsible than any other single measure for assuring water potability and preventing water-borne microbiological diseases. Typhoid has become so relatively rare in the cities of the developed countries that cases are reported as isolated incidents rather than an incidence rate (i.e., number of cases per 100,000 population).

By the mid-1970s, it was reported that the chlorine reacted at the water-treatment plant with organic chemicals present in the water either from man-made or natural sources to form trace amounts of reaction products called trihalomethanes (THMs). The National Academy of Sciences stated that these chlorine derivatives such as chloroform, bromoform, and dichlorobromomethane, have been demonstrated in animal testing to be carcinogenic with possible human implications, and their review of epidemiological studies suggested a possible association with increased human bladder cancer. Other water-disinfection methods, including ozone, boiling, ultraviolet radiation, and non-THM producing chlorine derivatives such as chloroamines and chlorine dioxide, are all more expensive or impractical substitutes. On any scale of balanced risks, it would appear that the proven record of chlorine in preventing and controlling serious water-borne diseases outweighs the more hypothetical risk of increased cancer cases and its replacement with a disinfection method of unproved long-term safety and reliability.

Antibiotics and Drugs

The discovery of penicillin by Fleming in 1928 and the synthesis and commercial production of it and successor antibiotics revolutionized the battle against infectious diseases during the twentieth century. The prognosis for victims in the pre-antibiotic era of such then common diseases as pneumonia, meningitis, rheumatic fever, endocarditis, and mastoiditis was often dire. The opportune administration of the antibiotics for many diseases drastically reduced or eliminated fatalities, the disease severity, communicability period, and the likelihood of recurrent epidemics. Within a generation, the wonder drugs were freely and indiscriminately prescribed for even the runny noses and high temperatures of an ordinary common cold and extensively fed to cattle, swine, and poultry to prevent disease and promote their growth. In a case of microbial evolutionary adaptation, the surviving pathogens developed resistance to the then current antibiotic. The development and prescription of a new antibiotic would work for a while but time and reproduction rates were on the side of the surviving microorganisms which developed a new generation of resistant and meaner strains. For example, the salmonella organisms commonly associated with food contamination would cause diarrhea and most victims without any complications would recover without antibiotics in a few uncomfortable days. Some particularly susceptible people, such as those who ran an enteric fever, those at both ends of the age spectrum, and people with other illnesses might require the antibiotics. By the end of the 1980s, about a third of these salmonellae were found to be resistant to the antibiotics so that the usual treatment was now often ineffectual resulting in greater morbidity and in some cases, mortality.

The tuberculosis organism which had been largely controlled by early diagnosis of the disease and prompt treatment with the antibiotics introduced in the 1940s has not only become largely resistant to the eleven antibiotics developed since but a more virulent form appears to have evolved. A fulminating tuberculosis epidemic with high fatality has developed in the 1990s among certain highly susceptible populations with compromised immunological systems such as AIDS victims, drug users and many long term prison inmates.

With fewer effective alternate antibiotics being developed while the microorganisms are gaining in resistance, it would seem that the antibiotic as a disease weapon has been a victim of both its successes and excesses.

Pesticides

Dichloro-diphenyl-trichloro-ethane (DDT) was developed in 1939 as a synthetic pesticide to kill a variety of insects on contact. Because it remains active for a long time after application and seemed virtually harmless to man, it provided a powerful new weapon in the battle against insect-borne diseases. During the Second World War, the U.S. military first used the powdered form largely to control body lice and then to contain a flea-borne typhus epidemic that erupted in war-torn Naples. It was later widely applied as a spray to control mosquito vectors for malaria and was, until the mosquitos developed a resistance, the prime control method for malaria in the developing countries as well as for containing yellow fever, encephalitis, and bubonic plague. The early and extensive success of DDT encouraged the development of related chlorinated hydrocarbon pesticides such as lindane, heptachlor, chlordane, and mirex, with more selective and persistent insecticidal power but with higher toxicity for man.

The level of insect-killing power and human toxicity was elevated by the later development of organic phosphate and carbamate pesticides intended primarily to control insect pests damaging to agriculture and as a supplementary weapon against the insects which developed resistance to the older chlorinated pesticides. Unlike the chlorinated compounds which persist in the environment long after they have been applied, the newer pesticides will decompose in a relatively short time but not soon enough to prevent serious accidental injury and death on acute human exposure. Some were so extremely toxic that they might have been considered for chemical warfare and were subsequently eliminated or banned. As an occupational hazard, many agricultural workers were seriously poisoned during spraying or even by contact with the residual pesticide. In one tragic accident, a young child died from dermal contact from a discarded bag of phosphate ester pesticide which served as a cover for a swing seat.

In another area of chemical attack, herbicides which selectively kill weeds were developed to enhance food production. Herbicides now account for almost 90 percent of the total pesticides sold and used in the United States, far surpassing the insecticides.

Analogous to the antibiotic treadmill, the utility of many of the insecticides is compromised as the target insects gain resistance to successive substitute pesticides. However, the benefits to human health of using all pesticides have exacted a price in environmental and health hazards with diminishing returns.

The adverse environmental effects of spraying of DDT as indicated by the increased mortality and reduced reproduction of bird life were popularized in Rachel Carson's *Silent Spring* in 1962 and with continuing supporting evidence, the Environmental Protection Agency (EPA) finally banned DDT in 1972. Carson did not oppose the use of chemical insecticides; rather, she felt, as industrial hygienists do regarding the use of toxic industrial chemicals, that the problems arise from the failure to use them safely and discriminately. Carson's primary concern about DDT, in particular, and pesticides, in general, was their possible effect on human health from a lifetime accumulation of even low levels in man suggested by the bioconcentration of DDT levels in animals and the appearance in man's food chain and in human fat tissue. Later animal studies of DDT metabolites and other chlorinated hydrocarbon pesticides indicated possible carcinogenic activity, and human exposures to the phosphate ester pesticides have been implicated in neurological, reproductive, and possible psychological effects. Despite having made great contributions to saving human life, chemical pesticides, at least in the developed countries, may ultimately be replaced by nonchemical methods because of the now more subtle threats to human health.

There are many examples of laws and regulatory actions in many of these public health issues in which the public could identify a self-interest and accept, but as indicated earlier, the enactment of laws to provide a safe and healthy workplace took a torturously long path well after the recognition of the toll on workers' lives and health.

Chapter 6

The Fight for a Safe and Healthful Workplace

The effort to bring about a legal requirement to improve working conditions in the face of the indifferent, if not antagonistic, attitude of employers and the courts started modestly and appropriately in England just after the turn of the nineteenth century. In focusing on child labor and specifically on the inhumane apprentice system which virtually kept poor—often abandoned—children in bondage, Sir Robert Peel, a social reformer and member of Parliament, appealing on moral grounds, was able to blunt any objection to his first proposal. The Health and Morals of Apprentices Act, which passed easily in 1803, puts an ambiguous twist on whose morals were at issue. The act fixed a daily maximum of twelve hours with no night work but curiously did not put an age limit for the apprentices. The factory walls had to be washed twice a year and work rooms had to be ventilated. In 1819, the first of what became known as the Factory Acts established a minimum age of nine and a maximum workday of eight hours up to the age of 13 for apprentices and children in the mills. In 1833, a twelve-hour daily work limit was established for children up to the age of eighteen, later charitably reduced to 10 hours, and all children under thirteen had to receive at least two hours a day of schooling, which assumed that after an arduous eight hour shift at a factory or mill they could pay attention. Without having any prior provisions for enforcement of the previous legislation, by far the most significant provision of this act was to establish inspectors to enter the workplaces to assure compliance with the regulations and the power to prosecute. Although these civil servants were not chosen for their technical knowledge or experience with workplace exposures, they may be regarded as the forerunners of the governmental industrial hygienist, which under OSHA (Occupational Safety and Health Act) today are called compliance officers. An amendment in 1844 enabled the factory inspectors to appoint physicians to perform qualifying physical examinations and age verification of child workers.

During this period of relatively modest and at times unenforced regulatory action and laws, social reformers and industrialists in England including Robert Owen, Jeremy Bentham, and the seventh Earl of Shaftesbury fought to improve working conditions and eliminate child labor. Picking up in the tradition of Ramazzini, Dr. Charles Turner Thackrah (1795–1833) dedicated his short-lived professional career to a more thorough and contemporary study of the specific work factors which caused ill health and occupational diseases such as lead poisoning and pulmonary dust diseases, and safety hazards with specific instructions for prevention and improving the work conditions.

In the next fifty years or so, workplace exposures were addressed by the general requirement for mechanical ventilation of injurious dusts, particularly in mines, and a specific regulation covered the prevention of lead poisoning in 1883, but there was no knowledge or thought given to how much constituted a safe exposure and "adequate" ventilation. In 1898, notification of industrial diseases was established and Dr. Thomas M. Legge was appointed as the first medical inspector of factories. Subsequently, periodic physical examinations were started first for young workers to assure that their work was not adversely affecting their health, and ultimately in 1937, initial placement and periodic medical examinations were established for all English workers.

In contrast to England's progressive actions during this entire period, there were essentially no regulatory actions taken to protect workers' health and safety in the United States. By the end of the century, the United States had surpassed England as the leading industrial nation, accounting for almost 25 percent of total world manufacturing production. This difference in regulatory response between the opposite sides of the Atlantic was made evident in dealing with what Dr. Donald Hunter cited as ". . . the greatest tragedy in the whole story of occupational disease."

Phosphorus, in the white or yellow form, is an extremely reactive element which glows in the dark (hence, phosphorescent) but will burst into fire when exposed to the air at slightly above room temperatures so that it is stored hermetically or inertly under water. Although discovered in 1674, it was not until 1832 that yellow phosphorus was first used in Germany and Austria to manufacture an easily ignitable match. About 12 years later, the first cases of "phossy jaw," which is a necrosis of the mandible, or lower jaw, were seen among the factory workers of the rapidly growing match industry. The condition, which is uniquely associated with exposure to the white and yellow forms of the elemental phosphorus and not to the red phosphorus polymorph or any of the phosphorus compounds, is unusually insidious and devastating. It takes about five years of exposure on average for the first signs—usually a toothache—to appear, the gums become painfully swollen and abscessed with foul-smelling discharge and the jaw bone deteriorates, leading to a horrifying disfigurement of the face with a mortality rate of about 20 percent. Workplace sanitation and effective controls to limit the exposure of the match workers to the toxic elemental phosphorus could have been implemented, but the substitution of the nontoxic, although less pyrophoric and ignitable, red phosphorus in the manufacture of matches would have eliminated the major source of phossy jaw. Finland and Denmark first banned the use of the toxic phosphorus by 1874, followed slowly by other European countries. A multi-European nation convention in Berne adopted a ban on the manufacture and importing of the white phosphorus matches in 1906. Perhaps because of more vested economic interests in the old-style match industry, England did not take similar legal action until 1910, and in the United States, elimination was directly instituted in 1931 by imposing a heavy tax on the manufacture of white phosphorus matches with an outright ban on imports and exports.

Federal legislation governing working conditions in the United States was jump started by a series of New Deal legislations beginning in June 1933 with the National Industrial Recovery Act—well known as the NRA—which set up under Title I, codes specifying maximum hours and minimum wages and banning child labor. In 1935, the Supreme Court declared Title I unconstitutional, but by then the beginnings of economic recovery from the Great Depression had set in, creating a more favorable climate for advancing social welfare and labor legislation. The Social Security Act of 1935 which is best identified in the public mind for an old-age retirement pension system also had provisions for unemployment compensation, income support to victims or their survivors of industrial accidents and diseases, and prepared the way for a national annual reporting system of occupational injuries and diseases through subsidies to the individual states. Without reliable data and statistics on workplace injuries and health conditions, it would have been difficult to convince the public and the legislators of the importance of addressing the health and safety aspects of working.

The Wagner–Connery act of 1935 which reinstituted the provisions of the NRA was later upheld in its Supreme Court review, and in 1938, the Fair Labor Standards Act established a forty-hour work week and a minimum wage of $0.40 an hour under its stated objective of ". . . the elimination of labor conditions detrimental to the maintenance of the minimum standards of living necessary for health, efficiency and well being of workers." The Walsh–Healey Public Contracts Act in 1936 was a preliminary effort to require compliance with generally recognized recommended workplace health and safety standards. In a carrot-and-stick approach, compliance was a condition for any company or business seeking or awarded a federal contract in excess of ten thousand dollars; however, there was no effective stick, namely, there were no federal inspectors, to enforce the compliance at the work site, particularly during the intense industrial activity of the Second World War. A federal Mine Inspection Act was passed in 1941 attesting to the well-recognized hazards of mining and the advocacy of the powerful mining unions. By the late 1960s, there had been sufficient public awareness of the deaths, disabilities, and diseases in the workplace, bolstered by impressive statistics, that a broad-scale legislative remedy had political and popular appeal. The Coal Mine Safety Act and the Construction Safety Act were passed in 1969 as prologues to the main act, the Occupational Safety and Health Act (OSHA) which was enacted in December 1970. It was, in fact, the most comprehensive and trailblazing regulatory action on workers' health and safety ever taken in the United States.

Chapter 7

It's Now the Law

To meet the goal of ensuring safe and healthful working conditions for their workers by virtually all employers, OSHA gave authority to the Secretary of Labor to promulgate "reasonably necessary and appropriate" workplace standards to help define these conditions. To get under way, OSHA conveniently adopted existing safety and health standards recommended by professional organizations and trade associations. For example, for airborne chemical exposures, OSHA largely adopted the airborne concentration limits of the more commonly used chemical substances that had been recommended in 1968 as threshold limit values (TLVs) by the American Conference of Governmental Industrial Hygienists. The TLVs are daily time-weighted average concentrations believed to be safe to breathe over a lifetime of work. For workplace safety, OSHA turned to the consensus standards and safe working practices from professional safety organizations that had proved to be workable and effective in reducing accidents and injuries. In this early attempt by OSHA to be comprehensive, the sections in the *Federal Register* covering these occupational health and safety standards for general industry and those mandated by the Construction Safety Act for construction consisted of well over a thousand pages, which are frequently supplemented by proposals for proposed additions, revisions, and interpretations of the regulations. Minor provisions of the consensus documents intended to be advisory were indiscriminately adopted in approximately six hundred standards which later proved to be nitpicking, if not silly, when presented as a legal requirement. Industry and political opponents of the agency angrily mocked these nuisance standards such as those requiring the precise wording and designation of the arrow in fire extinguisher signs, a holder for toilet paper, and a sexist provision for a room with a sofa only for tired female employees to rest. OSHA learned to accommodate to political and practical reality, and in November 1978 these six hundred or so *de minimis* (Latin for "trivial") standards were cleaned out. In a bow to free enterprise, employers were given the flexibility to select the method of their choice to comply with certain regulations, which are termed "performance" standards.

Health standards and safety codes were also incorporated from more than twenty government agencies and major acronymic trade and industry standard setting organizations such as American Conference of Governmental Industrial Hygienists (ACGIH), American National Standards Institute (ANSI), American Petroleum Institute (API), American Society of Mechanical Engineers (ASME), American Society for Testing and Materials (ASTM), Compressed Gas Association (CGA), National Fire Protection Association (NFPA), and one pamphlet each from the Institute of Makers of Explosives (IME) and the Fertilizer Institute, which passed on an acronym. There were also rules for employers of eleven of more employees to maintain and report injury and illness records, and all employers had to provide their workers with the requisite safety training and hazard information. For unsafe conditions or exposures that had not been explicitly covered in the regulation but were commonly recognized hazards in the industry, OSHA inspectors could cite the catchall general-duty clause which states that each employer "shall furnish . . . a place of employment which is free from recognized hazards that are causing or likely to cause death or serious physical harm to his employees."

The act authorized compliance safety and health officers to enter a workplace generally without prior notice to investigate an on-site death or serious accident, in response to a specific complaint from an employee, or at random at a workplace covered by the law. If warranted by the findings of the survey, the compliance officer could recommend to the OSHA area Director that the employer be cited for specific noncompliances. The Area Director could seek a court order to cease at once if the situation were judged to be immediately dangerous to life, assess fines with an order to take corrective actions with a time table, or possibly even dismiss the citations.

To employers and industry already antagonistic in the early 1970s to what they regarded as meddlesome and costly government intrusion into their business, the battle lines were soon drawn with little promise of a propitious debut for the new bureaucracy. To industrial hygienists, safety engineers, and occupational medical personnel, however, OSHA showed promise of being a full employment act.

It was considered fair game for industry to impede and then belittle the early inspection activities of the new agency created in the Department of Labor. The act provided for the prompt admission of an OSHA inspector into an employee's work site at all reasonable times upon proper identification to the person in charge. This apparently open-admission policy for inspection was anathema to some hard-nosed company officials and owners who were used to running their operations as restricted fiefdoms without outside interference. Sometimes they simply refused entry to the inspector, who then had to retreat to the regional office to obtain a court-issued warrant and return the next day or so to confront the next roadblock.

The recently hired compliance officers might have had textbook knowledge of workplace health and safety hazards, but they were hard pressed to undertake knowledgeable inspections of workplaces with which they had little or no familiarity. For example, large chemical plants and oil refineries are complex operations which are not generally open to any one outside of the industry or, more likely, outside of the company. Company officials smirked when the OSHA inspector, arriving at a refinery for the first time, had no clue of the functions or work health problems of the huge manufacturing structures they had come to inspect. On these early forays into the enemy's camp, the inspector was often cautious, if not intimidated, and the company was wary, if not antagonistic.

The act equitably provided that the employees and the management were each entitled to a representative to accompany the inspector during the survey and the inspector could ask questions of the workers en route. In an early challenge, a major corporation refused to compensate the employee representative for the time spent performing what they stated was not company business. The issue was brought to the Supreme Court, which upheld the company position in what may have been a judicial vindication but a public relations defeat. Very few companies today, including the original plaintiff—having made their point—withhold pay from the employee participating in the OSHA inspection.

A maturing decade or so later, the OSHA inspectors had developed into well-qualified, experienced, and confident professionals who were trained to encourage employers to maintain employee health and safety protection and loss prevention as a matter of self-interest rather than as a police action. As a sign of conciliation and trust, the agency has even encouraged and accepted self-policing programs by companies with good safety records. Industry has become more cooperative than confrontational, having spent large sums to comply with and sometimes exceed the requirements of the regulations. Even in OSHA inspections that are in response to a worker complaint, almost 60 percent during a recent four-year period failed to cite serious violations and almost a third had no citation of even a minor nature. This does not mean that OSHA is less resolute in achieving its objectives if the inspected company is uncooperative or willful in its noncompliance. Whereas the early fines levied for noncompliance were negotiable paltry sums that most employers would sooner pay than contest or remedy, the agency is no patsy. By proposing a *minimum* of $25 thousand for each willful violation that could result in death or serious physical harm and multiple citations, OSHA has not hesitated to sock recalcitrant and willful violators with multiplicative fines—one, in 1994, totaling almost seven and a half million dollars with civil penalties.

The Occupational Safety and Health Act has indisputably been a boon to the growth in the numbers and influence of industrial hygienists. In the five-year period just before and after enactment of OSHA, there were barely sixteen hundred members in the American Industrial Hygiene Association. A decade later, membership had more than tripled and then doubled in the next ten years to over eleven thousand. Although their total numbers are relatively small compared with other professional and technical occupations, industrial hygienists have assumed top leadership roles in administering OSHA and testifying or advising and, as experts in the field, have been influential in shaping the occupational health laws and policies.

Conflict Resolutions

Anticipating challenges to the citations from the workplace inspections, Congress established in the act an independent presidentially appointed three-member board called the Occupational Safety and Health Review Commission (OSHRC) to adjudicate contested inspections. Insulated by political appointment, the members of the commission did not have to have a judicial background or knowledge of workplace safety and health hazards, the lack of which, some critics of the commission assert, was evident in their decisions. To start the appeal process, an aggrieved company cited for noncompliance could contest the findings and the possible penalties in an informal meeting with the OSHA Area Director. Many such appeals are amicably resolved in the director's office with modified citations and penalties and the promise of the employer to schedule remediations, sometimes with the sweetener of reduced fines, but occasionally an employer refuses to acknowledge their malfeasance, and the appeal process starts its escalation with the OSHRC assigning the case to an administrative law judge.

Any party to the case—the employer, the government, or even the affected employees—can request a review by the OSHRC of the administrative law judge's decision, and the commission's ruling can, in turn, be appealed through the federal courts. To be sure, there is a point of diminishing returns for a company to continue to contest a fine or an order to institute expensive control measures. Of far greater significance in defining the new law via the judicial review process were the appeal cases brought before the Supreme Court by powerful interest groups contesting a new regulation or change in an OSHA standard.

The Benzene Standard: Reasonably Safe Versus Risk Free

No one questioned that benzene, a volatile aromatic hydrocarbon liquid largely derived from petroleum, is toxic, and breathing low levels can lead to serious blood disorders including aplastic anemia with fatal consequences. When epidemiological studies in 1974 and 1975 confirmed earlier studies suggesting that benzene at concentrations under 25 ppm causes leukemia, OSHA, responding to a National Institute for Occupational Safety and Health (NIOSH) recommendation, lowered the then 10 ppm permissible exposure limit to 1 ppm daily limit averaged over eight hours. If an existing standard is judged insufficient to protect employees from a serious threat to human health, OSHA can issue in an emergency temporary standard (ETS) effective immediately, which it did in May 1977. When the district Court of Appeals issued a restraining order of the ETS opining that OSHA had not justified its action with appropriate findings, OSHA responded with a proposal for a permanent standard and the battle to the Supreme Court began.

The act refers to workplace standards that are "reasonably necessary or appropriate to provide safe or healthful employment and places of employment." In proposing to lower the allowable limit to 1 ppm, OSHA argued that preventing leukemia as a form of cancer was their primary consideration and as no safe level of exposure had been demonstrated, they assumed there was none and emphasized that their limit was based on limiting exposure to the lowest feasible (i.e., achievable) limit. The industry opponents contended that OSHA had not proved that the current limit of 10 ppm caused leukemia and, therefore, lowering the level to 1 ppm was unjustified and, by implication, would impose an unnecessary financial burden on industry. The estimated cost to industry of complying with a more restrictive limit of 1 ppm was a numbers game depending on who did the estimating, but the sums were not inconsequential. A consultant for OSHA estimated a first-year initial capital investment and operating costs of approximately $450 million with annual recurring costs of thirty-four million. Although over two-thirds of the thirty-five thousand workers exposed to benzene at the lower levels were employed in rubber manufacturing, the projected costs of compliance were disproportionately higher to the petroleum and petrochemical industries, which explains why the American Petroleum Institute was the principal group contesting the new regulation.

Had OSHA exceeded its authority? A plurality of the Supreme Court, in effect, agreed by upholding the Court of Appeals stay while pointing out the Congress never intended that a workplace can be made entirely "risk-free" which is a distinctly reasonable difference from being made "safe." Only when further studies were reported which supported the likelihood of leukemia risk at the lower levels was OSHA in 1987 able to lower the permissible benzene exposure level. The net effect of the split Supreme Court decision was to restrict OSHA's authority to reduce permissible exposures or establish standards based on unproved assumptions.

The Cotton Dust Standard: Whose Cost? Whose Benefit?

Workers who handle dried raw cotton such as in the spinning of the fiber—not the cotton harvesting and ginning or the processing or handling of the finished textile product—often gradually develop breathing difficulties with chest congestion and coughs. The cotton spinning mills are notoriously dusty and no serious attempts were made at dust control or protecting the workers from inhaling the airborne particles. Almost three centuries ago, Ramazzini had reported similar asthmatic reactions with workers exposed to the dusts from other natural products used for textiles, namely, flax and hemp, and the condition became identified as byssinosis after the Greek word for flax. In an early stage of the disease, within an hour or so of starting the work week after a symptom-free weekend, the typical cotton spinning worker characteristically feels a temporary tightness of the chest, which often disappears before the end of the shift and invariably disappears by night time. The sequence and symptoms suggested a transient allergic reaction and, understandably, the condition was dubbed Monday Morning sickness by the workers. However, with day-after-day exposure to the dust at work, the breathing difficulties gradually extended over the entire day, appeared on successive days, and could eventually lead to a permanent pulmonary disability.

Industrial medical researchers had suggested that the causative agent for the disease was a biologically active agent in the woody portion of the plant containing a soluble broncho-constrictive protein material or possible a contaminant microorganism or endotoxin in the raw cotton dust. Judging that byssinosis constituted a life-threatening health hazard to an estimated 800 thousand cotton workers, principally in the Carolinas, OSHA proposed a detailed Cotton Dust Standard requiring compliance with a reduced dust exposure level preferably by engineering methods of control to the permissible limit or the lowest feasible level with personal dust masks allowed as a backup measure. The standard also mandated a list of work practices to minimize the dust exposures, annual medical examinations, employee education, and training programs and recordkeeping.

Representatives of the cotton industry, for a time, refused to acknowledge byssinosis as an occupational dust disease and implied that the mill employees were suffering the common respiratory disorders and bronchitis largely from their lifelong smoking habits. Even if "Brown Lung," as the victims chose to call their condition as a reminder of the compensable Black Lung disease of the coal miners, was accepted as an occupational disease, the mill owners fought to have the proposed new standard vacated. Bolstered by the executive requirement from the Office of the Management of the Budget (OMB) that a cost–benefit study of any new government regulation was required to justify the action, they argued that the projected costs to the industry of complying with the regulation were excessive and life threatening to *their* health. It is a difficult feat to balance two sides of a cost–benefit equation when the units of measurement are incommensurate. What dollar value could be placed on the human suffering and disability that resulted from an admittedly costly but controllable occupational exposure? The advocacy for the victims of byssinosis was taken up in hearings by unions and worker health activists, but the most telling and convincing testimony came from the poor, hollow-chested gasping workers themselves who spoke movingly of their despair.

In addressing toxic exposures, the act directs the Secretary of Labor to "set the [health] standard which most adequately assures, to the extent *feasible*, on the basis of the best available evidence, that no employee will suffer material impairment of health or functional incapacity." Feasible means "capable of being done" but satisfying the cost–benefit requirement of the OMB implies to some, only if the price is right. It was inevitable that the Supreme Court would have to establish the primacy between the conflicting goals of protecting human health from a demonstrable occupational health risk and the economic burden of prevention to the employer. A deeply polarized 5 to 3 decision of the Court upheld the Cotton Standard, but because the ruling applied only to that standard, there was no clear-cut resolution of the conflicting interests.

Industrial hygienists, whose view of the primacy of employee health was clear, have their own possible conflict of interests. A Code of Ethics adopted by the professional industrial hygiene associations succinctly recognizes "that the primary responsibility of the Industrial Hygienist is to protect the health of employees." However, the majority of hygienists are employed by industry or, as consultants, are paid by employers, which underscores the biblical admonition about serving two masters.

A Matter of Faith

The Occupational Safety and Health Act boldly states that employers must comply with their rules and regulations and, similarly, although less emphatically, that employees shall do so. It would seem then that the question of compliance is not "whether" but "how" and that would be that, except for the unique place that individual religious practice plays in the United States. Should an employer insist that his most capable and dependable workers wear hard hats in a construction area when their religious scruples forbid covering their heads or not doing so with profane headgear? Similar dilemmas were faced by employers dealing with the refusal by nominally law-abiding workers, who placed unassailable faith in their protection from their maker, to wear ear protectors in a noisy textile weaving plant. The conscientious objectors might be as dissimilar as Old Order Amish, the Sikh Dharma Brotherhood, orthodox Jews, and Christian Scientists, but their reasons were commonly based on sincerely held religious convictions rather than any libertarian challenge of government authority.

Their employers invariably extolled their work performance and would not consider firing them for their refusal, and unless someone was going to make an issue of it, the breach of the regulations among the true believers would remain more common than the observance.

A consulting safety engineer once cautiously warned the owner of the textile weaving plant in a Pennsylvania Dutch country farming community.

"You realize that those people will sue you when they learn they lost their hearing."

"That never entered by mind," the owner snapped, aghast that any one could cynically question the deeply held Amish beliefs and their motivation.

In 1978, OSHA reverently bowed to the religious noncompliants and their employers by providing hard hat exemptions specifically for the Amish and Sikhs. In 1990, when the Supreme Court did not buy the argument of an American Indian religious group that under the Free Exercise Clause of the First Amendment, they were free to use the illicit mind-altering drug, peyote, as part of their religious practice, OSHA rescinded the hard hat dispensation but not for long. The following year, OSHA reinstituted the exemption but, in a careful separation of church and state, tactfully directed the exemption to the individual religious belief rather than to any established religion.

Suppose the refusal of a worker to follow a regulation on religious grounds creates a serious hazard to a fellow worker or poses a demonstrably life-threatening risk to himself or herself? Does OSHA have the power to assert what they regard as the greater good or the lesser evil? The Religious Freedom Act of 1993 somewhat plays to both sides by saying that the government cannot restrict religious practice without a compelling justification and, in any case, should be the least restrictive to religious practice for attaining the greater need. Justice is not only blind; it can wink.

Chapter 8

The Prognosis for Staying Healthy at Work

As a status report and possible guide for future activity, the National Institute for Occupational Safety and Health (NIOSH) in 1983 issued its suggested list for the 10 leading categories of work-related diseases and injuries (Table 8.1). The selection of health and safety problems of the contemporary workplace is a mix of the old, the new, and the questionable. It might be disconcerting to occupational health professionals that some of the traditional occupational diseases and illnesses of the past persist as major problems today; most notably in the first category of occupational lung diseases which highlights silicosis (earlier called "Miners' Asthma, or phthisis), coal miners' pneumoconiosis ("Black Lung"), and byssinosis ("Brown Lung"). Similarly, the entries of hearing loss from high noise exposures, back problems from lifting, severe traumatic injuries from accidents, and skin problems are nothing new. Their staying power may have something to do with both our failure to communicate the dangers and precautions to all employers and the workers at risk, or *their* failure to take informed action.

In some measure, these factors account for the appearance of what should be well-known and preventable chemical hazards in the case stories of Part 2. These include the unreported chronic lead poisoning of the lead recovery workers in "The Workers' Right to Know," the death of the young oil refinery worker from hydrogen sulfide overexposure in "No Sense of Danger," and the dermatitis problems of the female trainees unaccustomed to working with liquid petroleum products in "The Girls in the Machine Shop." Although asphyxiation by either lack of oxygen or chemical poisoning did not make the NIOSH list, carbon monoxide is probably the most common cause of chemical asphyxiation in and out of the workplace, causing an estimated five hundred deaths annually in the

United States with at least one order of magnitude greater in near misses and unsuspected illnesses. Awareness of its sources and hazards *should* be better known; nevertheless, the stricken frozen food plant workers in "The Fire Next Door" case study failed to recognize that the carbon monoxide in the exhaust gases belched from the gasoline-powered fork lift truck passing in and out of their food locker was the inside insidious culprit.

Is the Illness Work Related?

A physical injury at work is usually evident, and if it results from an exposure or activity on the employer's premises or elsewhere as required by the work, it is presumed to be work-related and is reportable under the OSHA tally of work-related injuries. This covers the traveling salesperson who incurs a whiplash injury from an accident driving to make a sales call as well as the worker who gets injured on the job from some obviously work-unrelated fellow worker's horseplay. For occupational safety and health professionals concerned with prevention, the *reason* for the condition is more important than the location, which explains why the recorded statistics of workplace injuries and illnesses do not provide a true picture of their concern.

Whether an illness of a worker is caused by the workplace is less clear. First, the illness has to be recognized and reported by a qualified person—be it a physi-

Table 8.1. Ten Leading Work-Related Diseases and Injuries

1. Occupational lung diseases: asbestosis, byssinosis, silicosis, coal workers' pneumoconiosis	6. Disorders of reproduction: infertility, spontaneous abortion
2. Musculoskeletal injuries: disorders of the back, trunk, upper extremity; Raynaud's phenomenon	7. Neurotoxic disorders: peripheral neuropathy, toxic encephalitis, psychoses, extreme personality changes (exposure related)
3. Occupational cancers (other than lung): leukemia, mesothelioma; cancers of the bladder, nose, and liver.	8. Noise-induced loss of hearing
4. Severe occupational traumatic injuries: amputations, fractures, eye loss, lacerations, and traumatic deaths	9. Dermatological conditions: dermatoses, burns (scaldings), chemical burns, contusions (abrasions)
5. Occupational cardiovascular diseases: hypertension, coronary artery disease, acute myocardial infarction	10. Psychologic disorders: neuroses, personality disorders, alcoholism, drug dependency

Source: NIOSH, 1983.

cian or an employer—as an occupational illness. To complicate the matter of etiology, exposures or activities of workers *outside* the workplace may, in fact, cause or contribute to some of these "work-related" illnesses and health problems. The use of medications and drugs—controlled or otherwise—smoking, diets, hobbies, and sports activities, whatever constitutes the current life-style choices and, most notably, personal stress factors, have all been implicated in effects on worker health. These "non-work-related" factors also bedevil the industrial hygienist seeking a solution to the work health problem which will become evident in several of the story cases in Part 2.

Many of these cases deal with traditional workplace illnesses so that the cause and contribution from exposures outside the workplace may be easily overlooked, which puts into question the validity of the "work-related" statistics.

Problems Anew

The introduction into the twentieth-century workplace of new patterns of working and new applications of potentially health-damaging forms of energy such as radioactivity, microwaves, ultraviolet and infrared radiation and magnetism, literally thousands of man-made chemicals, and even man-made workers (robots) created health and safety problems that a Ramazzini could hardly have imagined. To be sure, many of the modern labor-saving procedures have moderated many of the physical stresses as in lifting and the installation of safety devices such as machinery guards and the wearing of personal protective equipment such as hard hats, safety glasses, and steel toe safety shoes have prevented many serious accidents. In other ways, the new work patterns have introduced different hazards or exacerbated those which were formerly of lesser concern.

Repetitive Motion Injuries

We are all well aware from practical experience that repetitive hand motion be it from piano practice, computer key punching, peeling potatoes, slicing meat, weeding in the garden, or using a manual screwdriver could lead to muscular and skeletal discomfort and possibly pain. In similar fashion, repeated physical assaults from any force on the body including pressure, noise, vibration and even auditory assaults were known to have a damaging effect which we now term cumulative trauma injuries. The occupational health professionals were caught off guard by a virtual epidemic of severe impairments of wrist motion accompanied by severe pain in the wrist joints, hands, and shoulders that resulted from extensive changes in industry work practices. The condition known as carpal tunnel syndrome (CTS) was not exactly unknown to professional musicians, waitresses, typists, and meat cutters in previous years, but the reported number of cases proliferated with large numbers of assembly line workers in the electronic and automotive industries, among others, performing repetitive wrist and hand motions. Repetitive trauma injuries were hardly acknowledged in the 1970s but by the early 1990s, the numbers of new cases in this category had accounted for more than 60 percent of all new occupational illness and continues to stretch the lead. The principles for diagnosing and applying ergonomic measures to prevent these repetitive traumatic injuries—as well as the major workplace health and safety problems—are, indeed, well known.

Chemical Burdens and Sensitivities

Consider the health implications to workers of the exposures to new chemicals that had never passed through the human body before. Among the hundreds of thousands of new chemicals that have been created this century, perhaps the ten thousand or so entries in *The Merck Index*—which according to its editor is "probably the most widely used chemical/biochemical index in the world"—represent the most commonly encountered chemicals. Although the synthetic chemicals are alien to our body, at the usual levels of occupational exposure, only a relatively small number have been associated with or suspected of causing the occupational cancers, adverse reproductive or neurological effects, or dermatological and asthmatic reactions that are categorized in the list. This may be analogous to reporting that only a relatively small proportion of the incalculable numbers of microorganisms that enter our body are pathogens capable of causing disease; but when they are bad, they may be very, very bad. Less than two dozen substances or processes, in fact, have been identified by OSHA or the American Conference of Governmental Industrial Hygienists TLV Committee as being confirmed human occupational carcinogens.

From the practical standpoint of complying with the OSHA regulations and surviving in the courts and the marketplace, industry has developed a more anticipatory approach to health problems of chemicals in the workplace and the environment. Chemicals manufacturers are required by EPA regulations to perform toxicological testing and evaluation, and report any adverse human health effects before a new product is permitted to be manufactured and distributed. These toxicological testing and evaluation procedures are not fail-safe, but the likelihood of unsafe exposures at work is greatly reduced, particularly with industrial hygiene surveillance of the workplace and medical monitoring of the workers.

These predictive laboratory tests usually evaluate only the effects of an individual chemical, whereas workers are commonly exposed to multiple-chemical exposures. We just do not often know what effects are caused synergistically by low levels of multiple-chemical exposures which individually are believed to be safe. For example, healthy workers continually exposed to Chemical A at levels well within its permissible exposure limit over a lifetime of work may reasonably be expected to be safe. Suppose they are concurrently exposed to Chemicals A, B, C, D, . . . and more at similarly low "safe" levels. It is possible that the net effects on the body are considerably greater than the sum of the parts; we often just do not know.

The TLVs or safe levels for lifetime occupational exposure are based on concentrations that are believed to protect nearly all health workers, but the matter of individual hypersensitivity or hypersusceptibility has to be addressed on a case-by-case basis. There are many volatile chemicals present at extremely low concentrations in the atmosphere of just about everybody's workplaces emanating from the many industrial, office, and personal use products containing them. The presence of these chemicals in a labeled bottle or container may be identified, if not smelled, by the user, but small contributions of chemicals to the work atmosphere emanating from furniture, newly installed or cleaned rugs and drapes, the photocopier and the photocopies, office and house cleaning compounds, cosmetics, and air "fresheners" may be invisible but no less implicating. Dermal reactions from chemical sensitizers can result from contact with tools or jewelry containing nickel and even from washing one's hands with a germicide-containing or perfumed soap. Fortunately, the bad-acting chemicals have largely been removed from most commercial products and relatively few people are hypersensitive or allergic to chemicals, and if they or their physicians identify the cause, they learn to avoid the exposures.

Recently, the occupational health professionals have been dogged with a condition termed Multiple-Chemical Sensitivity in which a worker claims he or she has a severe reaction—often asthmatic or incapacitating—to extremely low levels of any and all chemicals in the workplace that heretofore had never elicited reactions. If a fellow worker's perfume, or trace chemical of whatever happens to be in the workplace, is alleged to trigger a response, it would appear that the only solution would be reassignment of the employee to a chemical-free environment, which may not be feasible. Since many researchers believe there is no scientific or medical proof for multiple chemical sensitivity, they have concluded that the condition may well be psychogenic and clearly outside the expertise of occupational health professionals to solve.

In a similar vein, if a worker's health complaint is unsubstantiated by the findings from a thorough industrial hygiene survey, the industrial hygienist will wisely pass on any such judgment. However, the suspicion that their employees' health complaints are feigned is freely expressed in several of the story cases by the bosses in "Sick of the Job," "Our Son's Just Not the Same," "The Fire Next Door," and "Who's Itching Now?" Even the secretary to the investigating industrial hygienist in the "Sick of the Job" story implies that the young map reproduction workers have psychosomatic headaches.

The NIOSH list contains several nontraditional disease categories that are questionably work-related: most notably, cardiovascular diseases, psychologic disorders such as neuroses, alcoholism and drug disorders, and reproductive disorders. It may be argued that the workplace conditions aggravate a preexisting condition, but proof that working is the source of a heart attack, a nervous breakdown, or an addictive habit is far more tenuous. Establishing a workplace relationship for alcoholism may prove even more daunting, except, of course, in the case of brewery workers, spirit distillers, or bartenders.

Stress at Work: The Universal Ailment

Curiously missing from the NIOSH list may be a virtually universal cause of work-related illness and injuries, namely, stress. The omission is understandable and a definition unnecessary, as there is nothing specific in the workplace to measure as to cause and effect and yet virtually every person who has ever worked can tell you all about the stress of the job and how it affects his or her well-being and health. The symptoms may be headaches, nervous stomach, increased blood pressure, jumpiness, anxiety, chronic fatigue, and sleeplessness. Stress has been variously categorized as being blue collar, white collar, professional, and executive or just nondenominational job burnout with both distinctive and common features. Possibly because many of the causes for stress at work relate to psychological and emotional factors and interpersonal relationships, psychologists, social scientists, and employee relations counselors, rather than occupational health professionals, are faced with the problems.

Finally, for most people, working represents security and purpose, so that the stress or fear of losing a job or being chronically unemployed conveys a more comprehensive meaning to "work-related" illness.

The Ultimate: Murder at Work

About 6000 work-related fatalities have been reported annually. We expect to see the biggest representation of these deaths in construction, transportation, and public utilities caused topmost by falls, followed by electrocution, but we are the ones taken off balance and shocked by the fact that in many workplaces, *homicides* account for more deaths irrespective of the job title. In fact, the Labor Department's Census of Fatal Injuries for 1973 for the first time reported that homicides placed a close second (17 percent) after highway-related injuries (20 percent).

The committing of a murder at work is, however, part of the larger problem of dealing with violence and crime. Murder on the job is largely committed during a robbery and the location for the crime is simply, as Willie Sutton said about why he robbed banks, a place where the money is. More commonly than banks, the top job locations for occupational homicide include taxicab operations, retail facilities such as liquor, grocery and jewelry stores, and gasoline stations; public facilities including hotels, motels, and restaurants; and protective and enforcement services such as guards, detectives, and police officers. The service facilities in high-crime areas that are open all night and lack security are particularly accessible targets. Many women work in such facilities, which may explain why although more men are murdered at work overall than women, homicide is the leading cause of death for women.

As a summary observation, it is evident that the contemporary industrial hygienist is challenged with solving many new and sometimes unforeseeable problems in keeping workers safe and healthy. The work health problems may involve multiple-chemical exposures, physical agents of as-yet undefined human biological effects, biological agents that defy ready identification or measurement, ergonomic stresses from "poor fits" with tools or improper work procedures, stress from psychological factors, interpersonal relationships, and life-style habits on and off the job, and, strangely now, even senseless acts of violence.

Industrial hygiene has, indeed, evolved into a profession that calls for a sleuth at work.

PART 2 Case Stories in Industrial Hygiene

SECTION ONE

▪

Are These Complaints Work Related?

Case *1*

Just Two Beers

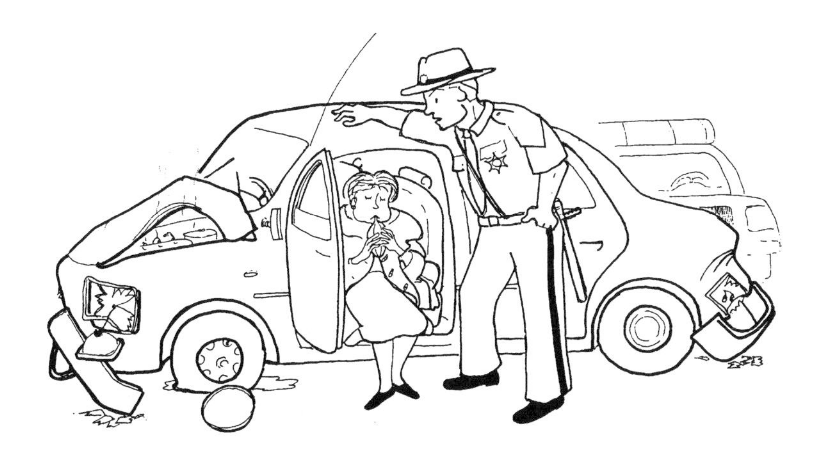

The telephone caller to Professor Lazar Davis sounded like a bilingual sports announcer alternating languages within the same sentence.

"You're Davis, right? The professor that knows all about how you get sick at work?"

"Yes, this is Lazar Davis and I am a professor of industrial hygiene. But, how did you know . . . ?"

"Lady that answered the phone at the college office. She said you're the health expert that could help me."

Davis often received unsolicited telephone calls from lawyers seeking his expert advice in representing employees alleging illness caused by their work, or from a consumer claiming injury or sickness from using a particular product. Just as likely, it could be from the lawyers defending an employer or a chemical product manufacturer, or from their insurance company. Davis would frequently serve as a consultant in these matters, but lately there had been a proliferation of these inquiries, so that he was now faced with the problem of deciding how much time he could spare from his busy academic responsibilities.

Most of his callers usually started by saying that Davis had been highly recommended by a colleague who had been helped with a similar problem. They would clearly and tersely describe their client's problem. Could the professor as an expert in the field have an opinion that would support their case? Davis would ask a series of pointed questions and, based on the preliminary information, he might agree that they had a case, but he could not give his professional judgment until he thoroughly investigated the matter. Would he be willing to serve as their consultant and expert witness with the case after he had done so? If he was too busy to get involved or simply did not believe there was a credible scientific basis for their position, he would decline the offer and they were free to seek out a more amenable expert.

For a lawyer without a referral, a university with a graduate program in industrial hygiene like Davis' was a logical place to start. But this man threw him off balance. Unlike the smooth delivery of most of his callers, this man was garbled and his manner was hardly professional. Davis questioned whether he was really a lawyer.

"Well, what's the problem?" he asked directly. "And by the way, who are you?"

"Name's Laguda. That's L.A.G.U.D.A. Oscar Laguda. I got this woman with D.U.I. in Jersey. She works evening shift at a food factory, and, of course, has no money. If she loses her license, she can't work."

D.U.I., or driving under the influence of alcohol or drugs, as the formal charge reads, is serious in or out of New Jersey mused the professor, but the cryptic reason for Laguda's call to him soon followed.

"Can ya get drunk from work, Doc?"

Davis restrained himself from quipping something about *workalcoholics*. Reflecting more soberly, he was not about to be a party to the defense of a drunken driver, but he did have a professional obligation to respond without prejudging.

"I guess it's possible, but I need a lot more information about what she does there. What chemical products does she use? I need to know about her exposure conditions and the workplace controls. I may even have to visit the workplace and. . . . "

"Of course, doc," Laguda interrupted, and as if he had rehearsed, he launched into a rapid fire narration. Davis prided himself on his ability to guess the nationality or regional origin of unseen voices by their distinctive speech patterns and nuances, but Laguda's novel pronunciation and staccato delivery of what seemed to be a hard luck drunken driving charge stumped him.

"Well, did she get drunk from work?" Laguda persevered.

"Mr. Laguda, it's possible," Davis answered cautiously, "but only after I review all the evidence and complete any investigation. And only then if I believe there's a scientific basis for a work-related cause for the D.U.I. charge."

"Right, professor. I don't expect you to lie. But if you find there's reasonable doubt, will you testify for her?"

"Let's take it one step at a time."

"Sure. I understand," Laguda interjected anxiously. "Remember, Doc, she don't have much. But if we do have a case, what'll cost for you to testify at her hearing?"

Davis was accustomed to a more delicate request for his fees and usually without negotiation. He started to explain that his charges would be based on the hours spent in preparation, consultation, and writing up any formal reports plus the time and expenses for travel, when he was again interrupted. In Laguda's world, price setting for his legal services was usually negotiated as a lump sum representing what his clients could afford. He asked Davis to take on the case for an amount that Davis would normally have charged just to travel to the out-of-state hearing.

"I promise to get you everything you ask for. She's a good person in trouble with no money. What d'ya say? Can you help her?"

Davis had to acknowledge that the novelty and implications of this off-beat case were now far more intriguing than the token fee. He really wanted to know for his own professional knowledge whether it was possible that chemical exposures at work could be contributory to a drunken driving charge.

"Okay, I'll do it," he reluctantly agreed and repeated his list of required information as if he was not sure that his listener had a full command of the language. "Mr. Laguda, her employer should have a form called a Material Safety Data Sheet, or MSDS for the chemical products she works with. That will tell me what's in the product and their hazards. I'll want a copy of each. And I want to see the accident report and the alcohol breath test."

"No problem, Doc. I'll send everything with my check."

Davis reminded him that he also wanted to talk to his client and might want to visit her workplace for an on-site evaluation.

"Gotcha," Laguda cheerfully agreed. "Her name's Kathy Grogan and I'll send you her telephone number. And I'll let the municipal prosecutor know we got an expert testifying."

"I didn't say that," Davis almost screamed. "Oh, forget it," he concluded, with resignation, and said good-bye.

To Davis' pleasant surprise, a package arrived a few days later at his office with all the requested materials and a check. More unsettling, however, was a notice of Kathy Grogan's hearing at 10:00 A.M. on April 15, scarcely one week later. Like most of the full-time faculty engaged in research, teaching, and consulting, Davis had an extremely busy schedule. Without checking his calendar well in advance, he might be lecturing in class, attending a faculty committee meeting, delivering a paper at a scientific meeting in New Orleans, or serving on a government committee in Washington reviewing research proposals. Fortunately, the hearing date was on a school holiday and he happened to be free, but the timing was an uneasy portent of Laguda's loose style.

First, Davis reviewed all of the requested materials and did a quick study on breath alcohol testing. He then spoke on the telephone briefly with Laguda, at greater length with a hapless Kathy Grogan, and then with the state trooper who had made the arrest and performed the alcohol test.

It seemed that Laguda operated a store-front legal services office in a blighted downtown urban neighborhood. His mostly blue-collar clients earn close to minimum wage and, according to Laguda, fall into hard luck legal problems more from trying to survive the vicissitudes of the city than from willful activity.

Kathy Grogan was a divorced forty-nine-year-old woman who worked the evening shift as an unskilled laborer at a large food processing and canning plant. One day in mid-February, she was given a new assignment scrubbing metal plates with a wire brush in a deep bath of a chemical solvent contained in a large dumpster. Kathy would then place the cleaned but wet plates in a drying oven. There was some kind of fan over the oven, but Kathy said it never worked right and she could smell heavy solvent fumes. When the plates were dried, she would remove and stack them for later use in the food preparation. Using the same solvent and brush, she also cleaned up the stained surfaces of the lacquer-coated machinery. Kathy reported that she was not given any information about the dangers of the chemical cleaner or safe handling procedures and, apart from rubber gloves, she was not provided with any protective equipment or respirator. There was no other exhaust fan or hood in her immediate area so that the solvent vapors evaporating from the chemical cleaner made her feel dizzy during the cleaning, forcing her to leave the area to get fresh air every fifteen minutes or so. As she lives fairly close to the plant, she often drove home at her meal break to grab a bite or take care of some chore. Getting into the car that evening, she could still smell the solvents on her clothes and hair. Her throat was dry and irritated, her eyes burning, and she felt tingling in her legs. When she got home, she immediately went to the refrigerator for a cold beer to soothe her raw throat. She heated up a slice of frozen pizza in a microwave oven for dinner and may have had a second beer with it. Less than thirty minutes later on her hurried way back to work, she was observed by the lady motorist immediately behind her as driving erratically just before she crashed into two cars at a stop sign, waiting their turn to enter a main highway. No one was hurt, but her car had to be towed. A patrolling police officer was dispatched promptly to the accident. Smelling what he suspected was alcohol on her breath, he noted that she had great difficulty retrieving her driver's license from her wallet and was very unsteady when she tried to walk to his patrol car. When asked if she had been drinking any intoxicating beverages, she said meekly, "A beer. Well, maybe, just two beers."

She was advised that she was under arrest for suspicion of driving while under the influence of intoxicating liquor, read her "Miranda" rights, and then taken to the police station for booking and a mandatory alcohol breath test. Kathy's unsteadiness and lack of coordination, her physical appearance, slurred speech and, even her surly behavior—all commonly associated with drunken behavior—were sufficient to warrant the breath testing. It was made clear to her that in New Jersey, her refusal to submit to the breath testing could be used, in effect, as proof of the charge. Two successive breath samples taken about four hours after Kathy's last drink gave identical values equivalent to 0.11 percent blood alcohol concentration (BAC). In most states, 0.10 percent or more BAC (0.08 percent in two states) is legally presumptive of intoxication. Some airline pilots and ship captains, most notably, the skipper of the run-aground *Exxon Valdez* oil tanker, accused of being intoxicated at work have maintained in their defense that they can "hold their liquor" and are, therefore, unimpaired, irrespective of an incriminating BAC. The motor vehicle laws do not allow for these alleged individual differences and, indeed, most medical and behavioral experts on the effects of alcohol believe that essentially all persons, including the heavy drinkers, with a BAC of 0.10 percent are too significantly impaired to drive a vehicle safely. If a traffic crash reported to the police involves anyone with a BAC of 0.10 percent or more, the National Highway Traffic Safety Administration defines it as alcohol-related.

At the police station, Kathy cried almost continually and vented her anger at the arresting officer by telling him she did not like him because he was going to make her lose her license. When the officer solicitously asked her if she was sick, she snarled, "I'm sick of you" in between her sobs.

As an experienced industrial hygienist, Davis had had little involvement with drunken behavior attributed to drinking alcohol on or off the job. Controlling drinking practices which impact on work performances was the concern of the worker's supervisor or, in the larger and more progressive companies, of an alcohol and drug counselor or physician rather than the company hygienist. Nevertheless, it was possible that Kathy's work exposure was responsible or, at least, contributory to her drunken appearance. Davis had a lingering unease at the prospect of defending a drunken driver if the facts were misrepresented, and for a personally experienced reason.

Davis remembered from about ten years earlier, in his only selection and service as a jury member, the severely injured, unemployed young man who hobbled slowly into the courtroom on crutches and painstakingly took the witness stand to testify in a personal injury suit involving a highway accident which had occurred almost a year earlier. He identified himself as Barry Green and related to a sympathetic audience that while walking along the berm of a well-lighted major highway late one August night, he had been struck by a reckless motorist. Barry admitted that he had been drinking "a few beers" with a buddy from work at a roadside bar for several hours before the accident. He maintained he had not been drunk despite the testimony of the defending motorist that he had been seen staggering by the edge of the road, but too late to avoid being hit. He had been treated in the emergency ward of a nearby hospital and because no tests for sobriety had been made and his drinking buddy was no longer in the area, there was no way to corroborate or refute his story. His plight seemed particularly pitiful when he said, between sobs, that since the accident, he had been unable to work, was depressed, and started to drink more. The defendant's attorney carefully had him affirm that he had drunk only beer that night, that he had no more than two or three servings, and that he had been in the bar for several hours watching the baseball game before he left to walk home by himself. Green was absolutely certain this was the truth and he was dismissed from the witness stand. After a brief recess, the defendant's attorney brought into the courtroom a brash looking young man, wearing jeans, a brightly colored cowboy shirt, and boots. He identified himself as Chuck Harris in taking the witness' oath, and said in answer to the interrogation of the defendant's attorney that he knew Barry Green as a fellow worker and remembered drinking occasionally with him.

"Yeh, that's him," he said, pointing in Barry's direction. Then noticing Barry's crutches, he added, "Jeez, what happened to him?"

Barry sat glumly next to his perplexed attorney.

In response to the defendant attorney's follow-up question, Chuck said he was unaware that his sometime drinking buddy had been in an accident because they had gone home their separate ways that night. He remembered he and Barry both had just been laid off from work earlier that week in August and that he, Chuck, had left the area the next day to look for work back home.

"What were you and Barry drinking that night?"

"Well, beer and stuff," he answered, casually.

"Stuff? You mean you were drinking more than just beer that night?"

"Yeh, we was drinkin' our usuals, you know. Double scotch boilermakers." Then, recognizing his need to educate his audience, he explained to the jury that boilermakers were shots of whiskey followed by mugs of beer.

"How many boilermakers did you each have that night?"

"Oh, at least five or six. I don't count 'em."

"Over what period of time did you both imbibe—that is, finish off the boilermakers?"

"Maybe, two hours. We didn't spend the night there."

"Were you and Mr. Green intoxicated when you left the bar?"

"I guess you might say we was feelin' no pain when we left. Somebody must of drove me home. Can't remember who."

The judge called for a conference with the attorneys and then gave a directed verdict to the jury to acquit the defendant so that Davis and his jury members never even had the opportunity to render their judgment.

Davis was understandably somewhat skeptical of the number of beers reported by Kathy when he called her at home. Although she had been told to expect his call, she sounded very tentative until she was sure it was the "professor." She was not tentative, however, about the lack of any warning information or training about the chemicals she used. No, she was definitely not given any protective equipment like gloves or respirators or provided with any kind of ventilation or fans. She was sure the fumes from the chemical cleaner made her feel dizzy and sick to her stomach. In fact, although she no longer was assigned to the cleaning detail, up to three weeks after her last exposure, she still felt some tingling in her legs, the veins in her legs were protruding, and after a pause, she said plaintively, "I just feel like I don't want to help myself."

Davis knew from his reading of the formal police report that it had corroborated essentially what Laguda had initially related but with more incriminating details about Kathy's unsteady behavior, including the results of the balance and coordination tests. For example, she was observed to have swayed and was unable to touch her nose with either hand and could not walk heel to toe, continually veering to the right. There were, of course, many common chemicals at work which could produce some degree of motor interference and movements similar to the effects of intoxicating alcohol. It was essential for him to know what specific chemicals were involved.

Laguda's packet of information indicated that Kathy used only one proprietary chemical product at work. He could determine the specific chemical components of the product from the Material Safety Data Sheet (MSDS), which must list all the hazardous ingredients and their amounts. Under a Right To Know regulation of the federal Occupational Safety and Health Administration (OSHA), a copy of the MSDS should have been made available to Kathy, and her supervisor or safety advisor should have explained to her the product hazards and instructed her in the precautions and protective measures for safe handling. To an experienced hygienist like Davis, the composition of chemicals revealed in the MSDS immediately suggested what health and safety problems could be anticipated under the described conditions of use.

According to the MSDS, the trade name chemical cleaner that Kathy used was comprised of four organic liquid chemicals, commonly used as solvents. During use, the solvents evaporate into the atmosphere, producing distinctive odorous vapors, or what are commonly, though incorrectly, referred to as "fumes." Inhaling these vapors, or fumes, above certain allowable or safe limits without adequate ventilation or respiratory protection will often cause headaches, dizziness, giddiness, confusion, mild narcosis or sleepiness, and physical instability; in short, the typical symptoms associated with drunken behavior and what Kathy had been describing and evincing. Some solvents exert more specific toxicological effects, particularly with long-term or repeated exposures, such as damage to the liver or kidneys; others may be highly irritating to the eyes or nose and throat. More recently, there has been a lot of concern about the more subtle and possibly more insidious damage from the neurological toxicity of solvent vapors, particularly from long-term cumulative or chronic exposures. Certainly, Kathy's solvent vapor exposure might have been implicated in her report of nerve tingling.

The MSDS describing the chemical cleaner reported the following composition:

methylene chloride . . . . 75 percent
normal propyl alcohol . . . . . 10 percent
methyl cellosolve . . . . 10 percent
petroleum naphtha . . . . 5 percent

Davis was very familiar with the health effects that might be expected from overexposure to these chemicals, individually and collectively. Methylene chloride, the predominant constituent, is also the most volatile and could very likely, by itself, produce light-headedness, dizziness, and nausea, and a depressed state of weakness or neurasthenia under the excessive vapor conditions described by Kathy. There have also been reports of associated nerve tingling in the legs and methylene chloride is somewhat unique among solvents, in that once inhaled into the lungs and absorbed by the blood, it is later metabolized to form carbon monoxide, producing symptoms of headache and light-headedness associated with carbon monoxide poisoning. It was confirmed later that no measurements of Kathy's workplace atmosphere had ever been taken for the solvent vapors, but expert industrial hygienists could testify on the likelihood of overexposure based on the known properties and conditions of the contaminants and their professional experience. In short, Davis was reasonably comfortable with his preliminary opinion that Kathy could have appeared to be drunk in consequence of her workplace exposure. The opinion had to be termed "preliminary" because the actual conditions at work, as reported to him by Laguda and Kathy, were not yet confirmed by his own observations or measurements. From his experience in providing expert testimony in court, he knew the value of stating that he had personally visited the actual workplace and that his survey and observations corroborated his preliminary opinion. Sometimes, to nail down the case, he would have had the exposure conditions simulated and then collect air samples on charcoal tubes placed in the breathing zone of a worker performing the same work under similar conditions. The air sample could then be analyzed by an accredited chemical laboratory for the specific air contaminants to confirm the exposure. The concentrations reported would then be evaluated with respect to accepted workplac exposure limits, such as those established by OSHA.

Kathy's breath alcohol test results from the police report indicated the manufacturer and model number of the analyzer used. Davis called the manufacturer to get information on how the breath analyzer worked. They told him when the alcohol in the breath is mixed in a glass ampoule containing yellow acid chromate reagent, a reaction involving a chemical reduction changes the yellow chromate color to green. The amount of this color change is correlated with and read directly as the amount present in the blood. For confirmation and record purposes, he requested that copies of the operating specifications and descriptive literature be sent to him as soon as possible. He then called the state police officer who had administered the test to confirm that he had used the specific analyzer named and that the instrument had been calibrated before use to make sure the results were accurate. He also raised questions regarding the specificity of the chemical reaction; that is, how did the police officer know that what he was measuring was only ethyl alcohol, the alcohol of intoxicating beverages. There are many other alcohols, such as, *isopropyl* alcohol, commonly present in the rubbing alcohol in the medicine chest, and the highly toxic *methyl* alcohol, or wood alcohol, which is used in antifreeze solutions The officer, who professed no knowledge of chemistry, assured the professor that everything was done according to the manual.

When he called Laguda to arrange for his inspection of the working conditions at the food plant only a few days in advance of the trial, Laguda said that Kathy was afraid of causing any trouble at work, which characteristically meant she was intimidated at the retaliatory prospect of losing her job and that they would have to make their case without it. Laguda added, almost as an afterthought, "Didn't my secretary call you? The hearing's been postponed to May 14."

Davis was again rankled by Laguda's evidently chronic loose style of operation. How does he even know I'll be available then without checking with me? Davis angrily asked himself. Although he now had serious misgivings about his continuing involvement with this lawyer of questionable professionalism, he knew he was committed to see the case through.

"Well, I'll see you on the fourteenth, Doc," Laguda said, without apology and hung up.

There were still those incriminating results of the breath alcohol tests which legally define the limits for driving at 0.10 percent BAC. Because Kathy's level was just above the limit at 0.11 percent, Davis knew he had a scientific basis for introducing reasonable doubt, as he had implied to the state policeman who had performed the test. He had recently read a newspaper account of an attorney defending a D.U.I charge, who argued that his then ailing client had been taking cough medicine, which contained ethyl alcohol, and that the breath measurements did not represent alcohol from liquor. Apparently, the judge did not accept this argument because the driver was convicted, as charged.

But suppose there were chemicals in Kathy's breath other than the ethyl alcohol from her beer which could be producing the same reaction in the test? Davis reasoned that if it could be established that there was a likely interference, the measurement results could be declared invalid. The MSDS for the chemical cleaner listed a content of 10 percent normal *propyl* alcohol. Thirty years earlier as a young analytical chemist working at a government laboratory, Davis recalled having to measure propyl alcohol vapors in air by bubbling the air sample through a small glass bottle containing the same absorbing chromate solution as in the BAC test and producing the identical color reaction as that given by ethyl alcohol in the BAC test. As the brilliant yellow color of the acid chromate solution was gradually transformed by the cascading bubbles of the air sample into a distinct green, he remembered thinking then that this demonstration was so startling and impressive that it would be a great addition to the "Chemical Magic" show that he awed the kids with at the local schools. It was also widely known that acetone, which is not an alcohol and is commonly found in the breath of diabetics, will interfere. In consequence of these problems of interference, the law enforcement agencies have widely supplanted the older nonspecific breath analyzers with high-technology analyzers employing more sophisticated and specific methods. These include infrared spectrometry, electrochemical oxidation, and solid-state sensing. Davis had, of course, confirmed that the older nonspecific analyzer had been used at the station where Kathy was tested. He also was confident from his own experience with exposures to normal propyl alcohol to testify that Kathy would be expected to have had sufficient levels of normal propyl alcohol vapor in her breath resulting from her work; in any case, enough to interfere with or cast reasonable doubt on the BAC test results. But, would a municipal court judge concur by accepting the professor's scientific testimony and dismiss the charge?

Davis arrived at the municipal court about a half-hour before the scheduled hearing and was immediately greeted in the waiting room by a tall, good-looking man in his mid-thirties dressed nattily in a bold pin-stripe suit, who pumped his hand vigorously.

"Professor Davis? I'm Oscar Laguda. Pleased to meetcha."

Laguda nodded to a thin, frightened-looking woman of about fifty, dressed in dark purple slacks and a pink flowered blouse. This was obviously Kathy, who was huddled closely to a slightly taller woman dressed similarly and who could have been either her sister or her best friend. Both women looked like chain-smokers at a funeral service who are unable to light up. Davis introduced himself to the women who were too nervous or intimidated by the courtroom atmosphere, or possibly by "the professor" himself, to make small talk. They retreated to huddle in a safe corner.

Unlike the marbled halls of county and state courthouses with their imperious statues of Blind Justice, imposing portraits of black-robed judges, and bronze dedicatory plaques, at which Davis was more accustomed to testify, this municipal court looked more like the assembly room of a country grade school. The floor of the small bare-walled waiting room was covered with heavily scuffed and faded vinyl tiles. There were seven or eight plainly dressed local residents, waiting patiently inside, or standing just outside the entrance, smoking nervously. Like Kathy, the litigants were largely there to contest traffic violations, to seek or avoid payments, or to defend charges of minor infractions of the local laws. It was, for Davis, a heretofore unexperienced venue for seeking and dispensing justice in what might have seemed, except to the principals, as mundane matters.

Laguda, who had left to check with the court clerk, came back to announce with an embarrassed grin that the hearing had again been cancelled and was now firmly scheduled sometime in June. Apparently, he was accustomed to such last-minute changes, but Davis, who was missing an important department meeting, tried to maintain his composure while firmly serving notice to Laguda that he might not be available to make any more appearances at court and left abruptly.

Laguda yelled, albeit pleasantly, "I'll letcha know the exact date, soon as I can, Doc."

About a month later on the rescheduled date, Davis entered the same crowded waiting room of the municipal building and was almost sure he recognized some familiar faces. Laguda greeted Davis expansively, with the assurance from the court clerk that they would absolutely be the first case to be called that morning. Kathy and her companion actually smiled at him.

Kathy asked him nervously, "Are we gonna win, professor?"

"I think we have a good case, Kathy."

Davis had prepared a suggested series of questions for Laguda to pose to him, as needed, during his testimony, so he did not expect to remain too long in the witness chair. Filing into the court room, in addition to the principals involved with the case, was a young woman whom Laguda informed him had been recently admitted to the bar and had been at the earlier postponed hearing. Apparently, she was the lady motorist who had been driving behind Kathy at the time of the accident and had been so disturbed by Kathy's apparent drunk driving that she was willing, as necessary, to provide her eyewitness testimony and was now again ready to do her duty.

After the usual formalities of reading the charge, the professor was sworn in. Laguda entered into the record Davis' resume and was about to verify in detail his education and professional accomplishments. The judge said it wasn't necessary to go through with all that and, with the agreement of the municipal prosecutor, they accepted the professor as an expert in the health effects of workplace exposures.

Without benefit of any histrionics, Laguda blandly asked the professor to explain how it was possible for his client to appear drunk from her work activities and why the breath alcohol samples were not valid. The professor, speaking clearly and with a minimum of technical terms, explained how an industrial hygienist was able to draw causal relationships between workplace exposure and conditions, and observed health effects. He described the physical and toxic properties of the particular chemicals that Kathy used and explained why the absence of ventilation and protective equipment exacerbated the exposure to harmful conditions. Contrary to his instinctive responses to inject qualifiers introducing his conclusions, which most lawyers do not like to hear but as a scientist he felt were indicated, his answers were simple and direct. Laguda read almost mechanically his versions of Davis' suggested questions.

Q. "Professor Davis, could my client's drunken behavior be affected by her working with these chemicals?"
A. "Yes, sir. The symptoms from overexposure to the solvent vapors are similar to those commonly seen in drunken behavior."
Q. "Does the breath machine just measure alcohol from beer or liquor, professor?"
A. "No, sir. It can also measure other chemicals such as other alcohols and solvents."
Q. "Would the alcohol in the chemical cleaner be in Kathy's breath a few hours after exposure, professor?"
A. "Very likely."
Q. "Would this alcohol be measured as beer alcohol in the test?"
A. "Yes, it would."
Q. "Would this screw up the results?"
A. "Yes, it would. The likely presence of propyl alcohol in Kathy's breath from her solvent exposure at work would interfere with the test used to measure the ethyl alcohol from intoxicating beverages. Certainly, it would cast doubt on the validity of the results."
Q. "Thank you, professor," Laguda concluded, with a look of triumph.

The judge, who gave no clues to his thinking during the testimony, called for a ten-minute conference with the police officer, the municipal prosecutor, and Laguda. He sifted through the material entered in evidence for several minutes. He asked the municipal prosecutor several questions, who looked puzzled and shook his head each time. Then almost matter-of-factly, the judge announced that the charges were dismissed on the basis of the professor's unrefuted testimony. The young female attorney who had not been given the opportunity to testify seemed startled at this unexpected defense and acquittal of the drunken driver. To Davis, it now all seemed so undramatic and foregone. Kathy cried and kissed Laguda. Laguda told the professor he was terrific and asked if he could call upon his help in other cases. Davis smiled without answering and waved good-bye.

Back on campus by noon, Davis checked into his office for his messages and then left to meet his usual lunch companion, Jack Miller, from the Civil Engineering Department, at the faculty dining room. It was already uncomfortably warm for mid-June and he casually picked up an iced bottle of beer from the bar to have with the Tuesday corned beef on rye special. He spotted Jack at their customary table and quietly sat down. The two friends were comfortable enough with each other not to have to talk. Or at least, not until they felt there was something worth saying. As Davis pensively etched the frosty coating of the beer bottle with his finger nails, he broke the silence.

"Jack, do *you* think a person can get drunk on just two beers?"

Case 2

Awash with Noise

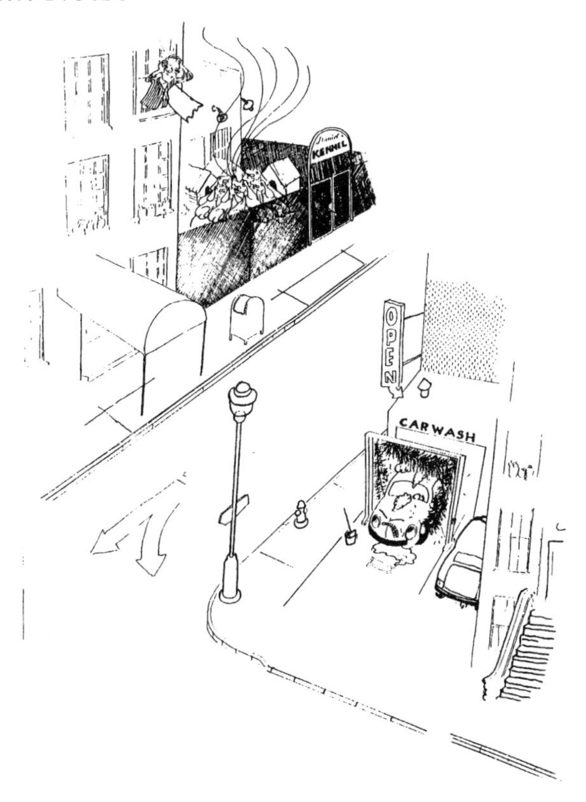

Long before we had instruments to measure the intensity of noise at work or conduct hearing tests, it was well known that certain workers exposed repeatedly to high noise levels gradually and permanently lost their hearing; hence, the designation of blacksmiths' and boilermakers' deafness. Even today, we instinctively describe noise from a thunderstorm or a rock concert—if you are not a fan—as deafening. At a dog kennel housing, among other breeds, a dozen or more yelping beagles, the hapless caretakers were more concerned with losing their minds than their hearing. It was difficult enough for Mr. Daniels, the owner, to placate his employees during the day, but the beagles kept up their periodic outbursts of howling until late evening so that his neighbors in the thin-walled apartments on either side, behind, and above him could not even fall asleep watching television.

Mrs. Gump, the usually dour and uncommunicating wife of the retired postman in the apartment above Daniels' place, stopped him in the hall one morning.

"Mr. Daniels, can't you stop them dogs of yours from howlin' night and day? Even my Albert, who can't hear so good, says their barkin' is getting on his nerves."

"I really don't understand what's got into them lately, Mrs. Gump," he replied, with a genuine air of puzzlement and despair.

Mrs. Gump was not satisfied. There's a reason for everything, she believed. "You ain't using your animals for tests or something, are you?"

The last thing Daniels needed was an animal rights issue. He took great pride in his dogs, really loved them, and was genuinely hurt by her implication.

"Absolutely not, Mrs. Gump. Really, I just don't know. . . ."

Unsatisfied, Mrs. Gump stalked away, leaving him in mid-sentence, while mumbling that the neighbors might have to do something about it.

Directly across the street from the kennel in this busy commercial and residential area, the attendants' ears at the recently opened drive-in car wash operation were also assaulted by periodic outbursts of other noises but of a different quality and source. The entering vehicles rattled over the treadles, were hydraulically raised, and mechanically moved by powerful and noisy forces through the prewash, shampooing, and final rinse/wash cycles. The final blow drying of the dripping vehicle with high-velocity, high-horsepower air blowers produced overpowering whooshing, which precluded normal conversation. Safely insulated inside the vehicle and oblivious of most of the noise, the customer could unembarassedly enjoy this functional version of an aquatic amusement park ride. Although the work noise exposure of the car wash attendants probably warranted ear protectors, the youthful workers sometimes masked this noise with even higher levels of self-inflicted, rock music through waterproof head phones. In their favor, their hearing damage risk, at least from the work, was minimized by their usually short tenure at the job.

If Mrs. Gump had not enjoined her fellow-suffering neighbors to register a complaint first to the police, then more formally by a petition to the mayor's office, the matter might have been dropped or, at least, tolerated. For his part, Daniels, who had spent over thirty years in the animal care and breeding business, knew that his beagles—characteristically, among the noisiest barker of the breeds—had never erupted with such frequency until the drive-in car wash people moved in. Unfortunately for Daniels, no one in the neighborhood, not even the residents next door to the car wash, had complained about the car wash noise. Because the mayor did not have the foggiest idea how to resolve the situation, he tried to get the adversaries to reach some accord at a meeting in his office. Daniels could not, or would not, relocate his dogs, or spend the money to soundproof his building. Irritated to a frazzle by the beagles' piercing yelps heard throughout most of the day and evening in their living quarters, his neighbors were totally unsympathetic. Rather, they were doggedly angry and unwilling to accept less than their normal evening quietude. Daniels responded defensively and more aggressively by filing for a cease and desist order with the local magistrate, claiming that the excessive noise from the new business across from him interfered with his business operations.

In an era of widespread business diversification, it was not surprising that the owner of the car wash facility was a major oil corporation, which was particularly sensitive to its corporate image as a good neighbor. Automated car washes, then, were innovative entries in the marketplace and the company was particularly concerned with establishing a favorable reception. Consequently, shortly after the noise complaint had been filed by Daniels, the matter was referred to the legal department at company headquarters. Lazar Davis, then regional industrial hygienist in the corporate medical department, was promptly contacted by George Halley, one of several company lawyers, who would frequently call him for help with environmental and occupational health problems.

"Hello, Lazar," began Halley cheerfully. "You know about the automated car washes the company opened last spring?"

"Yes, I remember reading an article about them in the last company magazine."

"We just opened a new one about twenty miles north of Philly."

Then jesting about a possible health- and safety-related reason for calling an industrial hygienist, Davis asked, "Did someone forget to close the car windows?"

"That would be easier to handle than this one, buddy. You know we always seem to get some crank in the neighborhood with an objection whenever we start up a new operation. Seems like some local business there resents the noise from the car washing. Or maybe he just doesn't like the extra traffic on the street."

"I wouldn't have thought a newly opened car wash would be particularly noisy. But then again, I wash my own, so I wouldn't really know what's not a noisy car wash."

"If you satisfied that complaint from our truck drivers, who thought the diesel engine noise affected their libido, Lazar, you ought to be able to solve a simple neighborhood noise complaint. We just have to prove to some magistrate that our noise levels are not unreasonable for their locale."

As George Halley knew from having read their reports, the company industrial hygienists had had plenty of experience measuring noise exposures of workers at refinery units, in the engine rooms of tankers, in paint and plastic plants, and at pipeline pumping stations, to name a few of the more typically noisy company operations. After evaluating the noise exposures, the hygienists would recommend measures to control the noise exposure within the regulatory safe limits. George rightly assumed that handling a neighborhood noise complaint required much of the same expertise.

"Sure, George, I have a file filled with noise surveys taken at company property lines—usually at night—in response to neighborhood noise complaints. In fact, I once had to testify on a ridiculously restrictive community noise code being proposed in Delaware, which would have shut down the nighttime operations of our refinery there. When we introduced tapes of the cricket noise in the fields outside the refinery which exceeded our noise at the fence, as well as their proposed legal limits, they tabled the proposed code indefinitely."

"Great," said George, with a sigh of relief. "I always knew we could count on you."

"Let's hope it's not a problem, George, but if the noise levels are higher than what's been generally recommended in community noise codes, we may have to make some modifications to lower the noise."

"Of course, we'll do what we have to," George said, followed by the familiar refrain that the company always wants to be a good neighbor.

Davis knew there was a significant difference, however, in the criteria used to evaluate a workers' noise exposure and neighborhood noise complaints. The hearing damage risk to workers of daily and repeated noise exposures has been developed from the correlation of the results of their ongoing hearing tests with extensive noise surveys of their actual exposures on the job. The federal Occupational Safety and Health Administration (OSHA) regulations define a continuous noise level of ninety decibels averaged over an eight-hour work shift as excessive and indicative of hearing damage risk for day-after-day exposure. Since ninety decibels is a level at which one would have to shout to hear ordinary conversation, most people would agree, hearing loss risk or not, that a continuous ninety-decibel noise is too loud.

It is a far trickier task for the citizens in a community to prescribe what noise levels are acceptable from their neighbors. Unlike hearing damage, there are no measurements relating cause and effect or, more accurately, response to the considerably lower noise levels encountered in the community. There have been studies which purport to predict probable community response to overall noise levels in qualifying terms ranging from "few or sporadic complaints" to "widespread and angry response." Accordingly, some communities have adopted some form of the model noise codes which specify noise limits, taking into account the type and duration of the noise, the time of day, and the makeup or zoning of the neighborhood; that is, whether it is industrial, commercial, residential, or hybrids. These noise codes may also address—or ignore—the noise from trucks, motorcycles, trains and aircraft, emergency sirens and factory whistles, domestic quarrels or celebrations, power mowers and saws, band and vocal practice, and yes, barking dogs. In most communities, there is no specific regulation governing neighborhood noise and such complaints are treated under a general nuisance code, enforcement of which judiciously depends on what is reasonably acceptable to the majority and feasible for the noisemaker.

Davis was pleasantly disposed to take on this assignment. He had heard about the diverse business activities being started up by the New Ventures division of the company and was curious to see what kind of occupational health and environmental problems they might have. With the noise complaint at the car wash, he was told only that a neighboring business objected but knew nothing of the initial complaints about the barking dogs from the nearby kennel, or that the complainant was the kennel owner. It was mid-fall, his favorite season, and he welcomed the opportunity to get away from the confines of the corporate offices to be challenged by an offbeat problem.

To the extent possible on such a busy main street, the new car operation was fairly unobtrusive. A large white sign discreetly displaying the familiar company logo simple stated DRIVE-IN AUTO WASH under which a fluttering banner announced the weekly special. Clearly painted directional arrows at the entrance led the uninitiated customer to a flashing indicator, further directing the driver to one of two bays. Davis parked on a side lot and walked over to identify himself to a smiling, nattily dressed man of about fifty, whom he suspected was the district marketing manager responsible for the "New Ventures" operations.

"You're Davis, the hygienist from Medical? Right?" the man began, vigorously pumping his hand. "I'm Bart Baker. I remember you gave that great talk on skin problems in machine shops at our managers meeting in New Orleans last year. It was really helpful."

Davis grinned politely. It both pleased and embarrassed him to meet strangers in the company who knew him by name or reputation.

"Thank you. So the company is now in the car wash business?"

"You bet. This is the first in my region and there are already plans for six more next year in the other regions."

Davis nodded. "What's next?" he added, not expecting a serious reply.

"Didn't you hear about the plans for groceries, sundries, and fast food at the new service stations? They call them convenience stores," Baker reported.

Davis recalled how inconvenient it was at one of the "newer" service stations last week during a rainstorm when the attendant told him that they don't replace wiper blades any more, or "stuff like that." Then he thought about suggesting to Baker a sign for the projected newest venture proclaiming "EAT HERE AND GET GAS," but he kept quiet.

"Well, I'll introduce you to the manager here so you can get started with this noise problem," Baker said. Then in a more confidential tone, "Personally, I think this noise complaint is political and totally unfounded. Why, there's a hell of a lot more noise on this road from the heavy trucks trying to beat the light than from our blowers."

In a more refreshing sign of the changing times, the facility manager was a very pleasant-looking, businesslike, and self-assured woman of perhaps forty, dressed in what could have been designer coveralls for the working woman. Introduced as Peggy Russo, she gave Davis a clear and concise tour of the car wash, emphasizing at each stage what kinds of noise were generated, how long they lasted, and whether anyone complained about them. When she could not answer Davis' detailed questions about the horsepower of the two high-volume air blowers which did the final drying, she promptly looked up the information for him.

"The blowers are rated at sixty-five horsepower each, Lazar. Is that a lot?"

"Judging by the high velocity and volume of the air flow, I'd say so. By the way, Peggy, which businesses have been complaining about the noise from our operations? And at what times?"

"Officially, just one, as far as I know," she answered. "That's the dog kennel place directly across the road from us. The owner, Mr. Daniels, claims he can hear our blowers from the time we open until quitting time at night, which is about eleven."

"Daniels is the only complainer about noise in the neighborhood?"

"Well, I've also heard from the deli owner next to us that the neighbors of the kennel have been complaining about their dogs barking, but that's not our problem."

Davis and Baker were both surprised to learn from Peggy's on-the-scene version of the noise problem that there were two different, and probably unrelated, noise complaints.

"Thanks for your help, Peg," said Davis. "I'd like to start with some random noise measurements inside the facility. That'll tell us where the main sources of the noise are, and whether there's a hearing damage risk to your workers."

As the car washing operation was largely automated, the attendants' main activity was to perform an energetic cosmetic wipe of the draining windshield with a lint-free cloth at the exit, collect the payment due, and, hopefully, a gratuity when they delivered the receipt and the change. Both Baker and Peggy accompanied him as he began his survey.

He used a small hand-held sound-level meter in which a microphone starts vibrating in response to the sound waves it "hears" from a noise source. Like a telephone, the instrument converts these vibrations to electrical energy, which can be read on the meter scale as decibels. Our eardrum similarly vibrates in response to sound. The energy from the vibrations is transmitted through the fluid in our middle ear and converted to nerve impulses in the inner ear, which are then carried to the auditory center of the brain. There they are discriminated as meaningful sounds of communication or gibberish, melody, or cacophony, or the recognized inflections of familiar voices or those of strangers.

"Is that what you measure the noise with?" Baker asked, pointing to the meter.

"Yes, this gives me a quick measure of the noise in decibels."

Baker nodded, reflectively. "I heard about decibels but I don't really know what they are."

"They're a measure of the intensity of the noise. Simply, it's how loud the noise is. Decibels—or dB, as they're abbreviated—are sort of difficult for most people to deal with because they are based on logarithms; actually, a logarithm is a ratio of two quantities, rather than a quantity itself. Because decibels are ratios, they don't have dimensions, like feet or pounds so you can't add and subtract them in the usual way. The bottom part of the ratio is always some reference sound level."

He paused, to make sure Baker and Peggy were still with him. "Do I confuse you by talking about logarithms?" he hesitantly asked.

Peggy had been listening attentively during their conversation. "That's the exponent of a number, when the number is expressed as a power of some base number."

"It's been a long time since I studied math," Baker said, defensively. Then, looking quizzically at Peggy, "How come you know that?"

Peggy almost apologized, explaining, "Before I went to work for the company, I was a high school math teacher."

"Well, maybe decibels will be clearer if I give an example," Davis tactfully interjected. "If you have one blower producing a noise level of 80 dB by itself and turn on another blower, which also produces 80 dB, the noise level from both blowers is not 160 dB, but 83 dB. In other words, doubling the noise intensity increases the sound level by only three decibels. You see, small differences in decibel levels can represent enormous difference to our ears."

"I get it, but give me some examples of what the decibel numbers mean," Baker said, cautiously.

Davis knew that the numbers would not mean anything without another background lecture, so he tried not to sound too pedantic.

"We can hear a tremendous range of sounds starting at zero decibels.* That's our threshold of hearing, or the least amount of sound we can detect under quiet conditions. The upper range, which can be physically painful, and sometimes cause deafness, might be the rocket launch at levels of 140 dB. In between, a soft whisper close by may be only 20 dB and traffic at a busy freeway may register 60 dB. Below the hearing damage level, most people become most aware of noise when it interferes with their conversation or sleep. Let's see what the inside levels are."

The two attendants occasionally looked up at him when he pointed the sound-level meter close to the rotating brushes lathering the car body and, then, by the air blowers.

"Do the air blowers ever get any noisier?" Davis asked, trying to engage one of them in conversation.

The young man shrugged. "Hard to tell. I keep my Sony on."

He turned to the other attendant and repeated the question.

---

* The decibel (dB) is the dimensionless unit which expresses the relative sound power level (L_w). By definition, the sound power level is: $L_w = 10 \log$ of $W_s \div W_0$, where W_s is the sound power of the source and W_0 is the sound power of a reference sound power. Because the sound level of the reference sound power by convention is taken as the threshold of normal hearing and the log of unity is zero, the scale measuring the values of sound intensities starts with an anomalous zero value.

"I don't know. I just started here on Thursday," he answered, evincing no interest in why the question was even raised.

Davis thought back, in sharp contrast, to an incident in his career when he was covertly assigned to evaluate the noise exposures of marine transport workers under strict conditions of secrecy. Before the law required monitoring and reporting workers' noise exposures, management commonly feared that employee access to any information of potentially damaging exposures would set off labor unrest, demands for hazard pay, and possibly a flood of compensation claims for any injury or illness. Consequently, Davis was instructed not to talk to any of the crew, to keep his noise meter out of view, and surreptitiously record his measurements of the intense noise levels inside the engine room of the oceangoing oil tanker. He had arrived on board under cover of darkness and was met by the first mate, who served as his guide and watchman and who again reminded him that the crew was not to know why he was there.

Although the philosophy of keeping workers ignorant of their own workplace hazards was professionally repugnant to him, Davis had to follow orders. The first mate assured him it would not be too difficult to keep the benighted sailors unaware of his activities because the foreign crew spoke little English, or anything else, for that matter, and were certainly ignorant of the effects and measurements of noise. As Davis pretended to study the inscription on a boilerplate while awkwardly manipulating the dials of his survey meter under his jacket, an impassive looking engine room mechanic, observing him for several minutes, disarmingly asked, "How many dBs are you getting, mate?"

As Davis completed recording the car wash levels, he found that with the exception of the air blowers, the noise was neither alarmingly high nor continuous in output. At worst, the air-blowing part of the cycle, which peaked at about 91 dB close up to the blowers, could last for several minutes with the downtime intervals of 5 to 10 minutes, depending on the number of cars passing through. Most of the time, the noise levels inside the car wash bays were less than 80 dB.*"

"It looks like the attendants' average exposures are well below the allowable OSHA 90 dB limit," Davis reported to Baker and Peggy. "That means that they're not at risk of getting hearing loss from their work, but it might be a good idea to issue them ear plugs or acoustic ear muffs. Although the blowers are not on continuously or for very long, they are pretty darn noisy."

"It's good to know the noise here won't harm the workers' hearing," said Baker, "but what about the dB levels the neighbors are complaining about?"

"I was just getting to that, Bart. That's more complicated and hard to pre-

---

* Because humans do not perceive low and middle frequencies linearly, sound level meters used to evaluate noise have been designed to discriminate against the low and middle frequencies. Thus, the frequency weighted scale of a sound level that simulates human response to noise is termed the A-scale, and measurements so taken are represented as dBA. OSHA and most community noise codes specify A-scale measurements for compliance purposes.

dict," Davis answered, shaking his head. "Noise is produced by sound pressure variations caused by something vibrating, measured in frequencies of cycles per second, or hertz. So in addition to the intensity of noise in decibels, we have to measure and take into account the many frequencies which make up the kind of noise we usually have at work. We can hear frequencies from about 20 cycles up to, perhaps, 20,000 cycles per second. Low frequencies sound like hums and are basslike in quality. High frequencies, we say, are high pitched and often irritating to our ears. We speak using frequencies in the 250 to 3,000 cycle range, so from a practical standpoint, they're the frequencies of most importance. If you lose hearing sensitivity in those frequencies, you have trouble understanding speech and with more extensive loss, you can become deaf." Davis paused, noting that his attentive audience now even included the attendants, thanks to a lull in the car washing.

"Why is my dad hard of hearing now?" Baker asked. "He was an accountant all of his adult life and never worked at any noisy job."

"His hearing loss is probably due to aging. The tiny hearing receptors in the inner ear start to deteriorate slightly at about thirty and gradually increase more rapidly with the years thereafter. Obviously, some people, like your dad, are more affected than others. Not much you can do about that. Noise deafness from work, though, is largely preventable today."

"Lazar, I can tune out to a lot of noise, but some noises can make me want to jump out of my skin," said Peggy. "Like scratching on glass or whistling through the phone. If you say noise is made up of many frequencies, why do some bother me more than others?"

"Because the predominant frequencies comprising the noise determine how we react to a specific noise," he answered. "At the same intensity, or dB level, we hear the middle high frequencies—say, from 750 to 3,000 cycles—much more easily than the lower or higher frequencies at the same intensity level. From an annoyance standpoint, a noise mainly made up of many high frequencies would be very shrill and probably irritating. Like a steam kettle whistle, or metal scratching on glass."

"Now I understand why the blowers are the main problem here," Peggy said. "They're definitely high pitched and extremely loud. That's the only noise that you can identify at any distance from here. Can you show that with your instruments?"

"I can measure both the intensity and the distribution of the frequencies making up the blower noise using this," he said, pointing to a larger noise-measuring instrument in a black leather case. "It's called a frequency-band analyzer. Then, I'll measure and compare the noise levels and frequencies outside at the entrance and across the street, when the blowers are operating."

Davis confirmed with his frequency-band analyzer what his experience and ears suggested; namely, when operating continuously at high speed, the high horsepower air blowers produced an ear piercing level of 91 dB, which was made up predominantly of frequencies ranging from 4,000 up to 20,000 cycles per second, the maximum measurable with his instrument. The overall noise level dropped off sharply with distance, so that at the street entrance to the car wash, the reading would average about 62 dB or slightly above the normal background of busy traffic. Across the street in front of Mr. Daniels' kennel, it was hard to get an overall decibel reading appreciably different from the same background level, with or without the blowers operating. Significantly, however, with the blowers operating, he was able to pick up here some of the characteristic high frequencies measured at the source of the noise.

"You can hear the blowers here alright if you listen for them," Davis told Baker and Peggy in front of Daniels' place. "You were on the right track, Peg. My instrument shows the same high-frequency component of the blower noise like matching fingerprints. But the contribution to the overall noise level doesn't seem overwhelming when you consider the intermittent noise from that airplane flying overhead, or the sirens from the ambulances, police and firemen, and. . . ," he paused, with sudden awareness. "Yeh, even the barking we hear from this kennel."

Davis did not know that the dogs howling was intermittent throughout the day until late evening, that it had only recently erupted, and that it was violating the tranquility of the people living nearby like an unrelenting intruder. As Davis was recording the last of his measurements, Baker nudged him vigorously aside. A short, elderly woman with a frosted bouffant hairdo and pink sneakers had been cocking her ear in their direction, obviously intent on learning what they were up to.

"I'm starved. Let's first have lunch at that deli," Baker said firmly, directing them across the street. "We can continue our discussion in Peg's office later."

Ben, the affable owner of Quality Deli, who was skillfully slicing a roasted turkey, looked up and smiled at Peggy, a regular take-out customer. "Would you like a fresh shrimp salad sandwich today?" he suggested.

"We'll be eating in today, Ben," Peggy explained. They found a corner booth in the restaurant, ordered their food, and in the kindest and social sense of the word, made conversation during their repast as befitting three disparate company employees with very different job functions and interests. During his many investigations of problems, Davis had been accustomed to bifurcate his thought processes during countless company business meals. The conversation dealt with weather, company gossip, sports events, and, occasionally, personal history and nonpolitical news. Privately, his mind now was sorting out the incomplete data and observations acquired during the morning search for the missing pieces needed to solve the current problem.

He reflected that the noise from the blowers reaching the kennel during the day could hardly be differentiated from the normally noisy background of this busy neighborhood. Possibly by evening when traffic died down and many of the local stores had closed, the noise from the blower would be more obvious. It was also likely to be louder than the level recommended by the model noise codes for a commercial and residential neighborhood at night. But only one business owner in the entire neighborhood had actually complained about the car wash noise and his place was not even adjacent, but was across a wide, busy street. Other conflicting factors flashed through his mind. Fewer cars were washed at night, particularly as the weather got colder. Windows were closed. External noises are usually masked by blaring television sets and overwhelmed by dish washers and vacuum cleaners. The car wash noise should not be a problem at night either, he concluded.

"Was everything okay? Another cup of coffee?" Ben asked, interrupting his internal monologue.

Ben's sudden appearance prompted Davis to ask him, casually, "Do you ever hear the car wash next door?"

"What do you mean?"

"Can you hear any special noise coming from the car wash? Like the cars driving over the treadles. Or the blowers."

Ben looked puzzled. "I'm pretty busy here, thank God. I guess if I stopped to listen, I might hear something. But nothing, really, to make me take notice."

"Let's get back to Peg's office, Lazar. I'd like to know where you think we stand. This lunch is on me," Baker said, picking up the check.

As they were waiting at the cash register for Baker to pay the bill, the little elderly lady, who had seemed so inquisitive about their discussion in front of the kennel, pushed past them to get to the display counter.

"I want six ounces of boiled ham and don't cut it too thick this time."

"How's this, Mrs. Gump?" Ben said, offering her a generous sample for a taste test.

"Not bad," she admitted, "if you don't mind it salty."

"How's Mr. Gump these days?"

"Ornery as all getout," she said. "The beagles next door are still making such a racket, day and night, he can't hear the TV, or me for that matter. If we can't get no satisfaction, we got to move."

No one said anything as they made their way back to Peg's office. In about twenty minutes, they regrouped in Peg's office to hear Davis' initial appraisal of the situation.

"Doesn't seem like we have the problem, Lazar," Baker began.

"It would seem so," began Davis, guardedly. "My measurements indicate that our operations don't contribute significantly to the noise level in front of the kennel, at least, during the day. The fact that nobody else in the neighborhood has complained, or that, like the owner of the deli, they are hardly aware of our blower noise suggests we're not causing an unreasonable disturbance. I need some nighttime measurements as proof, but my gut feeling is that the noise then might be only slightly more noticeable."

"Sounds good to me," said Baker. "Can you put this all up in a report for the magistrate so we can put the matter to bed?"

"Sure, Bart. Since someone in the community believes we're at fault, it may strengthen our case if we offer some 'good faith' measures."

"Like what?"

"Well, for example, since not being able to sleep at night is always a sensitive matter, maybe you could consider closing an hour or so earlier. But, let me think about it. I'll discuss it with you before I put anything in writing."

"Closing earlier would be fine with me, Bart," Peggy agreed. "I've been plotting our hourly throughput and it's hard to justify staying open after eight o'clock, particularly with the cold weather coming on."

"I'll study your numbers and let you know," Baker cautiously considered. "What else?"

"Well, sometimes, erecting a sound absorber or baffle helps to lower the noise level, or direct the noise away from the complainer. I'd have to get an associate of mine—a top-notch acoustic engineer—to help with that."

"Sounds good, if it takes care of the complaint and doesn't cost too much. Or set a precedent."

Lazar nodded, mechanically. Then, after a short pause, he confessed. "To tell you the truth, there's still something missing to explain this situation. It doesn't make sense why the noise from the car wash measured in front of the kennel property should elicit this complaint, particularly when it's pretty clear that no one else within the same, or close, earshot, has complained, or even noticed. It's like the missing key to a Sherlock Holmes mystery in which the cause is so obvious, nobody but Holmes considers it."

"The guy's a crank, or some kind of nut," Baker concluded. "He's like my father-in-law. He always finds something to bitch about that nobody else notices or cares about."

"I've been thinking about that little old lady we heard in Ben's deli complaining about the beagles barking," Peggy said. "Ben mentioned to me last week that several of her neighbors had the same complaints. Might there be a connection, Lazar?"

Peggy's suggestion was like telling Lazar that he was wearing the eyeglasses for which he was searching.

"Beagles? Yes, of course," he said excitedly. He remembered that years ago a neighbor kept two beagles in their backyard and every time the siren from the volunteer fire station nearby summoned the firemen, the beagles howled liked crazy. His wife said that if the sirens didn't wake the volunteers—and everyone else in town—the beagles would.

"It seems obvious now that the beagles were being driven crazy by the high frequencies from our blowers. You probably could plot their cycles of howling whenever the blowers went on," Davis exclaimed, with growing confidence. "There are even dog whistles which emit frequencies beyond our hearing that are easily heard by the dog. Many animals are very sensitive to these ultrasounds."

In fact, Davis knew of several fascinating studies by animal behaviorists which indicated that several species mysteriously communicate or get their information at frequencies inaudible to the human observers. Davis had become aware of this phenomenon at high frequencies following a request he had once received for a noise survey from a research scientist at an animal laboratory. The scientist was concerned from reports in the literature that many of the smaller laboratory animals, such as rats and mice, can be adversely affected by their detection of high-frequency sounds up to about 80,000 cycles per second. One study reported that very high-frequency exposures had induced convulsions in mice, rats, and hamsters. The scientist was aware of the many extraneous sources of continuous high-frequency noise in his laboratory from mechanical and electrical equipment, besides occasional emissions from running taps and squeaky furniture.

Katy Payne, a trained musician turned field biologist, reported a somewhat quirky inverse sensitivity by the world's largest land mammals to very low frequencies of fourteen to thirty-five hertz. Ms. Payne was intrigued to learn how the female elephant, which goes into heat for just a few days every four or five years and otherwise lives independently from the males, manages to let the bulls know of her availability. By observing mother elephants with their calves in the Portland, Oregon zoo and analyzing their audiotape recordings, she cleverly deduced that although *she* could not hear them, nonaudible low frequencies generated in definite patterns and sequences were sensed by the elephants. In 1986 at an elephant-frequented wilderness in Namibia, she broadcast a recording of a female African elephant's rumblings in heat over a mile away from a couple of bulls drinking at a water hole near her observation point. She reported that the bulls suddenly stopped drinking and trotted off, gallantly, in response to the cow's invitation.

Baker's animal interest, however, was focused only on beagles. "Can you really prove that our blowers are causing the dogs to howl, Lazar? And, if so, why would *we* have to do anything if it's not really our problem?"

"We could easily turn off the blowers for a while and see if the dogs quiet down. If they start up when we do, that would pretty well establish a cause and effect. As to your second question, I think if you lived next door to the kennels, you would be pretty upset by the barking. Since our blowers are very likely the off-stage initiator of the problem, I think we owe it to the community to do something about it. Remember our good neighbor policy? Anyway, I believe we can solve the problem at the source by modifying the blowers to reduce the high frequencies as well as the decibel level. But that's for a noise control expert to figure out, which will probably take some time to change. In the meantime, we can buy some time with Daniels if we agree to close earlier in the evening so, at least, his neighbors won't lose sleep."

"Okay, Lazar, I'll arrange for a meeting with Daniels and the magistrate. I want to show them that your measurements prove we are not producing excessive noise in the community. I'll lay it on that as a good neighbor, we are offering to shut down earlier in the evening until we are able to make permanent changes to lower the noise level—even though we don't have to."

Davis was satisfied and correct that the noise problem could be resolved to everyone's satisfaction. The magistrate agreed that the company was, indeed, acting responsibly and in good faith, and Daniels agreed to give the company time to effect the changes. Even Mrs. Gump was more conciliatory when Mr. Gump was able to sleep and watch his evening television as soon as the nighttime operations were curtailed. A few weeks later, the expert acoustical engineering friend of Davis' suggested replacing the high-horsepower blowers with a pair of considerably lower-horsepower blowers, which were much quieter with markedly reduced high frequencies and airflow. It might take a little longer for the car to dry but the attendants would be happy at the opportunity for more tips. Bart Baker was delighted to recommend to his boss his idea for incorporating this change in the design specifications for all the projected new car washes, nationwide.

Davis learned in his years of experience as an industrial hygienist that there were always new and unpredictable twists to the environmental problems that challenged his professional expertise and interest. And not unexpectedly, about ten months later, he heard the familiar voice of Bart Baker.

"Lazar, remember we were opening more car washes this year? Well, we have a new noise complaint with the one we just opened last week out on Long Island."

"You're across from a duck farm, this time?"

"It's the town church. With the windows open in the warm weather, the minister says we're interrupting his Sunday morning sermon."

Case 3

Sick of the Job

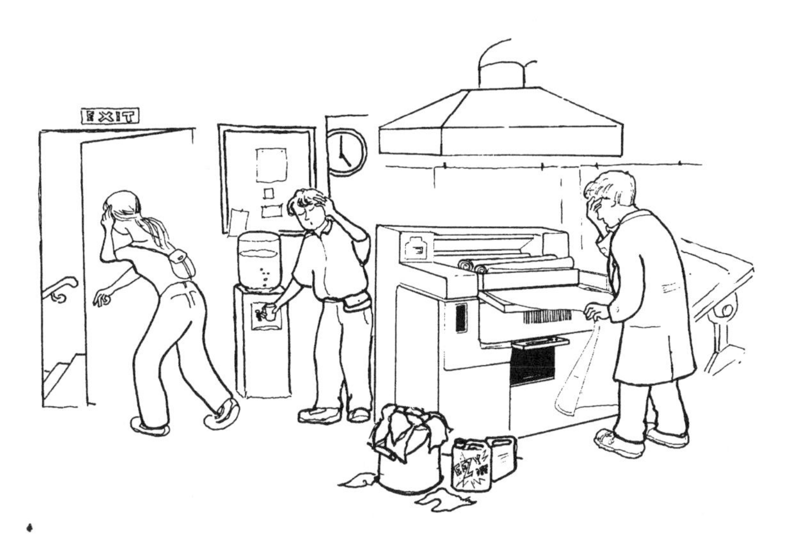

Marge Brody had been a secretary for the corporate industrial hygiene group for most of her 24 years with the company medical department. In contrast to the indifferent attitude of the younger secretaries, she had made it her business to learn about the work health problems with which her scientifically educated bosses were dealing. She more than compensated for her lack of formal training by having a sharp and retentive mind, and in time she developed a practical knowledge of what causes workers to get sick on the job. She went even further. In her not always subtle manner, she would freely express her untutored opinions about the cause of a newly reported problem. Lazar Davis, the senior industrial hygienist, for one, never took umbrage at her unsolicited advice. One summer Tuesday morning as Davis was returning from a meeting of his group, she greeted him, waving a familiar pink telephone memo slip.

"Lazar, you got this call from the employee relations manager in the Denver headquarters. Three office employees working in a small, inside office claim they're getting headaches."

"You said the headquarters building, Marge?" Lazar asked, somewhat incredulously. "Isn't that the brand new skyscraper that was just on the cover of the company magazine?"

"Yes. That's what he says. No one else in the building is complaining," she said, pointedly, and waited while Lazar read the brief message.

"What exposures do *they* have there to cause headaches? They don't even work with chemicals in a high-rise office building, do they?"

"Probably not."

"If you ask me, they're just bored and sick of the job so they imagine the work gives them headaches."

Lazar was somewhat amused, but hardly influenced, by Marge's psychosomatic interpretation of the problem. There were many familiar work operations presenting, almost ad nauseam, recurring problems with the same predictable causes and cures. For example, he knew before he went to a machine shop where newly hired trainees were developing skin problems using cutting oils that he would invariably find that the rookies had not been properly instructed in washing and keeping their oil-contaminated skin and clothing clean. At automotive repair garages where the mechanics were suffering from headaches, he would routinely confirm that they were breathing excessive levels of carbon monoxide from the engine exhaust, which had not been properly ventilated. Sometimes, it seemed to reduce his professional diagnoses to a simplified word association game in which a duo of symptoms and work activity would immediately define the cause of the problem.

However, the causes for serious health problems in white-collar settings, like offices, are fewer and usually less obvious, so that solving a health complaint there is more challenging. It was particularly frustrating to Davis when the causative agents were elusive or unidentified because he had to regard the workers' complaints as being no less genuine. The information in this report of three cases of headaches and malaise in an office building was too scant even to suggest a possible cause. Davis promptly called the Denver office and was referred to Joe Daily, the manager of reproduction services for the oil exploration division.

"We make photocopies and blowups of the topographical maps used by the geologists in searching for oil," Daily explained to Davis. "It's just the three employees working in the map reproduction room who say they get headaches almost every day."

"Only at work?"

"Right. Two young men and one female college student on summer employment."

Earlier, Davis' word association technique had immediately suggested a suspect. Ozone, or O_3 in chemical symbols, is a highly reactive and severely irritating form of oxygen which contains one more atom of oxygen in the molecule than ordinary di-atomic oxygen. It is often formed around electrical equipment which produces electric discharges, or arcing of the current. In nature, we can often smell its distinctive, pungent odor after a violent electrical storm, in which case it rapidly dissipates and causes no problems. An electric field in electrostatic photocopiers is generated to charge and discharge the photoconductive materials, which produce the photographic images, or copies. If the photocopier is used extensively in a small, poorly ventilated indoor space, it can readily produce concentrations of ozone as low as 0.1 ppm, which can initially cause irritation and dryness in the throat. With extended use of the photocopier, the worker's exposure to ozone can increase to the point of causing headaches, dizziness, and burning sensation in the eyes of the workers.

"Do you know what ozone gas smells like?"

"Sure. It has a sort of sharp smell. But since we've been getting our copiers services and the filters replaced regularly, we can't smell any."

Davis could never be confident of a lay person's identification or report of an odor. Many workers would report smelling hydrogen sulfide when they meant sulfur dioxide and one worker would swear he or she smelled "something funny," whereas others in the same locale would deny the presence of anything unusual. He knew he would have to verify the presence and amount of the exposure for himself.

"Do they use any inks or solvents?"

"Not now. The photocopying is practically a dry process. We used to use a duplicator with methyl alcohol, which took a while to dry and the fumes would irritate our eyes. We changed the process just before we moved into the new building to make sure we didn't have to deal with that. We even have an exhaust fan over the work table so you can hardly smell anything."

In answer to his specific questions relating to possible sources of carbon monoxide, or other chemical exposures or contributing factors, Davis was informed that there were no other processes using chemicals in or near their offices, no manufacturing in the building, and no bothersome noises or vibrations. The lighting, air conditioning, and ventilation all seemed fine. It was a showcase modern building, he was reminded. Oh yes, Daily confirmed that all three employees were moderate smokers.

Headache is probably the most commonly suffered human ailment with as many possible causes as there are kinds. Many of the chemical causes of headaches associated with working are well defined and controllable; for example, breathing excessive concentration of chemical substances like paint solvents, gasoline vapors, and, of course, ozone or carbon monoxide. Physical stresses like excessive heat, noise, or vibration have also been causally implicated with headaches on the job. Davis was invariably successful in solving health problems associated with most common chemical and physical agents at work because they can be measured and compared against known health standards. Headaches and illness due to stress related to emotional and psychological factors on the job are far less demonstrable. These might include pressures from overwork, antagonistic bosses and fellow workers, insecurity, and, above all, fears of job loss. Employees are similarly burdened on the job with their worries and anxiety brought on by personal problems from home.

If the complaining employee is a hypochondriac, is feigning the complaint, or is reacting in a sympathetic fashion to the illness of others, the hygienist might just as well stay home. The latter situation, which usually involves a group of workers or people, has been judgmentally termed "mass psychotic syndrome" and often disappears as mysteriously as it erupts, without conclusive identification of a causative agent.

"How do they describe their sickness, Joe?" Davis continued.

"Well, they all agree the headaches seem to come on late in the day. One guy said it felt like a steel band around his forehead and the college student says she feels a little nauseous and has no appetite. But you know women."

"Do they feel okay by morning?"

"They say they feel better when they start work and they're fine on the weekends. It seems strange to me that they're the only people here at work to get headaches, but you're the expert."

Because he could not be the expert at a distance, he told Daily he would fly out tomorrow evening and to expect him early on Thursday morning. He had not the slightest idea of what could be causing the problem.

Before leaving work, Davis made a rush request to the technical information group in the library to do an abstract literature search for recent reports of headaches in offices and nonindustrial buildings and then brainstormed the problem with two younger colleagues in the industrial hygiene group. They all immediately agreed that ozone from the photocopier was the obvious and prime suspect despite the denial. However, the absence of any odor and a characteristic, but hardly conclusive, report of a sensation of tightness on the forehead were compatible with carbon monoxide poisoning. But where and how did this gas, which is largely associated with the burning of fuels, get into just one room of a high-rise office building at levels high enough to cause daily headaches? Could it be automotive exhaust from an inside parking garage, or from heavy street traffic somehow infiltrating into the building ventilating system? But why only one office among hundreds? Was it a space heater, like an inefficiently operating kerosene stove, which can emit carbon monoxide? An auxiliary heater was unlikely to be needed or even allowed in the building. Was the air heavily contaminated due to cigarette smoking in a poorly ventilated inside office? That was possible, but it was unlikely that the ventilation system in an ultramodern building would only be deficient locally in just one room. Furthermore, cigarette smoking, particularly among white-collar workers, had been on a downward trend, and recent restrictions on smoking in the workplace were now common in many office settings. Each suggestion was countered with improbabilities and discounted or dead-ended, Davis said it was enough to give him a you-know-what.

On the long plane ride across the country on Wednesday, he reviewed the case reports provided by the library of headaches and malaise in offices, now reported under the rubric of indoor air-pollution problems. Although expecting to get some clues of what to look for, he found no new or unsuspected causes that he had not already considered. Early Thursday morning, Davis entered the latest stainless steel and glass architectural contribution to the Denver skyline. In New York, the building would be virtually indistinguishable from its crowded neighbors, but here in the West, it was a gleaming and stunning new attraction. He joined several well-dressed and important-looking people carrying briefcases, waiting impatiently in a mirrored elevator. After the door had closed, an uncomfortably saccharine voice from an intrusive loudspeaker announced the floor stops.

"Twenty-nine, next," it reminded him, "Watch your step, please," and it parted with an especially mindless, "Have a nice day." He wanted to tell this mechanical larynx to mind its own business, but he was afraid it might invite an embarrassing rejoinder.

Joe Daily thanked him for being so responsive to their call for help and offered him a cup of coffee before they started their tour. Daily had nothing new to report other than to confirm that either aspirins were effective or the kids, as he called them, might be getting used to the headaches and weren't complaining as much.

Just as Marge had predicted, the reproduction room was an inside windowless room about the size of a large family living room. Large aerial photographs of vast, unexplored terrains were stacked in a pile on the center worktable, and drawings derived from the photographs were hung like the newspaper scrolls in a public library reading room. Sophisticated scanning devices and computers had converted the photographs into multicolored plats with concentric lines, shadings, squiggles, and cryptic markings, which to the petroleum geologist were important clues in their prohibitively costly and chancy quest for oil. The job of the staff was to reproduce enlargements of sections or entire copies of the photographs, maps, and drawings with the high-technology photocopier at one end of the room. Although Daily stated there was no solvent used in their process, there was a slight odor in the room, possibly from some volatile materials in the toner. Occasionally, some tiny particles were released, so that it was necessary to allow the sheet to dry completely to avoid any smudges. Consequently, the copies were pressed through rollers and placed on a large table to dry, above which was a slotted ceiling exhaust vent.

One of the group would operate the photocopier while the other two were busily working at a desk or a small worktable on the other side of the room, carefully cutting out sections of the drawings or maps, or filing and recording information in manilla folders. They barely looked up at Davis from their work, as if they were not supposed to acknowledge the presence of a stranger or deign to ask why he was there. Davis had told Daily earlier that he would like to interview them whenever it was convenient, so he purposely made a point of saying good morning to each of them.

Walking around the room, he could not smell any unusual odors or see any other activity that might suggest a significant source of chemical exposure. He did notice a two-ounce bottle of ink eradicator, a half-dozen, or so, small bottles of different colored inks, a vial of Hot Pink nail enamel, a jar of a protective skin cream, and a half-gallon metal can of a proprietary liquid desk-top cleaner called E-Z-OFF. The precautionary label on the can which is required to warn the user of the principal hazards of the product used the archaic double negative "NON-INFLAMMABLE," meaning that it does not burn, and generically described the contents as "CHLORINATED SOLVENT," which covers a broad range of toxicity. It also gratuitously advised the user not to breathe the vapors. Davis asked Daily if they kept a file of the Material Safety Data Sheets on the chemical products that they used in their work, such as E-Z-OFF cleaner.

"What's that?"

"It's a form prepared by the chemical manufacturer which tells you what's in the product, what the hazards are, if any, and how you should safely handle it."

"No. Never heard of it."

Joe Daily's unawareness of the Material Safety Data Sheet was understandable since there was no legal requirement at that time for the manufacturer to provide such information to a user.

"Well, I'll get the information later myself. Meanwhile, I'd like to start out by taking some measurements for air contaminants and checking the ceiling exhaust vent."

"Fine, you need anything from me?" Daily asked, somewhat impatiently.

"Do you have a small stepladder?"

As Daily nodded, Davis tactfully suggested that he could work on his own, to which Daily readily acquiesced. He instructed one of the young men to get their visitor whatever he wanted and told the group that they would be interviewed later about their complaints.

"I'll pick you up around noon for lunch," Daily said, obviously gratified to get back to his desk.

Davis had done research on ozone detection while at graduate school and could readily detect its presence well below the allowable occupational exposure limit of 0.1 ppm. He could not smell any ozone around the photocopier or anywhere in the room. He took several air samples with a direct reading tube indicator in the work area and close to the copier and, not unexpectedly, found no measurable ozone. So much for the prime suspect.

Although Davis had seen nothing to suggest a source of carbon monoxide in the work area, having transported the carbon monoxide detector a few thousand miles, he felt obliged to check for its presence. The instrument was a direct reading survey meter containing a chemical sensor, which is specific for the gas and sufficiently sensitive at low concentrations to establish unequivocally whether it was present. After making some operating checks and adjustments, he placed the instrument probe over the large table for his initial reading and waited for the blower inside the instrument to draw in the room air for measurement. Glancing around the room, he smiled in acknowledgment at the three pairs of inquisitive eyes tracking his activity. The instrument needle barely moved past the zero point. When he subsequently placed the instrument probe in the corners of the room, at the ceiling vent, by the room air inlet, close to the photocopier, or randomly in the adjacent areas, the levels were similarly low. These readings of only a few parts per million in the room indicated that carbon monoxide was present at normal concentrations expected in a workplace with casual smoking and could now be reasonably eliminated as the cause of the reported health problems.

He climbed up on the stepladder to measure the airflow drawn into the ceiling grill above the worktable, using a device called a velocity meter. As originally designed for the older photocopying method, most of the vapors or odors from the photocopying and the drying copies would be captured and exhausted away from the breathing area of the workers. Any uncaptured or fugitive vapors, in any case, would largely be diluted by the room air so that there should not have been any significant exposure problem.

Davis was somewhat surprised to find that the exhaust airflow into the grill was almost negligible. Although there were adjustable louvers which allowed one to regulate the airflow, nobody had bothered to make sure the louvers were, in fact, open. According to what Daily had told him, this new process did not produce any significant emissions, so a ceiling exhaust was hardly necessary. It probably had been retained because nobody remembered the original purpose of its design or thought it was worth changing. Davis found it ironic that the two human errors neutralized each other in that with no apparent contaminant in the room, the ventilation defect was not a critical finding. Nonetheless, as Davis consoled himself, at least, he had found something to report.

The dictum in medicine which says that if you pay attention to the patient, he or she will tell you what the diagnosis is, was equally applicable in industrial hygiene investigations. Davis decided it was a propitious time to interview the employees, which is to say, at this point, he did not know what else to do.

"I'm Lazar Davis from the company medical department," he said, extending his hand to each of them, who identified themselves as Brad, Mitch, and Susan. They looked at him impassively and said nothing. Davis was attuned to the inherent caution with which the field employees regarded any representative of the corporate headquarters.

Starting with one of the two young men, he asked, "What can you tell me about your sickness, Brad?"

Brad hesitated for a minute or so, as if he were waiting for his fellow workers to give him some sort of supportive signal.

"I usually get headaches by the end of the day," he began. "It feels real tight here," he said, pointing to his forehead.

"Every day?"

"Well, not every day, but most. Sometimes, it's not too bad and goes away when I go home and take a couple of aspirins. And I'm fine over the weekend."

"Anything else?"

"Yeh, I sometimes feel a little sick to my stomach and dizzy."

His two fellow workers confirmed that they had similar symptoms but admitted that it seemed not to be too bad on some days, but it had been going on ever since they had moved into the new building. The no-smoking rule in common work areas had not yet been established and both Brad and Mitch lighted cigarettes.

"How much do you smoke, Brad?"

"Maybe half a pack a day here. I only smoke at breaks and lunch, so why should it bother me?"

"It could be a factor. What about your smoking, Mitch?"

"About the same. But, I got to have three or four with coffee to wake me up in the morning."

Susan giggled, nervously. "I chain-smoke when I study, but here I only join these guys socially at the breaks."

Brad shrugged and offered her a cigarette, which she gingerly accepted and lighted.

"Okay, I want to show you something," Davis said, to get their attention. He placed the probe of his activated carbon monoxide detector several feet away from where they were smoking.

"This instrument measures the carbon monoxide gas, or CO, in the air," he explained. "Before you started smoking, I could detect only trace amounts here, but take a look."

The instrument needle was now reading only about 4 or 5 ppm of CO. As he brought the probe closer to their cigarette smoke, the needle gradually climbed higher. When he placed the inlet of the probe directly over the smoke from a burning cigarette, the instrument reading increased dramatically and soon the needle went off the scale.

"See. You're inhaling several hundred parts per million, or ppm, of CO every time you inhale," he demonstrated. "And all of us are breathing in the carbon monoxide that's emitted into the room air while you smoke."

"But not enough to give us a headache," Mitch quickly retorted.

"Not from the smoking alone," Davis acknowledged. "But if the CO in the background air averages much above 50 ppm during the day, it's likely to cause headaches."

"Why is that?" Brad asked.

"Most of the oxygen our body needs to function is delivered by the hemoglobin as oxy-hemoglobin in our blood," Davis started to explain. "CO preferentially ties up the uncombined hemoglobin in our blood, forming carboxy-hemoglobin, so that the hemoglobin can't combine with oxygen. If we breathe in more than the usual amounts of CO, it can make us sick."

"Like the headaches?"

"Sure, Brad. If about 15% of the hemoglobin is tied up with CO, headaches are common. You smokers may already have up to 10% or more carboxy-hemoglobin in the blood, so any additional amount in the air will make you more susceptible to headaches than nonsmokers. That's why I had to measure the background CO levels in the room air."

"But you just showed there's practically no CO in the air here. I didn't think my headaches had anything to do with my smoking," Mitch said, defensively.

"Maybe not," Davis had to admit.

"But there's definitely something here that's making us sick," Brad insisted. "I've been feeling a tingling in my leg lately, but I haven't said anything."

Susan suddenly perked up. "That's funny. I've felt some tingling in my fingers too but thought it was my imagination."

"Anything else different, Susan?"

"I sometimes feel nauseous by quitting time and don't have any appetite for supper."

Mitch eagerly joined the group confessional. "I've been feeling a little groggy some times. Daily thinks we're faking it, so I just stopped complaining to him."

Davis focused on what might be present to cause the problems. "Do you use any special chemicals or smell any unusual odors here?"

They thought about it a while and said there was nothing new here that they had not been using before they got sick. There was a slight odor from the copies as they came out of the copier and sometimes there were little flecks or dust particles from the toner but that had been around before they had their headaches. Brad was sure that the problem was caused by something else in the new building and Mitch complained about their close quarters and lack of a window, but unless Davis had not been listening carefully enough, they did not fulfill the promise of the doctor's dictum. He was unable to match their reported symptoms with any suspected causes, and, so far, there was nothing indicated by his survey that would give him a reasonable lead.

"By the way, do any of you ever feel any burning in the eyes?" he asked casually, still thinking about ozone.

"My eyes get irritated every so often," Susan said, "but I wear contacts and it really has nothing to do with work."

The two young men both agreed that they could not feel anything bothering their eyes at work.

Davis asked them if they liked their work.

"I'd rather be skiing," Mitch answered, immediately.

"It's a job and it pays the car installment and that's as much as I want to think about it," Brad contributed.

Susan said it was just a summer job, so she did not have to like it.

Davis thanked them for their help and then made some notations of the interviews and survey in his notebook. It was a few minutes past noon and he tried to think of something substantive to report to Daily. He knew that many indoor air-pollution complaints are eliminated by simply increasing the among of fresh air added to the recirculated air without identifying a specific cause for the employees' health complaints. This may be due to the dilution of the unidentified contaminant by the additional airflow to a no-effect level. Or, if there really is no contaminant present but the employees are convinced that their complaints have been acknowledged and acted upon, then they may respond favorably to the placebo effect. If so, well and good, he thought. Recommending an improvement in the building ventilation was something he could usually do with some justification.

He was uncomfortable with the conversation at lunch. When Joe Daily asked him outright if he had found out what was causing the problem, he said he had eliminated a possible cause or two but he had not yet completed his survey. He casually mentioned the ceiling exhaust which had been closed and suggested that once opened, the better air exchange might eliminate the problem.

Daily was less reserved about the cause. "If you ask me, I think those kids are imagining they're getting sick. Or, maybe just sick of the job."

"I have to assume their complaints are legitimate, Joe."

More accurately, he was beginning to wonder if Marge Brody, his secretary, had acquired some special ability to divine the truth where his scientific training and instruments had failed. Was it possible that these young people were so bored or unhappy with their work that they had psychosomatically developed headaches, malaise, and tingling sensations? Even if that were the case, as an industrial hygienist, he was not professionally qualified to make that kind of judgment. He intuitively felt that the young workers were reporting the illnesses truthfully. Headache complaints are universal, but the report of a tingling sensation in the limbs or fingers was not the sort of symptom that one would likely conjure up. There must be something there that he had missed.

He returned with Daily from lunch and went directly back to the reproduction room and sat down in a chair placed away from the working desks. His game plan was to wait patiently and observe exactly what the workers were doing for the rest of the afternoon. It appeared that all the reproductive and editing work was completed before lunch. With the exception of emergency or priority jobs, any requests for reproduction jobs received after one o'clock were scheduled for the following morning. The young workers concentrated on getting the job requests packaged for mail or courier delivery that went out by mid-afternoon.

Because the maps and copies had to be scrupulously free of any smudges or dirt, they all spent almost an hour cleaning up the surfaces of their desks, worktables, and the equipment. They used a lint-free wipe cloth which had been liberally wet with the commercial liquid cleaner from the metal container labeled E-Z-OFF. Susan and Brad poured several ounces of the solvent on their desks and vigorously swabbed the entire surface until there was only a thin liquid film, which they dried with a clean rag. They were particularly assiduous in cleaning the trays and the rollers of the photocopier, which had been stained by the marking inks, toner particles, and the incompletely dried copies. Davis smelled a fairly mild odor in the room similar to chloroform. He examined the back panel of the E-Z-OFF container more carefully for an identification of the contents. The designation as a "chlorinated solvent" was too general a description to be of any value. He jotted down the name and address of the manufacturer, which was on the container.

As the workers finished using the cleaning rags, they placed them in an open 5-gallon-size metal trash container, which was hidden under the worktable.

"When do you empty this?" he asked Mitch, pointing to the container.

Mitch looked puzzled. "When it gets full, of course."

"Was there a lid for the container?"

"There was, but it was hard to get the rags in it under the table with it on so we took it off."

"You can see how tight for space we are her," Brad explained. "We have to keep the can under the table."

Davis could now point to several aspects of their work activities which were not good practice with respect to their possible exposure to the liquid cleaner. First, they were all getting appreciable skin contact from handling the solvent-wetted rags without any skin protection. Some organic solvents of this type can be absorbed through the skin and get into the bloodstream. All of them can dissolve the protective natural oils of the skin, rendering it dry and more susceptible to skin irritation. Dermatitis did not appear to be a problem here. He noted that they all carefully washed their hands and face in the room sink immediately after they finished cleaning. Susan and Brad, in particular, applied a lot of the emollient skin lotion.

By another route of entry into the body, the workers were inhaling fairly high levels of the solvent vapor during the actual cleaning. Because the wet rags in the open trash container were allowed to evaporate directly into the room, they were also probably inhaling low levels of the solvent for much of the rest of the time they were in the room. The closing-off of the ceiling vent and the generally confined conditions of the room further exacerbated their exposures. Davis had seen many similar exposures using the same type of chlorinated solvents with more intense odor levels but without this degree of almost daily headaches and ill feelings. He knew that any evaluation of the safety of an exposure based on smell can be very misleading, as the threshold level of odor detection may be well above the safe level. Furthermore, it was necessary to know which specific chemical was involved before he could evaluate the expected health effects.

By late afternoon, the young workers had finished their cleanup detail and all of their outgoing mail had been collected. Apart from the use of the solvent cleaner, Davis had seen nothing else in their final activities which could suggest a possible cause of their illnesses. Even their smoking of one or two cigarettes, as they waited for quitting time, was too inconsequential to be a significant factor.

Davis searched out Joe Daily in his office to give him his admittedly limited findings with some safe recommendations.

"Joe, your people are getting unnecessary exposure to the solvent cleaner they use in the Repro room."

"How's that?"

"They're storing their waste cleaning rags in an open container. Could you replace it with a locking sealed metal can? That'll help contain the vapors."

"That's easy. What else?"

"When they're finished cleaning up, have them empty the container daily into sealed plastic bags and dispose of them safely."

"Okay."

"They should also be wearing protective gloves to prevent skin contact."

"Tell me what to get and I'll order it."

"I have to find out from the manufacturer what chemicals are in the cleaner so I can recommend a glove that's impervious to them. And of course, I want to know if there's any special toxic properties or hazards."

"Sounds good to me."

Finally, Davis told Joe Daily that he would send him a report of his findings with recommendations for improving the room ventilation after he had a chance to sort out the information back at his office. Daily nodded and thanked him for his visit. Uncharacteristically, Davis left feeling uncomfortable because he had failed to identify a specific causative agent, if indeed there was one, for the workers' complaints. What he had suggested to Daily was perfectly valid and useful industrial hygiene advice, but it was in the brush-your-teeth-daily category that did not specifically address the problem.

He flew back on a late afternoon flight and dutifully, though bleary-eyed, reported into work on the following Friday morning. Marge Broody looked up quizzically at him above her eyeglass rims.

"Was I right about Denver? Can we swap jobs, now?"

"Sorry, Marge. My typing isn't up to speed yet."

Marge sensed that her boss was not ready to discuss his trip. "Don't forget the weekly staff meeting at two," she reminded him.

"Can you place a call to this company in Duluth, please?" he asked, handing her his scribbled note containing the name of the E-Z-OFF cleaner manufacturer.

While she called the long distance operator, he scanned his mail and a half-dozen telephone messages.

"It's ringing, Lazar."

He picked up the phone and poised a pencil on a notepad. He identified himself to the friendly operator, who had announced an unfamiliar name of a small chemical specialty company.

"I'd like to get some information on the composition of your E-Z-OFF cleaner which my company buys from you."

He was referred to Mr. Adrian Snyder, their Products Manager.

"Sorry, sir, I can't tell you. Our formulations are proprietary," Mr. Snyder said politely, but firmly.

Davis said that he represented the medical department of his company and his inquiry related to a possible adverse health effect from the employees' use of the product.

"Well, I really don't believe. . . ."

"The information on composition will be held strictly confidential, Mr. Snyder," Davis quickly interjected.

Snyder had recognized Davis' company as one of the major corporations in the country. "Well, if it's for health reasons, I guess I can tell you. E-Z-OFF is mainly methylene chloride," he revealed.

"Anything else?"

"Not really," Snyder admitted. "It's almost 100 percent methylene chloride."

The chlorinated hydrocarbon solvents, of which methylene chloride is a member, are widely used in industry and consumer products as highly effective cleaning agents with the distinct advantage over the petroleum-based solvents like mineral spirits, or ordinary paint thinner, of being essentially noncombustible. They are fairly volatile, which means they have to be used with good ventilation because inhaling too much of the vapors can lead to dizziness, nausea, and headaches. Their main toxic effect from chronic exposure above the recommended workplace levels, or Threshold Limit Value, involves varying degrees of liver damage. At one extreme, carbon tetrachloride, one of the simpler and more volatile members, was found to be so potently hepatotoxic that it had long since been effectively eliminated from consumer and most industrial products and replaced with less toxic chlorinated hydrocarbon solvents. This liver damage also plays a role in making people who drink particularly susceptible to the toxic effects from exposure to the chlorinated solvents, notably carbon tetrachloride and methylene chloride. It was later suggested from animal toxicity tests, human case reports, and epidemiological studies that they also have a strong potential for causing human cancer.

Davis only knew at that time that methylene chloride was considered to be one of the "safer" solvents with a fairly high Threshold Limit Value of 250 ppm as compared to 10 ppm for the highly toxic carbon tetrachloride. It was widely used, in particular, as a component of paint strippers, and he himself had recently been using this product on a furniture refinishing job at home. He had followed the manufacturer's advice on the can to use the product with protective gloves and good ventilation, which simply meant he did the job outside on a slightly breezy and sunny day to avoid inhaling the solvent vapors. He had no problems and was not unduly concerned about any unusual health hazards in using it. He certainly would not have expected methylene chloride then to be a health problem at workplaces, if used correctly. In fact, because of its generally established low toxicity, it had been approved by the Food and Drug Administration for use in the manufacture of soluble coffee and other food products. It had also been touted as a desirable substitute for the fluorocarbons, commonly referred to by their trademark designation of "Freon," as the gaseous propellant in aerosol cans. Fluorocarbons escaping to the upper atmospheric layers had been strongly implicated in contributing to the chemical breakdown of the stratospheric ozone layer, which serves to absorb ultraviolet radiation and thereby protect life on earth from harmful ultraviolet radiation.

It was only years later that the evidence of lung and liver tumors from mice studies, and suggestions that it may also be a reproductive toxin causing testicular atrophy in test animals, were reported. Consequently, methylene chloride is no longer used in food manufacturing and both OSHA and EPA have designated it as a suspect or probably (but not proven) human carcinogen. More recently, there has been a report of testicular pain and reduced sperm counts among a few unprotected male workers using rags soaked with the solvent. This not uncommon experience of discovering belated and untoward toxicological and health effects should temper any absolute statements by occupational health professionals of the innocuousness of using any given chemical substance.

Mr. Snyder promised to prepare and send him a Material Safety Data Sheet for the E-Z-OFF product. Davis requested his own company's technical information services to do an updated literature search on the toxicological and health effects of methylene chloride. Based on his sense that the exposure conditions he had observed at the office were not unusually high, he honestly did not believe the methylene chloride was likely to be solely responsible for the reported health complaints. Davis had not rushed to any prejudgment; he was, in fact, acting in good faith based on the then best available information. In preparing his preliminary report, he included suggestions for increasing the amount of fresh and total airflow in the Repro room and improving the ceiling exhaust ventilation over the worktable to capture the main sources of the vapor exposures. This and his recommendations for containing the solvent vapors from the waste container and wearing protective gloves to eliminate skin contact, he felt, should effectively remedy any problem.

About a week later, he received a large folder from the technical information services containing the abstracts of the scientific literature search he had requested on the recently reported health effects from exposure to methylene chloride. He put them in his briefcase for later reading on his regular hour-long train ride him but he was so tired from his travels that he fell asleep before he even opened the folder. It was only on his Monday morning return trip to work, and sometime after scanning the headlines and almost finishing the crossword puzzle of his morning paper, when he started his review of the abstracts. He rapidly scanned the abstracts and felt that most of what he read was already familiar and predictable toxicological information. About three-quarters of the way through the pile of abstracts, he felt there was nothing to implicate the methylene chloride solvent as the cause of the headaches and began to think that ozone gas, the most commonly associated exposure then associated with photocopiers, was the most likely cause and he just "blew" it.

His failure to confirm the presence of ozone was probably one of those quirky circumstantial happenings when the levels were too low for detection. The copier could have been recently cleaned, or the work load was low, or the air exchange in the building ventilation system had been turned up, or the louvers of the exhaust grill had been opened. Perhaps two or more of these conditions happened to coincide around the time of his visit, which could account for the low or nondetectable level of ozone. Anyway, the train was approaching his station, so he put the pile of papers back in his briefcase and made a fast-paced attempt to finish the crossword puzzle.

A new crisis reported from the marketing department dealing with an outbreak of skin problems at a customer's machine shop using a new and highly promising metal working fluid immediately occupied his attention for the next several days. By the end of the week, he had almost forgotten about his unfinished review of the solvent literature search. Only the train ride home afforded him the luxury of uninterrupted reading so he dutifully and somewhat fecklessly returned to the research papers. He finished the review of abstracts without finding anything particularly noteworthy or, rather, useful to solve his problem.

He happened to have the most recent issue of a research journal in occupational medicine—which had not yet been abstracted for inclusion in his review—and glancing through the articles, he was jolted to read about some experiments with men and rats which confirmed that methylene chloride was metabolized in the liver to, of all things, *carbon monoxide*. Once released into the blood, this internal carbon monoxide would bind with the hemoglobin in the blood, thereby interfering with the normal uptake of oxygen. In short, a person sufficiently overexposed to methylene chloride vapors or with skin contact to the liquid could develop the characteristic headache symptoms of carbon monoxide poisoning. Of course, this was what had caused the inexplicable headaches in the reproduction room. The poor work practices and lack of effective ventilation would certainly have created an excessive exposure. And the worker's sometime smoking not only would have exacerbated the exposure but would account for the inconsistent complaints.

Davis could at least console himself that his early failure to identify the culprit was understandable. It was, indeed, an inside job.

SECTION TWO

■

Unsafe to Breathe

Case 4

The Fire Next Door

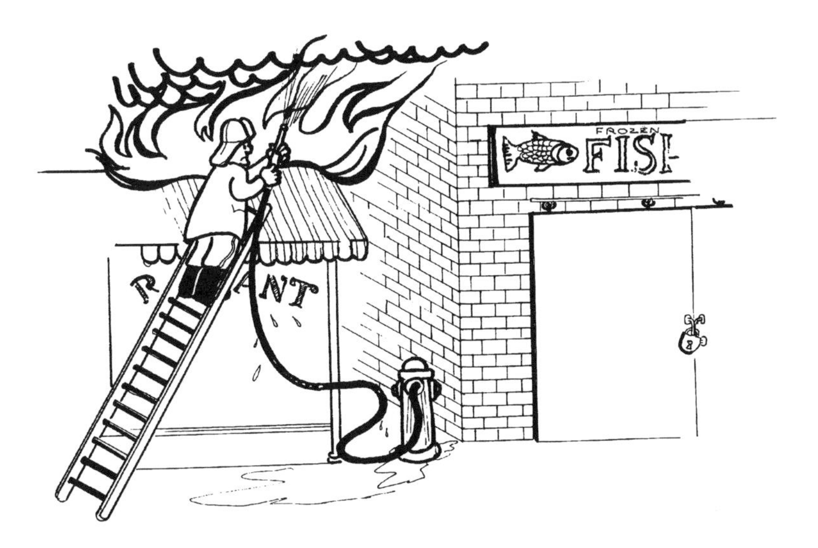

As Professor Davis drove north on the New Jersey Turnpike to the frozen-food warehouse to begin his investigation, he tried to picture several million dollars of frozen lobster, shrimp, and fish stacked in the freezer. The food-locker owner was unnerved by the suggestion from a consultant for the insurance company that the stock might have been fatally tainted by a poison carried downwind from a neighboring restaurant fire. The consultant had visited the warehouse the morning after the fire and warned that the potential liability from marketing the food was too great to risk. As proof of the toxic hazard was a report that two or three workers at the warehouse had recently been taken ill at work. It seemed prudent for both the warehouse owner and the insurer to call in Davis, an expert in identifying workplace illnesses and environmental contamination.

Davis had been informed that the fire had apparently started in the restaurant kitchen by a careless cook around 6:30 on a Wednesday morning, spread quickly, and was extinguished shortly by the local fire department after the food-warehouse workers had started their shift. Several hours later, only the two men at the warehouse working inside the frozen-food storage area complained of feeling nauseous and headachy. Davis was called on late Thursday with an urgent request to investigate the situation as soon as possible when it became apparent that the workers in the freezer area were still getting sick.

It was farfetched to believe that a toxic contaminant from a distant fire could be sucked into a building, penetrate the waxed or plastic wrapper of a frozen-food package, and be absorbed by the food. In that unlikely scenario, the Food and Drug Administration would classify the food as adulterated, meaning unfit for human consumption. Furthermore, it was somewhat incredible that this same unknown airborne contaminant would cause only a few—not all, or even most—of the workers inside the warehouse to get sick after several hours at work. In most of his workplace investigations of sudden illness, given sufficient background information, Davis was able to anticipate the most likely cause of the problem. On this one, he was stymied trying to think of even a tentative hypothesis with such contradictory information.

Exiting the Turnpike at a light industrial and commercial area of contiguous small municipalities, he drove a few miles to the warehouse and paused in the parking lot to look around. About one hundred feet directly across from the warehouse lot, he spotted the vacant, fire-gutted structure of the restaurant building. The three-story food warehouse had an exterior facing of corrugated metal with no evidence of any fire or heat damage. There were a few scattered small offices or light manufacturing buildings nearby but no stores or markets, scant traffic, and no one in sight. Suburban sterility, he thought, as he entered the warehouse to join a group of three men waiting for him in the clearly marked office of Mr. Sal Armenti, the owner-manager.

Smiling weakly, Mr. Armenti rose from his desk chair to introduce himself and the two men seated around him. George Evans was his foreman and J. Rodney Ryan was the loss control consultant called in by the insurance company. Ryan, a large effusive man conspicuously dressed in a maroon linen jacket, forest green slacks, and white deck shoes, initiated the obligatory business card exchanges.

"I see you're a professor," he said to Davis, with a slight raising of his eyebrows. "I got my degree in industrial management but I was always interested in science. Would you believe I passed a course in organic chemistry?"

Davis nodded in acknowledgment of Ryan's academic accomplishments but politely turned to the business at hand.

"I understand you think the locker food may be contaminated as a result of the fire," he directed to Ryan.

"Yeh. I was just explaining to these gentlemen about pyrolysis and thermal decomposition. That's how the heat from a fire can break down the synthetics in a building into very toxic chemicals," he translated for the lay audience. Davis listened patiently while Ryan expounded on his theories to account for the probably contamination of the food. First, there was phosgene, he began, which is so toxic it was once used for chemical warfare during World War I and is emitted during a fire involving plastics like polyvinyl chloride, commonly known as PVC. Or possibly, it could have been hydrogen cyanide, which every one knows is used in the death chambers and is given off when polyurethane plastics are burned. These poisons could have come from the restaurant fire itself, carried by the prevailing winds directly across to the warehouse parking lot, where it was sucked into the air intake of the food storage side of the building. When Sal Armenti mentioned that the warehouse was a fair distance from the fire and nobody outside, including the firemen, was reported to have taken sick during or for some time after the fire, Ryan had a ready answer. The intensity of the heat from the fire could have caused the insulation inside the warehouse to break down, thereby releasing the toxic gases. George Evans looked puzzled, explaining that the insulation on the walls and under the roof was not the decomposable type to which Ryan was alluding. Rather, it was a rock wool material, which is highly fire resistant, and, furthermore, there was no evidence of any heat damage inside the building from the fire. Undeterred, Ryan confidently asserted that irrespective of the mechanism, the fact that the men working inside the storage area got sick shortly after the fire proves that there was definitely something toxic released as a result of the fire. It was only logical that this toxic infusion would have also contaminated the packaged food, he concluded.

Such implausible nonsense, Davis thought, and this guy is ready to condemn the food lot with no direct proof for a projected loss of well over a million bucks. He restrained himself from expressing his opinion about Ryan's flexible theories and quietly asked if he could take a walk-through tour of the facility. Then, he would like to interview the workers who had been taken sick on the job.

George Evans had been waiting to take the professor around and promptly provided him with an oversized, thickly insulated, cover suit with a hood, because the temperature inside the food storage area was maintained at about ten to twenty degrees below freezing. Walking around the warehouse before inspecting the frozen-food storage area, Davis looked unsuccessfully for possible sources of workplace exposure or contamination. He noted that the man languidly filling refrigerated delivery trucks at the loading dock drove a nonpolluting electric fork lift truck. Business was uncharacteristically slow that day, George informed him, and the worker knew that if he did not stretch the assignment to the lunch break, he would be pushing a broom.

They entered the freezer through an outer, heavy canvas curtain and a thick, rolling steel door. Cartons of shellfish were stacked on steel-framed shelves almost to the ceiling of a room as large as a city high school gym. Although several dollies rested cater-cornered at the end of aisles, no one was seen working in the area. They started the tour with George explaining that maintaining the subfreezing temperatures was essential to protect and preserve the food.

Davis was interested in the presence of any chemicals or conditions which could generate a hazardous exposure, primarily in the frozen locker of the facility. George identified only two chemicals used in the freezer storage area. Davis sniffed the air for some telltale sign, although detecting the presence of an odorous chemical does not generally tell you much about the level of concentration other than it exceeds its "odor threshold," or the least concentration that can be smelled by someone with normal olfactory sensitivity. In this case, he could detect none of the characteristic odors of the two chemicals that Ryan had identified, which both had odor thresholds significantly well below the concentrations likely to cause ill effects.

The refrigerant in the cooling compressors was a chlorofluorocarbon liquid of a trademarked numbered series called "Freons" and now generically referred to as CFCs. These compounds are nonflammable, nonexplosive, essentially stable with a mild, nonirritating, ethereal odor and are generally regarded as having low toxicity. It would be hard to imagine a home or factory anywhere in the United States in which CFCs were not present in the refrigerators and air-conditioners or as components in cleaning fluids and as the propellant in aerosol cans. Stable at ground level, any escaping CFC molecules which diffuse up to the atmosphere some thirty to fifty miles above the earth's surface are broken down by solar radiation into chlorine which then acts as a catalyst to decompose the stratospheric ozone to oxygen. Since this ozone absorbs and thereby prevents a large portion of cancer-promoting solar ultraviolet radiation from reaching man's habitat, CFC production has been banned in the United States since 1979, and under a multinational agreement in Montreal in 1990, it has been gradually scheduled for ultimate elimination in the year 2000 by the signatory nations.

With a relatively high threshold limit value (TLV) of a thousand parts per million, an unusually high airborne concentration of CFC vapors would have been required to produce any adverse health effects from overexposure, let alone those reported by the warehouse workers. Practically, this would require the leakage of such a large quantity of liquid refrigerant that the loss would be indicated either by a noticeable drop in the fluid levels of the gauges or by an obvious increase in the storage room temperature due to a drop in cooling efficiency. George confirmed that no makeup of fluid had been required for the past several months and the temperature recorders showed practically no more than a few degrees variation from day to day.

The only other chemical used in this area was another organic chemical liquid called propylene glycol, which serves as a water-absorbing antifreeze bath around the cooling coils to prevent the buildup of ice. At very low temperatures, the liquid has negligible volatility, which means that only trace amounts of the liquid would evaporate as gas into the air and certainly not enough to produce any meaningful exposure to the workers.

Davis walked up and down the aisles quickly, occasionally stopping as if he were returning the seemingly watchful stare from an unusual specimen of unpackaged frozen fish. Rather, his practiced professional eye was searching for some clue of a causative agent for the illnesses. He would return later to take some standard measurements of the air quality, including the carbon dioxide and carbon monoxide content, but so far he saw nothing even remotely suggestive of a culprit. He gratefully left this oversized, walk-in freezer with the hope of getting some plausible clues from the sick freezer workers. George left to round up the men for their interviews and said they would all meet back in Armenti's office.

Sipping a cup of black coffee, alone in the office, Davis reviewed his handwritten notes and while his mind was still fresh, he made legible some of his more obscure script with an air of affected concentration. He did not want to encourage any conversation with Ryan or anyone else until he had something substantive to report. If Ryan pressed his case, Davis would be tempted to ridicule his cockamamie theory. Sal Armenti returned to his office a few minutes later, expressly, as it became apparent, to share some of his private thoughts with the professor.

"Doc, I think you should know that one of the men you'll be talking to, Mike Nolan, has been a complainer and a goof-off since he started here. I have my doubts about him really being sick."

This was not an uncommon suspicion by the management at many plants, particularly when there are just a few isolated cases or complaints or work-related sickness.

"Possibly, Mr. Armenti," he granted, "But let's assume his complaints are valid until proven otherwise."

"Of course, if there's something in my plant that's making them sick, I want to know and straighten it out," Armenti quickly added. "But I know my men. They've been blowing it up. There's even some talk about refusing to work in the freezer room unless we get this thing settled. Jeez, don't they realize I could be ruined if my fish is spoiled and the insurance don't cover the loss?"

George entered the office with two young men in their twenties, briefly introduced them as Ray Kovacs and Mike Nolan and then he and Sal tactfully excused themselves. Both Ray and Mike gave similar accounts of the chronology and description of their sickness at work. About 10:30 on the morning of the fire, Mike, who had been stacking cartons at the upper levels all morning, began feeling queazy. Just before noon, he had a headache and felt so dizzy every time he bent down to pick up a carton, he had to leave, almost groping his way back to the main warehouse floor, and barely made it to the men's room before vomiting. He did not return to work in the freezer area in the afternoon.

Ray said he started out operating the fork lift truck on that Wednesday morning, transporting stock into the warehouse. By noon, he had a slight headache and, although not feeling hungry, he ate his lunch, albeit, as he reflected, with little appetite. By mid-afternoon, working alone at the upper levels doing what Mike had been doing earlier, he began to feel dizzy and sick in the stomach. He managed to finish the shift, took two aspirins when he got home, felt awful in the evening, and took two more aspirins just before going to bed at ten o'clock.

On Thursday, the next day, Mike was operating the fork lift in and out of the freezer area while Ray remained inside, stacking the shelves in the upper levels. Although neither man recalled feeling ill at the start of the shift, they were not feeling particularly chipper, either. By the first coffee break, Ray felt weaker and had a headache which felt as if there was a steel band around his forehead. By lunch time, unable to eat, he sat outside with his head down and complained of numbness in his legs. Mike, on the other hand, did not feel the queasiness return until just after lunch, but by mid-afternoon he was dizzy and had a headache. Both men complained to George Evans that the work was making them sick and they refused to go back to the freezer area until the problem there was solved because they knew no one else working in the main warehouse or offices was getting sick. Davis learned later that when Sal Armenti heard of their revolt, he quietly asked his son, Nicky, to fill the orders which had to go out by that evening. Actually, Sal was still somewhat dubious of the validity of Mike's illness and sensed that Ray might be a psychosomatic victim of suggestion. What better way to prove that the sickness thing was trumped up than by having Nicky, whom everybody trusted, spend a few harmless hours there?

Davis recapitulated his understanding of their experiences and raised some points for clarification and more detail. When he asked Mike, almost casually, whether Wednesday morning was the first time he took sick, Mike thought for a while and then said, "Well, I left work early on Tuesday because I wasn't feeling great."

"Not feeling great? In what way?"

"Sort of the same thing. Sick to my stomach, you know, with a lousy headache. Thought it could of been a hangover, but I wasn't out drinking Monday night. Besides, I don't often get sick like that."

Davis, who had been fairly certain that the restaurant fire was not the cause of their sickness, was now pretty well convinced that their exposures originated from somewhere within the building and that what probably made Mike sick at work on Tuesday before the fire, and was what had made them both sick on Wednesday and Thursday. Based on the symptoms reported, he now had a fairly strong candidate in his mind for the probable cause of their illness, but, first, he had to confirm his hunch by showing it was present and in sufficient concentration to cause sickness. Then, if successful, he had to find the source in order to solve the problem.

Bundled up in his arctic space suit, he returned to the freezer section with George to take air measurements for the suspect contaminant using a direct-reading sampler. For purposes of quickly identifying whether there may be a problem with an exposure to a gas contaminant commonly found in the workplace, industrial hygienists have come to rely on the direct-reading indicator tube. This is a specially prepared sealed glass tube, less than a quarter of an inch in diameter, packed with a gas-absorbing powder or gel impregnated with chemicals which react, more or less specifically, with a particular airborne contaminant. If an air sample containing the contaminant is pulled through an opened tube with a small hand pump, the presence and amount of the contaminant is indicated, within seconds, by a color change or stain along a concentration scale printed on the tube.

Standing a short distance inside the freezer area at ground level, Davis first snapped off the glass tips of an indicator tube for carbon dioxide gas, inserted it snugly in the inlet of his hand pump, and pulled an air sample through the glass tube. Because the chemical reaction is slowed down below room temperatures, he had to warm the tube by wrapping his palm around it.

We are constantly exposed to fairly high amounts of carbon dioxide in our environment, without any apparent adverse effects. For example, carbon dioxide can be found at 3.5 percent concentration in our own exhaled breath, and higher concentrations are released from the tail pipes of our cars and trucks, from the combustion of oil or gas in home heating, and from the stacks of industrial plants and processes. There are also huge amounts emitted from natural sources, including forest fires, volcanic eruptions, and the eventual decomposition of all living matter. We are even exposed to carbon dioxide from the bubbles escaping from soda pop and beer. These emissions of carbon dioxide are greatly diluted by the time they become part of our breathing atmosphere. In short, we expect to find measurable, but low and tolerable, amounts of carbon dioxide just about everywhere. Normal occupied room air with adequate ventilation will average about 400 parts of carbon dioxide per million parts of air, or 400 ppm. Davis measured about 800 ppm of carbon dioxide in the freezer room air, well above the normal range, but not of any serious concern for health reasons. He said nothing to George, who was following his activities with great interest and seemed intrigued by Davis' facility to get information from the markings on a glass tube.

He then tested the air in the same way, only this time he used an indicator tube manufactured to respond primarily to carbon monoxide (CO) gas, also a naturally occurring compound associated with combustion but toxic at fairly low concentrations. If the combustion is inefficient as in a poorly tuned car engine, fork lift, or a malfunctioning home heater, then CO is produced in greater amounts. When the amount of CO gas released into the air we breathe exceeds tolerable concentrations, we can then become ill and possibly collapse or die, depending on the length and intensity of the exposure. Our body produces low concentrations of CO internally from our metabolism and, as such, it presents no problem to our health. The hemoglobin in our blood combines with oxygen and releases the oxygen wherever it is needed in our bodies. However, when oxygen and CO are both present, the CO will preferentially combine with the hemoglobin, to form the compound called carboxy-hemoglobin. This unwanted combination not only inactivates the hemoglobin, but it also restricts the useful oxygen-carrying hemoglobin from releasing its oxygen, producing a type of chemical asphyxiation. The most common early signs of overexposure to CO include nausea, headache, weakness, and dizziness.

As the air coursed through the narrow diameter of the glass indicator tube, a telltale coloration slowly developed along the bed of reactant chemicals. Davis nodded ever so slightly as he completed the requisite number of squeezes on his hand pump, warmed the tube again with his palms, which finally registered a concentration of about twenty parts per million, or ppm, of CO in air. Normally, the background concentration of CO in an office or home is only a few ppm and barely detectable with a direct-reading tube. If there are smokers or an open combustion source in the area, or the building is close to a heavily trafficked road where there is likely to be some contaminating air infiltration from outside, the CO level can be slightly higher. Davis told George he would like to get a similar set of air samples at the upper level, and spurred on by the nippy air, they quickly made their way up to an elevated platform. Davis obtained his samples, which not only confirmed the presence of both the carbon dioxide and CO at above normal background levels but were actually even higher than the ground-floor measurements. He recorded the results and they were on their way back to Armenti's office in just under ten minutes.

Mike Nolan, who had been unobtrusively watching them when they entered the freezer locker, was waiting for Davis, while managing to look busy collecting the empty shipping cartons strewn in the area.

"Find anything?" he asked Davis cautiously.

George Evans interjected, "The professor will give his report to Armenti and you'll be informed, Mike. We won't hide anything."

"George, do you mind if I ask Mike a few questions?"

George nodded.

"Mike, are all the fork lift trucks you use electric?"

Mike looked slightly puzzled. "We got a gas truck."

George interrupted to explain. "That's an old unit we keep as a spare in the warehouse or on the loading dock, for emergencies only."

By gas truck, he was referring to a fork lift truck, which burns a hydrocarbon gas, not a liquid, like gasoline or kerosene. Stored in a pressurized cylinder on the fork lift, the gas fuel may be propane, butane, or a mixture of hydrocarbon gases, called liquified petroleum gas, or LPG. The combustion products would always be high in carbon dioxide, but the amount of CO produced depends on the completeness of the combustion. A well-tuned LPG-burning fork lift burning efficiently and equipped with a catalytic after-burner to assure complete combustion will produce very low but safe levels of CO.

"George, two of the electrics have been in the shop for over a week now. We had to use the gas unit," Mike said. "Besides, it's more powerful than the. . . ."

"Mind if I see that gas truck in operation?" Davis asked George.

In a few minutes, Davis was taking CO measurements of the air around the elusive gas fork lift. Even at a distance of several feet from the discharge, the CO readings were so abnormally high they were off the scale of the indicating tube, or well above 500 ppm. With Mike seated at the operator's position, the CO levels in his breathing zone were over 100 ppm, which is in excess of the then federal government's workplace exposure limit of 50 ppm as an eight-hour daily average. The pieces of the puzzle were starting to come together.

Back in Armenti's office, J. Rodney Ryan was uncharacteristically quiet as Davis and George entered. Armenti looked up cautiously at Davis.

"Well, Professor, did the butler do it?"

"I don't think it was the cook," Davis retorted, with only the slightest tilt in Ryan's direction. "It seems very likely that your men were overexposed to carbon monoxide from your gas fork lift truck."

"The old gas unit? In the freezer room? Damn it, I gave orders they're not supposed to. . . . "

"Sal, I just found out about it myself," George said.

Davis' explanation of the sequence and causation now seemed perfectly obvious. The gas fork lift was spewing excessive levels of CO in consequence of neglectful maintenance. Because the air inside the freezer area was largely recirculated without makeup or fresh air, there was little dilution of the contaminant. Thus, the CO would rapidly accumulate to dangerous levels inside the freezer and the fork lift operator would also be exposed from the exhaust outside of the freezer. Even the observation that the CO concentrations seemed to be higher at the upper work levels was supported by the fact that the hot combustion gases from the fork lift would quickly rise to the roof in the cold room. Both of the stricken men were also smokers, which would have an added, exacerbating burden of carboxy-globin in their blood from their inhalation of CO in the cigarette smoke.

The restaurant fire next door? Only a coincidence, and Mike's claim of getting sick before the fire, concurrent with the use of the gas fork lift truck inside the freezer area, was believable. And as for the contamination of the food stock, well, no one even mentioned this charge. Ryan quietly left, muttering something about an appointment in East Orange. Davis told Armenti that if there were still any doubts of the role of CO in causing the illness of an exposed worker, he could indirectly estimate the carboxy-hemoglobin content in the blood by measuring the CO in the worker's breath with a technique similar to the breathalyzer check used by police on suspected drunk drivers.

"Nope, that wasn't necessary," a smiling Armenti said. He hardly had to be told the corrective measures which Davis recommended. The freezer area would be purged of the residual CO with large circulating fans before anyone returned to work there. Only electric fork lifts could be used in the freezer room, without exception. The spare gas fork lift would be restricted to outside use and would be serviced on a regular maintenance schedule to assure it was operating at optimum efficiency. As he was thanking Davis for his help, Nicky, his son, entered the office.

"You feeling okay, Nicky?" Armenti's cautiously asked.

"Yeh, I'm fine, Dad," he answered, hesitantly. Than after a slight pause,

"Well, not really, I think I feel a little dizzy and maybe I'm getting a headache and. . . ."

Armenti nodded knowingly and waved the professor on his way. He could smile now that he knew his fish could be shipped out safely and that things were under control.

Davis knew in a few days that the matter was really solved. They only call you when they have problems.

Case 5

The Tank Farm Tragedy

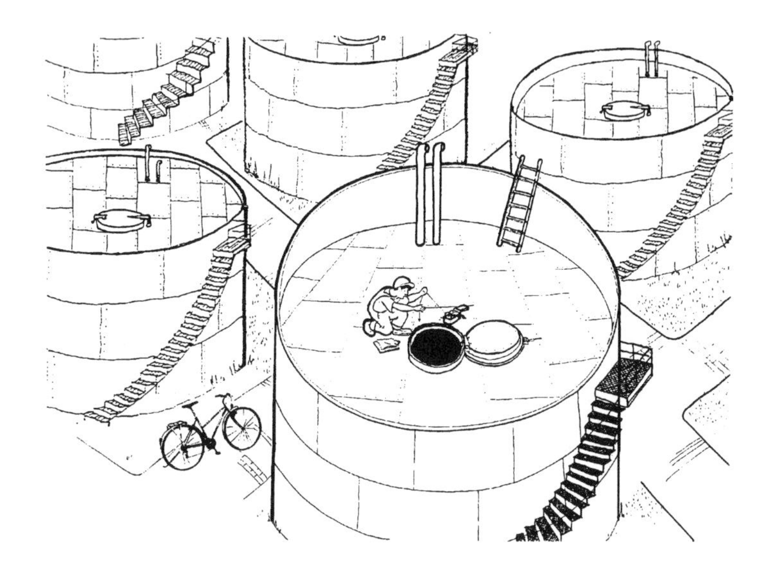

Every day in the United States, our cars, buses, and trucks, which keep us moving and supplied, consume almost 300 million gallons of gasoline, or more than a 100 billion gallons throughout the year. Between the time the gasoline is manufactured from the crude oil at the refinery and is delivered to a local terminal or service station, it is stored, along with the crude oils and other refined petroleum products, in high rise, cylindrical, steel tanks, often aligned in an area close to the oil refinery. The gasoline vessels can be as high as 48 feet with a diameter of 140 feet and a capacity of over 6 million gallons. The land on which they are located, although uncultivated, free of livestock, and otherwise barren, is called a tank *farm*. And possibly in an attempt to soften the assault to our aesthetic sensitivities at this antilogy, many of the refineries have whimsically decorated the storage tanks with baseball insignias or cartoon characters, often against pastel-colored backgrounds. From an aerial view, they might suggest giant children's blocks, or checker pieces.

Denny Moore was thirty-three years old and had been a full-time tank gauger at the tank farm for almost seven years. His father had retired from the company refinery next door after thirty-eight years as a pipefitter, and one uncle and a cousin still worked there.

The tank gauger indirectly measures the volume of product in a tank by lowering a weighted measuring tape, similar to a carpenter's plumb bob, to the surface of the liquid to obtain the product depth. In effect, the manual gauger is taking inventory of the stock. Today, electronic devices relay the measurements from an automatic mechanical gauge to a control center, and, thereby, have largely supplanted the need for full-time manual gaugers. But limitations of the smart electronic instruments to gauge certain viscous products like asphalts, and the need to validate measurements, particularly in product transfer between companies, occasionally require the services of a Denny Moore. In like fashion, only a human gauger may be able to collect quality control samples by dropping a weighted bottle, accusingly called an oil thief, into the storage vessel.

There are basically two types of liquid petroleum storage tanks. The conventional storage tank has a fixed roof which is not constructed to withstand any appreciable buildup of pressure or vacuum that might result from the expansion or contraction of product vapors as the product levels and temperatures change. Product vapors released by normal evaporation inside the tank would have to be allowed to escape into the atmosphere through pressure relief valves, or, reversibly, air would have to enter through vents to maintain equilibrium with the atmospheric pressure. Relatively low volatile products like kerosene and home heating oil, which do not evaporate appreciably at normal or room temperature, are usually stored in conventional or fixed roof tanks with little danger. With the more volatile products like gasoline, the constant release of highly flammable and toxic vapors could present a significant safety and health problem to the tank farm workers as well as appreciable contribution to the community air pollution. A *floating-roof* tank was, therefore, developed specifically to contain volatile product vapors. The roof, which rests on pontoons, rises and falls according to the level of the liquid product. By capping the liquid, the floating roof eliminates any "head," or air space and effectively prevents any appreciable release of dangerous vapors. To prevent the roof from sinking to the ground level at which level refloatation might be difficult, support legs were installed inside the shell at the three-foot level. All the gasoline and light products at Denny's tank farm were stored in tanks with floating roofs.

At the start of each work shift, Denny would be given his assigned list of tanks. On conventional fixed-roof tanks, he would climb up steep, outside stairs, often the equivalent of a five-story building, to the roof of the tank and open the hatch to get a liquid level reading. With the floating-roof types, he would climb down stairs inside the tank shell to the roof level and take his reading accordingly after opening the hatch. Illuminating the tank interior with a flashlight beam, he would carefully lower the measuring tape and record the scale reading when the weight made contact with the liquid product. The gauger's safety guide says that the gauger should stand so that the vapors will not be inhaled, but it doesn't say how. It also advises wearing a gas mask if toxic gases are present, but it doesn't identify what these gases may be or how the worker would go about identifying their presence. Denny understood the intent of the warnings and was particularly careful not to get any closer to the inside of the tank than was necessary to get his reading. He had heard that the men who filled barrels with gasoline would sometimes experience headaches, nausea, or sleepiness from the well-known narcotic effects of inhaling too much of the vapors. He had never suffered from the gasoline vapors or any other petroleum product vapors or, at least, had never complained about them.

Standing upright over the open hatch of a tank roof, Denny could easily smell the characteristic odor of the gasoline vapors escaping from the tank, although at this location the concentration is usually low. But sometimes, if it was dark or there was poor contrast, it would be difficult to see the liquid surface without kneeling directly over the hatch opening. If he then had to peer into the opening where the vapor levels were considerably higher, his nose and throat would be irritated and his eyes might burn despite the safety glasses. So warned, he might then hold his breath and try to get his reading as soon as possible. When he finished recording the result, he would promptly call in by walkie-talkie to his supervisor that he had finished the job and identify where he was headed for his next assignment. His boss, or a fellow worker, would routinely call him back later to check on his status or to make changes in his schedule; addendums might include comments about the weather, the Mets' loss the night before, or a reminder that it was his turn to drive for the bowling league game tonight. Thus, his supervisor or fellow workers always knew where he was or where he was heading. Since the tank farm covered almost one hundred acres, he got plenty of exercise riding his bicycle, or walking in all kinds of weather. The job was not particularly challenging or interesting; rather, as Denny preferred not to think about it, it was boring.

"I'll have seven years of seniority soon. And no other company gives you so many benefits," he would offer in response to Betsy, his wife, when she suggested that he might look for a more satisfying job with better opportunity for advancement.

"Your only news from work is Hal Berger's retirement party and whether being third in seniority, you can live long enough to become a group supervisor. Maybe you should think about going back to community college at night to get your associate's degree."

"You have to be realistic, honey. I'm almost thirty-four and would have to start at entry level pay in another job. We can't afford it, and besides, no other company has a better pension and stock savings plan and. . . ."

He didn't have to recite the litany to Betsy. She was very appreciative of the company-paid medical coverage, the new dental plan, the scholarship and interest-free college tuition fund for their kids, and, above all, the job security.

Denny's reminder of his forthcoming seventh anniversary with the company provoked Betsy to volley with the more pressing reasons to change her complacent husband.

"I always worry about a fire or explosion there."

"Honey, there hasn't been a serious fire in all the time I've been there."

"And your climbing all those stairs. Especially when the weather gets so beastly hot."

"The refinery doctor says I'm in great shape. You know I don't have to catch my breath climbing to the roof like some of those younger guys with the beer bellies."

"What about breathing in all those fumes all day long? They can't be good for your health."

He sighed, with slight exasperation. "You know you can smell the fumes before they can hurt you."

"Well, it just doesn't seem like a safe or healthy place to work," she summarized, sensing that the dialogue had run its course.

As an intelligent and perceptive woman, Betsy's instinct about the hazards of Denny's work at the tank farm were well founded. Apart from the common traumatic work injuries, like falls from ladders and unguarded elevated walkways, or even on level but slippery floors, and bruises and cuts from tools and machinery, with millions of gallons of oil, the tank farm was one vast tinder box.

Denny's high regard for the oil company's commitment to safe and healthy work practices was as similarly defensible as were Betsy's apprehensions. At least, for the record, the company required their employees to adhere to the work safety requirements spelled out in detailed regulations by the federal Occupational Safety and Health Administration (OSHA). Just one section of the OSHA safety regulations dealing specifically with flammable and combustible liquids of the type represented by gasoline covers almost thirty-three pages in the Code of Federal Regulations. In addition, the American Petroleum Institute (API), which is the trade organization of the industry and the National Safety Council's Petroleum Section had developed specific guidelines and procedures for the safe gauging and sampling of petroleum products upon which the OSHA regulations are based.

Even before a federal law required it, the refinery and tank farm employees were regularly instructed on the life-threatening dangers at their workplace. Their safety advisors and supervisors were generally implacable about insisting that the employees comply with the safety rules and procedures; that is, when they were on site to observe the workers. When unwatched, the workers might be somewhat less diligent. Nonetheless, the accident and injury rates of the oil industry are among the lowest of similar heavy industries and its employees are among the healthiest of all workers. This may be due, in part, to the industry's high standards for hiring well-qualified and initially healthy employees and then providing them with ongoing medical surveillance and safety training.

It was an overcast, windless Monday morning with high barometric pressure in mid-October. Denny was returning to work after a one-week vacation, purposely dedicated to personal and household chores in lieu of the usual family outings of a summer holiday. Traveling with his wife and four rambunctious sons to the seashore or the zoo during his earlier summer vacation was hardly restful or self-serving. Understandably, Denny planned his week after the boys returned to school. He did manage during the week to go to a football game with a neighbor, read most of a paperback detective story, and went to a dinner theater with Betsy. The last few days he devoted to the annual ritual of cleaning out the basement and garage, and seasonal activities like fertilizing and seeding the lawn and emptying and storing the children's large plastic swimming pool. It was during this last chore on a Friday morning that he had one of those quirky accidents that are cited by work safety proponents as proof that accidents can happen anywhere when the victim is not cognizant of or responsive to the hazard.

Denny had been well indoctrinated in safety at work and did not need to be convinced of doing the right thing at home. In this case, he and millions like him, working at home with chemical products available in any hardware store or supermarket, was simply unaware of the potential dangers of the indiscriminate use of these products. The federal labeling law on hazardous household products requires adequate warning with instructions for their safe use, but many people do not read the label or follow the advice. Notwithstanding the law, some manufacturers or suppliers, particularly a small company with limited or no technical resources, may have provided a label with insufficient information. And sometimes, despite the well-intentioned efforts of industrial toxicologists, industrial hygienists, and product safety experts, the hazard has yet to be discovered or publicized. We may never know just why Denny did not know of the danger in his seemingly harmless act of cleaning out a swimming pool with a mixture of household products.

Working inside his garage, he was suddenly seized with intense burning of his eyes, nose, mouth, and throat and began coughing unremittingly. His wife heard his coughing and panicked when she saw him lying on the ground, gasping for breath. She screamed, alerting the retired couple next door, and together they dragged Denny out of the garage and then called the local hospital emergency squad. At the hospital, Denny was given oxygen, a mild sedative, a bronchodilator, and an antibiotic. He responded very well to the treatment and although he felt somewhat weak, had a raspy throat, and some residual chest pain, he was able to go home, unassisted, several hours later. Despite some intermittent coughing, he slept through the night. He rested comfortably in the morning and by afternoon, he felt well enough to complete some light chores. By Sunday night, preparing to return to work, he practically forgot about the incident. Denny Moore was not a complainer.

He certainly said nothing about it at work when, dutifully and fecklessly, he returned on that dreary Monday morning. He was unabashedly delighted, however, to rejoin his pals, Ed Stanko and Stan Love, in the locker room. He and Ed had grown up together as neighborhood kids and had remained close friends.

"How was your parole?" Ed asked, playfully.

"Just stayed home, but it was fine, Ed. Maybe next year we'll go to Disney World. Anything new around here?"

"So what should be new?" Stan reflexively answered. At forty-three, and the leading man and mentor of the group, Stan had recently been awarded his twenty-five-year service emblem at a company luncheon, which he described as one of the more depressing events of his life. "I hate to think that I've been climbing up and down those damn tanks for a living. But to be reminded of it with a lousy silver-plated pin as an award, no less, is too much."

His two pals nodded in empathetic agreement. More accurately, as a group leader, Stan was mainly responsible for supervising the gauging operations of the regular gaugers. He only climbed the tanks for routine surveillance or to instruct a trainee from the labor pool as a backup gauger. They finished putting on the company-issued oil-impervious coveralls, nonsparking, nonskid, steel-toed safety shoes, impact-resistant polycarbonate hard hats, and then picked up their chemical safety goggles and walkie-talkies. They were ready to start their workday. They also had access to an explosion meter for checking the combustible gas concentration and an oxygen-level meter for confirming that there was sufficient oxygen in the air before entering inside the storage tank shells. For emergency entrance into an oxygen-deficient space, they had self-contained breathing masks. From experience, they felt there was little need for this equipment in routine testing, so they rarely carried the detectors and masks on the job.

At 7:35 A.M., on their leisurely walk to the manager's office for their weekly briefing, the trio confabulated on the more personally rewarding discussions of whether the Mets still had a chance in the final pennant race, why Ed should not trade in his vintage Camaro this year, and after mowing, do the uncollected grass clippings help or kill the lawn. When they entered the office, Hal Berger, the soon-to-retire, sixty-year-old tank farm manager and their boss, was dictating a letter to Bonnie Bray, his secretary of more than thirty years. Everybody joked that, like the Pharaoh's widows, she would have to be buried with him. They knew he was finished dictating when he mumbled the final of a series of "Et cetera. Et cetera," and Bonnie, knowingly, filled in the gaps and closed her steno pad. He greeted them curtly but pleasantly, and immediately got down to business. He briefly reviewed the previous week's mundane chronology and said something about the current percent of storage capacity relative to last year's figures, which was of no particular concern or interest to his audience.

"There's an announcement about an opening for a couple of unit operator trainees in the refinery," he directed to Denny and Ed. "If either of you guys are interested, I'll be happy to recommend you. Not that I want to get rid of you." He hardly had to reassure them. He was a good and fair boss, and they not only worked harmoniously together but they genuinely liked each other.

They said they would think about it but, as they had often privately concluded about such moves, the refinery was just a much bigger pond with more sharks and more of the same boring jobs. Besides, there were too many long-term refinery workers with seniority to expect better chances for advancement there.

Hal also announced that all operations employees were scheduled for refresher courses in fire-fighting and CPR. And the regular safety meeting, usually held on the third Tuesday of the month, would be held on Thursday afternoon because Rick Brown, their safety advisor from the nearby refinery, had to go out of town. They all listened politely and asked no questions. So much for their weekly briefing. Hal then retreated into his private office to mull over the dubious import of the latest formidable batch of company mail.

Stan handed Denny and Ed a single sheet containing their respective assignments, reminding Denny that the employee relations department at the refinery wanted him to stop by sometime during the day. He thought they said something about a payroll deduction form for Denny's credit union loan payment. Glancing at his work schedule, Denny said he would go there directly, as his first assignment was closest to their office.

It was now 8:10 A.M. and the three co-workers went their separate ways. They did not have to be reminded that they would rendezvous for a coffee break by the refreshment truck, stationed just outside the south gate at 9:30, give or take ten minutes. At noon, they would have their lunch together under one of the few trees on the tank car property near their locker room, weather permitting.

Denny headed on his bicycle for the employee relations office in the adjacent refinery, about a half mile away. The sky had darkened, so he had to turn on the bicycle light.

Most of the company workers suspiciously regarded their employee relations advisors as advocates for the company rather then the employees. Denny, as his Dad before him, never shared this adversarial feeling about the company. He might not love his job, but he felt the company was fair and decent to the employees, and he was particularly quick to remind his fellow workers that no one was ever laid off in almost forty years. There had only been one strike in all that time, which lasted less then three days over some minor seniority incident, and any bargaining over wages or benefit issues was invariably undermined by the company's generous offers before the negotiations even began.

By 8:45 A.M., he had finished his business at the employee relations office and headed for his first assignment, tank 409 containing regular gasoline. Shortly before nine o'clock, Denny called Hal's office on his walkie-talkie to report that he was ready to gauge tank 409.

Like the fuel oil tanks that many of us have in our basements, there are small graduated glass tubes called sight gauges on the outside or on top of the tank which conveniently provide an approximate reading of the product level inside the tank. Denny proceeded to take a sight gauge reading and noted that the product level was so low that it had fallen approximately one foot below the leg support level, which is only two feet from the bottom. Most importantly, there was now a one-foot-deep air pocket between the gasoline surface and the suspended roof, into which vapors from the liquid gasoline would rapidly collect. In keeping with his usual practice, Denny tried to call back to the office to tell them of his finding and that he was going to transfer sufficient gasoline from an adjacent tank to raise the level above the leg support level in 409. For one brief moment, no one was there to take any calls. Stan had spotted two of his labor crew passing by his window and hurriedly left the office without his walkie-talkie to tell them that there was a change in their assignment after lunch. Bonnie was using the photocopier across the hall. Denny started the gasoline transfer shortly after nine. Around 9:10 A.M. Stan returned to the office and was about to call Denny on a routine status check when the telephone rang with a message for Stan to call his wife. Employees could not get incoming personal calls directly and could return a call only when their duty allowed. Sue, his wife, reminded him to pick up a chair that had been reupholstered on his way home, and they discussed briefly whether they should eat the meatloaf again tonight or send out for Chinese food, as Sue had promised to babysit most of the day for her sister who had an appointment with her obstetrician. Stan hated detailed telephone conversation particularly at work so he politely terminated Sue's call. He reached for the walkie-talkie. There was no immediate response, which meant that by this time Denny was probably enroute to the next assignment and was in an area with poor reception or had stopped in the men's room. Nothing of immediate concern, though. In the meantime, on a separate walkie-talkie frequency, Stan called Ed, who was returning from the quality control laboratory in the refinery. He had just delivered a crude oil sample that he had collected from a tanker.

"Any chance you can referee my kid's Little League game tomorrow night, Stan?" Ed asked. "I forgot I promised my daughter I would go to her swim meet and I disappointed her last time."

They bantered about it for a minute or so and Stan good-naturedly agreed to help out his friend. Before hanging up, Stan asked Ed if he had seen Denny on his way from the lab.

"Haven't seen him since he left to go to employee relations," he answered. "Anything wrong?" he asked.

"I don't know. It's just that I haven't heard from him since he got to 409. That's not like Denny. Tell him to call me."

"Sure, Stan. I'll head right over there."

A few minutes after Stan hung up with Ed, Hal came out of his office with the mail. Stan casually asked, "Hal, did you hear from Denny while I was out?"

Hal shook his head, and pointing to his paper, said, "Nope. I was mesmerized in my office with this crap."

"Bonnie, did you hear from Denny when I was out?"

"No, Stan, I may have been making copies or. . . ."

"When did we hear from him last?" Hal asked.

"Gee, I guess it must have been about. . . ." Stan hesitated, not really sure of the time. He momentarily froze with a worried expression and then grabbed the walkie-talkie.

"Denny," he yelled into the speaker. "Can you hear me? Where the hell are you?"

There was no response. Just the usual background noise. Both men's eyes remained fixed on the mute receiver. It was now 9:40 A.M., or almost forty-five minutes since they had last heard from Denny.

They waited a full minute, when Hal urged, "Try him again."

Still, no response.

It was not that a forty-five minute interval of incommunicado was necessarily critical, but it was very unusual that there was no response from someone in the field to more than one follow-up call.

"Hey, Denny. Can you hear me? Answer me, please," Stan now implored.

When there was no response, Stan screamed at Bonnie, "Get the emergency squad over to 409 tank," and he sped off in a jeep.

He spotted Ed at the top of the stairway, flailing his arms and pointing downward into the tank, ominously gasping for breath. Stan raced up the 99 steps to join Ed at the top of the tank, climbed down to the floating roof, where he peered into the tank shell and spotted Denny about forty-feet below the tank top. Denny was lying face down over the hatch, motionless. Instinctively, and despite the protestations of Ed, Stan without a respirator started down the ladder, breathing hard from his physical exertion. Climbing down a few feet from the entry, he immediately smelled the characteristic gasoline odor and before he was halfway down, he was enveloped in a dense choking concentration of gasoline vapors forcing him to climb back up the ladder, holding his breath. He was vaguely aware that the piercing assault on his ear drums was from a shrieking ambulance siren.

"I . . . I . . . I called . . . the police," Ed explained.

Two members of a heart resuscitation squad arrived equipped with a resuscitator and a body harness with ropes and quickly joined them at the top of the tank. They tried to start down the ladder without any respiratory protection but were exhorted by Stan to stop.

"The fumes'll kill you. We need air packs to go down there."

A few minutes later, two corpsmen from the Emergency Services unit from a local hospital arrived—also without adequate respiratory protection—and actually climbed down onto the floating roof, where they quickly sensed the victim was lifeless. They were fortunate to escape just when two firemen arrived wearing air packs used to enter smoke-filled buildings. When they reached Denny, they felt no pulse, but were able to lift his body out of the tank with the rope harness and then down the outside ladder to the ground.

It was now 10:40 A.M., or about an hour and a half since Denny had entered the tank shell after the gasoline transfer. Perhaps unaware of the hospital corpsmen's findings, the heart resuscitation squad valiantly tried mouth-to-mouth resuscitation and CPR in the ambulance on the way to the hospital. The emergency ward intern confirmed that Denny had been dead on arrival.

An accident is considered to be an unexpected and undesirable event. When it involves a fatality, multiple serious injuries, or significant property loss at work, an investigation is mandated to find out why the unexpected occurred, largely to prevent repetitions. There are approximately four thousand work-related fatalities in the United States reported annually by the Bureau of Labor Statistics, although even the government acknowledges that an estimate of, at least, ten thousand by the National Safety Council and other safety experts is probably closer to the true picture. Whatever the total number, each individual death at work remains an unmitigated tragedy for many of the survivors, who believe that the death could, and should, have been prevented. By law, OSHA must be notified of the fatality within twenty-four hours.

According to oil industry safety records, no one had ever been overcome to the point of asphyxiation by gauging a gasoline tank. In a published survey of occupational gasoline vapor exposures, tank gauging was mentioned but was not judged significant enough to warrant exposure measurements. Everybody knew that working or going inside an enclosed space, like an empty tank that had contained gasoline, is a life-threatening situation and unprotected workers doing so have been fatally overcome. Strict safety rules require flushing, or purging, of the remaining gasoline vapors with fresh air before any one can enter, and only then with full respiratory protection and a backup crew.

Denny, like every gauger, knew from long experience that you could easily detect gasoline vapors well before the danger level. Your nose and eyes and throat were more sensitive to the vapors than the gas detector instruments. As for descending into a tank shell, there was an increasing gradient of concentrations. Since gasoline vapors are higher in density than air, the gasoline vapors tend to remain closer to the ground. In fact, at the very top of the shell, particularly as on the day of the accident if there were little wind and high barometric pressure, the vapor concentration at the top would be low but certainly sufficient to provide ample warning. Thus, in the minds of Denny's fellow workers and, indeed, within the industry, it was just assumed that Denny had suffered a heart attack, or some kind of stroke. "These things happen," they regularly intoned, to account for the inexplicable; notwithstanding that Denny was a young, nonsmoking, active, and apparently physically fit man, with no personal or family history of any serious health problems. They were shocked when they later heard that the autopsy indicated no evidence of a precipitating heart failure or stroke. It clearly showed extensive edema in Denny's lungs and congestion of his liver and spleen, entirely consistent with an asphyxiation due to hydrocarbons. For unknown reasons, Denny had no forewarning of the danger and in a matter of probably less than a few minutes, had, indeed, been overcome by breathing the gasoline vapors at a dangerously high level and was unable to escape.

Ironically, many injuries and deaths recorded officially as accidents, in retrospect, would not have been unexpected and would not warrant the time and energy for a formal investigation; for example, a highway crash involving a legally drunk truck driver exceeding the speed limit in the wrong lane. Denny Moore's death at work was unanticipated and clearly justified an investigation by experts.

When the floating roof at tank 409 dropped below its support level, the air space was rapidly saturated with gasoline vapors. Considering that the diameter of the circular roof was approximately 120 feet, the volume of air space when the roof was only 1 foot below the critical support level was over 11,000 cubic feet. When Denny transferred gasoline into the near empty tank, the air space saturated with gasoline vapors was displaced, pushed into the breathing space above the floating roof as if by a giant piston. For this reason, there was a safety requirement that at least four hours should lapse before employees could enter to gauge or work inside the tank shell to allow for dissipation of the vapors. The OSHA investigators used a checklist of the regulatory requirements and gave the company citations for numerous infractions of the gauging regulation. No checks for explosive gas levels or oxygen content had been made before the entry. The victim wore no self-contained breathing apparatus. There were no backup workers with respirators on hand and there was a critical lapse in communication. Most significantly, Denny had entered the floating tank shell immediately after making a partial transfer of product probably just to assure by gauging that the pontoons of the floating roof were afloat.

Rick Brown, the refinery advisor with thirty-five years of practical experience in refinery accident prevention conducted his own investigation by observantly walking around the accident scene, reviewing all the safety procedures used or abused, and asked a lot of questions of Denny's fellow workers and supervisors. A team from the corporate safety department conducted an even more formal investigation with dozen's of interviews and consultations with many safety experts in the industry. The absence of any prior gasoline vapor overexposure in gauging tanks—let alone, a death—stymied the industry experts.

When pressed, all of the investigators, by whatever method used, had to admit that they simply did not know what critical factor led to Denny's death. The failure to explain Denny's premature death only intensified his survivors' personal anguish and guilt feelings over the tragedy. Hal Berger wanted to cancel his retirement party and agreed to have it only when his fellow workers convinced him that that would have been Denny's wish. Ed Stanko was devastated and shuddered every time he passed by tank 409 or looked at Denny's locker. Within a month, he had applied for an opening at the refinery, was accepted, and had transferred. Stan Love, ultimately the lone and lonely survivor of the group, continued to perform his job conscientiously, seeming to chat only with Bonnie in the office, where he now ate his lunch. As Stan made plans to recruit and train a new gauging crew, John Del Monico, Hal's replacement and his new boss, informed him that an automated electronic gauging system would be installed throughout the tank farm and full-time manual gauging would be discontinued.

After higher management at the company headquarters had reviewed all the safety reports and conclusions, Roger Young, the senior vice president in charge of operations, was particularly dissatisfied with the uncertainty of the findings and felt that the company should continue to investigate the case. He knew the importance of conveying to the public and the employees the company's continuing concern for the accidental loss of human life. Implicit in his thinking was also the anticipation of a worker compensation inquiry or possible litigation by the employee's widow. Furthermore, he was a very astute and well-informed executive who had some questions of his own to raise. In early November, Roger Young arranged to meet Dr. Scott Robertson, the company medical director, for lunch in the executive dining room to discuss his concerns.

"Scott, I understand that the fatality we had last month at the tank farm was due to asphyxiation from gasoline vapors. The worker was a tank gauger, I think."

Dr. Robertson nodded. "Yes, we reviewed the autopsy findings. All the classic symptoms, as I remember."

"You know our safety people can't explain why it happened. They tell me there has never been an incident like that in the industry. Sure, we were somewhat lax with our safety rules, but why didn't the man sense he was in danger before getting overcome?"

The doctor was taken off guard. His department had not been a part of the corporate investigating team so he had not given it much thought. He answered cautiously, "It's possible that the man was particularly susceptible to an exposure that would not normally be expected to cause any problems. Perhaps he was on some medications or was a heavy drinker and there was a synergistic effect. That could account for it."

"What about other toxic exposures on the job? Or at another job?"

"Other chemical exposures at work? Yes, we can look into that. Fortunately, we don't see many chemical asphyxiations."

Dr. Robertson was not comfortable with his equivocal responses to a senior vice president, who might be the CEO some day. Before they had finished their dessert, Dr. Robertson offered to have a senior industrial hygienist on his staff perform a survey at the tank farm. He had in mind Lazar Davis, who was particularly adept at evaluating and considering all the causative factors, both on and off the job, which could be implicated.

"Sounds good," Roger Young agree. "I'll be anxious to see what you come up with."

In less than an hour, Davis, the senior industrial hygienist in the medical department, was told to drop what he was doing and see his boss, Dr. Kenneth Snyder, the Associate Medical Director. Davis knew nothing about the fatal accident at the tank farm nor would he be expected to. The company industrial hygienists performed ongoing surveys of the workplace exposures and conditions to assure compliance with the occupational safety and health standards. If they were not met, the hygienists would recommend the appropriate control measures. Since the emphasis in industrial hygiene is to *prevent* any adverse health effects rather than to have to respond to them, they might also participate in the planning and design of any new proposed operations or major changes with the existing operations. Unfortunately, a workplace death is after-the-fact and the hygienists are rarely involved or consulted then. The company managers, their safety advisors, and, sometimes, the company attorneys take over the fatality investigation.

"Lazar, the boss says Roger Young wants us to do a retrospective survey of the tank farm to find out why a tank gauger was asphyxiated by gasoline. Everything has been cleared for your visit ASAP and Corporate Safety will give you a complete briefing when you leave here."

Davis was well attuned to the crisis response within the company hierarchy which a request in the name of an "uppermost" manager could produce. Actually, some of the upper middle managers diluted the effect by indiscriminately incanting the big man's name for anything they wanted in a hurry. Davis knew that his boss was more prudent with his use of executive clout and he responded appropriately.

"I'll get right on it, Ken," he answered. By late afternoon, he had had his briefing from the safety department, but they said they weren't authorized to let him see their formal report of investigation. He nodded, as if that was expected, but he was rankled that turf protection between company departments took precedence over full cooperation. From his own medical department, he was given a summary of Denny Moore's medical history and from the employee relations department, a copy of Moore's work history. The library ran a rush computer search of the scientific literature for articles and reports dealing with gasoline vapor intoxication and came up with the printed abstracts of seven cases, none of them suggesting any unsuspected contributing factors.

He knew he would be doing a "walk-through" survey of the gasoline gauging operation, meaning he might take a few environmental samples, but mainly he would use his senses to gather information—particularly, by careful listening to Moore's fellow workers and their supervisors. The dead man's exposure was a singular event which could not now be surveyed. Nonetheless, he took a direct-reading survey instrument for some representative measurements. The values would only be approximate, but that would be good enough for his purpose of getting ballpark concentration figures to confirm the potential for asphyxiation, as reported. At the tank car farm the following morning, he was introduced to Stan Love, the gauging operation group supervisor, who was assigned to accompany him on his walk-through survey.

Stan described the tank gauging operations as they toured the facility on their way to tank 409, laconically answering the specific questions raised by Davis. In his twenty-five years at the tank farm, no gauger had ever been overcome by exposure to product vapors. Sure, gasoline was the most dangerous product stored there, but they were careful not to breathe the stuff more than they had to. No, they didn't have to use respirators because they never went deep into the tank. Headaches, sometimes, but doesn't everybody get headaches? No, the gaugers were not exposed to any other chemicals. Just the standard high-volume petroleum products.

After this background explanation, Davis felt slightly uncomfortable as the two men continued their walk to the tank site and climbed onto the roof of a typical floating-roof tank storing gasoline. Stan Love, looking sullen, volunteered no supplementary information, asked no questions about his visitor's background or procedures, and would not respond to Davis' friendly overtures of small talk.

With the tank hatch cover closed, Davis obtained a background-level reading of the gasoline hydrocarbon vapors on the roof top. There was a barely perceptible odor of gasoline wafting about the area. The vapor concentration was below the limit of detection of his gas detector tube, which he estimated to be appreciably less than fifty parts of the gasoline hydrocarbons per million of air, or 50 ppm. Stan then opened the hatch and Davis waited about ten minutes for the vapors to diffuse into the atmosphere. Then, standing upright directly over the opened hatch, Davis got a reading at his nose level of 100 to 200 ppm. This is a typical upper concentration to which a gasoline service station attendant or a customer at a self-service filling station might momentarily smell following some drippage from the pump nozzle.

The then OSHA permissible exposure level to gasoline vapors averaged over an entire eight-hour shift, called a time-weighted average exposure (TWA), was 500 ppm. Years later, OSHA lowered the TWA to 300 ppm averaged over eight hours but with a short-term exposure limit (STEL) of 500 ppm for a maximum of fifteen minutes. OSHA's reason for lowering the TWA and establishing a short-term limit was intended to prevent any narcotic effects because there was evidence that workers became dizzy at exposures of 500 ppm for an hour. Even in the unlikely event that Denny Moore had stood over the open tank hatch several hours, his eyes and throat might bother him somewhat, but it is improbable that he would feel sleepy or get dizzy at breathing levels well below the allowable limits. When Davis kneeled over the open hatch, as Denny would have had to do with poor visibility, the detector indicated levels of 1,000–2,000 ppm just above the floor level. Inserting the inlet of his detector tube slightly inside the tank, however, the reading went off the detector tube scale, or well above 13,000 ppm. For Davis, all these measurements were fairly predictable, based on the known physical properties of gasoline and his own monitoring experience.

Stan had been impassively observing the instrument readings until the indicator went off scale just inside the tank. "How do you get a reading on that?" he asked.

"You don't. But I know that is more than 13,000 ppm."

"Suppose you breathed that for a couple of minutes. What would it do to you?"

"Probably knock you unconscious or at least, disorient you."

"I once dropped the damn tape in the tank and I tried to fish it out with my head almost inside that hatch for about five minutes. But the fumes were so damn strong, I couldn't keep on breathing them without getting fresh air every thirty seconds or so."

"Of course. Nobody would voluntarily continue to breath that level of vapors."

"Then why did Denny continue to breath those fumes if he didn't have a heart attack?" Stan shouted.

"I just don't know why," Davis, sadly had to admit. "It doesn't make any sense."

He walked around the roof for several minutes as if he were looking for, but not expecting to find, some other clue. From what Stan had told him and what he saw for himself that morning, Davis suspected that the critical contributory cause of Denny Moore's bizarre accident had to be exogenous to, or outside of, the workplace. For an industrial hygienist, this means exposures or injuries away from work at a moonlighting job, or from hobbies, or at prior jobs including armed forces service. He knew the company doctors and toxicologists were looking into another kind of exogenous factors related to life-style, such as Moore's use of medications, tobacco, alcohol, or hard drugs.

Davis reasoned that there were two possibilities to account for Moore's particular vulnerability at both the high and low ends of the exposure concentrations. First, Denny Moore's sense of smell could have been insensitive to the incipient warning signs of a relatively safe gasoline vapor exposure, such as when he just started to descend into the contaminated tank shell. Simply, if he could not smell the vapors or sense their irritating effects, he would unknowingly subject himself to the higher and more toxic and narcotic levels as he descended further. Second, similar to the responses of an allergic or incapacitated person, his lungs or body defenses could have recently become particularly vulnerable to a normally safe and permissible exposure level. Davis was aware that it would be exceedingly difficult to prove either condition.

"I think I've seen enough here, Stan. We can head back." Disconsolately, they returned to John Del Monico's office.

"Find anything new, Mr. Davis?" Del Monico asked, as they took seats around his desk.

"Nothing yet, Mr. Del Monico, but I would like to talk to your people who knew Denny Moore, if I may."

"Of course. Stan, you know who Mr. Davis might want to talk to. Take care of him."

Davis explained to Stan what kind of information about Denny Moore, on and off the job, he wanted to know and why.

"Nobody knows more about Denny than Ed Stanko and me. Ed works over at the refinery now. No chance we can get Ed released to come over here."

Del Monico nodded in agreement. "Yes," he said, "the refinery bosses won't let anyone leave there just to talk. No chance of that."

Davis suppressed a look of triumph as he looked at John Del Monico and casually said, "We're doing this investigation at the personal request of Roger Young."

"Our vice president?"

As Davis nodded, Del Monico asked Bonnie Bray, now his office secretary, to call the refinery manager for him. In a little more than an hour, Davis, Ed Stanko, and Stan Love were having lunch together at a nearby diner. The two friends would alternately confirm what the other had said about Denny. He had no outside job or hobbies involving exposures. They were unaware that Denny had any recent injuries or complaints of physical or emotional problems. He was straight as an arrow. Never smoked or boozed, took no pills or any drugs. And they would know. Stan boasted that he had hired Denny seven years ago, spent practically every working day together, and they often went fishing or to a ball game. Ed said that he and Denny had been close friends since elementary school and had served in the same army unit for a year. Even their wives were friendly.

Davis was about to thank them for their help and call it a day when Ed suddenly remembered something that his wife had told him last week after she had met Betsy Moore, Denny's widow, for lunch.

"Betsy told my wife that the week before the accident, Denny got some kind of chemical poisoning, cleaning out their kids' plastic swimming pool, and he had to be treated at the hospital emergency room."

Davis almost jumped out of his chair. "Really? Do you think I could talk to her? It could be important."

Neither man responded. They were hesitant to subject Betsy to a possibly painful inquiry, particularly from a representative of the company management, as they regarded Davis.

"I really think it may be a clue to why your friend died. Please," Davis entreated them.

"All right. Let me call her and see if it's okay," Ed answered, softly. He returned in five minutes to say she would see them.

Betsy Moore embraced both Ed and Stan and smiled politely to Davis as they entered her comfortably furnished and attractively decorated colonial-style living room. Davis explained who he was, expressed his condolence at her loss, and thanked her for her willingness to talk to him. He emphasized that he had come only to hear her account of her husband's chemical poisoning from cleaning out their swimming pool.

Betsy told them how orderly and neat Denny was with his house chores. Maybe a shade compulsive, she added. When he was cleaning out their plastic swimming pool in the garage, he noticed some algae or rust stains, or whatever. When he couldn't remove them with the swimming pool disinfectant, he asked her for the toilet bowl cleaner. When she handed it to him, he remarked that it had removed all the persistent rust stains in the wash tubs so he figured that a mix of the two chemicals should do the job. He went back to the garage and about ten, maybe fifteen minutes later, from the kitchen, she could hear him coughing horrendously. Rushing to the garage, she found him, gasping for breath on the ground. She screamed to the retired couple next door for help. The husband helped drag Denny out of the garage while his wife called for the emergency squad, which took him to the hospital emergency room. He responded well to the treatment there, seemed to recover in a matter of hours, and was able to get home without too much trouble, but he still had a cough. By Sunday night, he felt much better and good enough to return to work. No, she did not know if he had planned to mention it at work. It just never came up.

"Do you have the packages for the swimming pool disinfectant and the toilet bowl cleaner?" Davis asked. "I'd like to see them."

"Sure, they should still be in the garage. I haven't touched anything there."

On the back of the labels, Davis confirmed his expectation that the disinfectant was calcium hypochlorite, a white powder, sometimes in tablet form, which in water solution gradually releases chlorine gas, a powerful disinfectant and oxidizing agent. In a treated swimming pool, people often complain of the irritation to their eyes from the chlorine dissolved in the water and its characteristic odor. Similarly, due to the residual chlorine in drinking water, people will complain of the antiseptic taste and smell.

The toilet bowl cleaner was, as he suspected, almost pure sodium bisulfate crystals, a highly corrosive and potent acid. Davis jotted down some notes from the product labels and thanked her again for her hospitality and cooperation and, signaling the men, said his good-bye. The entire visit lasted less than twenty minutes.

On the ride back to the tank farm and refinery, Davis told the two men he thought the home accident might be important, but it would be premature to say anything at this point. He knew that the normally slow release of chlorine gas from the hypochlorite pool cleaner is rapidly increased by the addition of any strong acid, like the sodium bisulfate in the toilet bowl cleaner. He had even read reports in the medical literature and consumer safety advisories that mixing these two chemicals, particularly in a confined space, like a bath tub or a garage had caused serious respiratory problems to unwitting housekeepers. Elderly people were particularly vulnerable. One woman who persisted in cleaning up stubborn stains in her bath tub with a similar mixture had to be hospitalized after her exposure for several minutes to chlorine concentrations estimated at approaching a near fatal level of 500–1,000 ppm.

The OSHA short-term exposure limit for chlorine of fifteen minutes or less is only 0.5 ppm, and concentrations of 14 to 21 ppm are judged to be dangerous. Denny Moore's exposure concentration, like that of the elderly woman, probably exceeded this level for several minutes.

Davis had deep respect for the dangerous properties and hazards of chlorine since his high school chemistry days. He remembered how the class watched in awe when Mr. Roman, the teacher, bleached a red rose inside a glass chamber filled with chlorine from a small gas cylinder. The teacher noticed that the cylinder was leaking slightly so he irresponsibly asked two of the students to take it outside and allow the gas to dissipate in a nearby isolated woods. When the boys did not return in fifteen minutes, they were found vomiting, coughing and sneezing, their eyes tearing, and their noses and throats burning.

In hospital studies of victims overcome by chlorine, the treating physicians invariably note tracheobronchitis, or inflammation of the mucous membranes in the windpipe, and pulmonary edema. In the latter stage, the lungs fill with fluid which would understandably account for breathing difficulties, and often develop into an inflammation, or pneumonitis. Some studies have indicated that victims overcome by chlorine had pulmonary impairment lasting for several weeks. Although none of the studies addressed reduced olfactory sensitivity, Davis opined that the highly corrosive and oxidizing action of the gas might well be expected to disrupt or diminish this capability in a severely exposed victim.

Davis' requirement of conditions to explain why Denny Moore could have succumbed to the gasoline vapors seemed to fall logically and convincingly into place with the reported facts. As a forerunner, even the weather that day had contributed ominously to the tragic sequence. The windless sky had been darkly overcast and sighting the gasoline level in the tank would have required him to bend over close to the hatch, where the gasoline vapor levels were potentially dangerous. His chlorine overexposure at home just days before the accident could have rendered his olfactory senses incapable of detecting the increasingly excessive vapor levels as he descended further into the tank shell. He had even been wearing chemical goggles which would have protected his eyes from another irritant warning of the gasoline vapor presence. Thus, his reliance on sensory warnings from his experience was now a deceptive guide. The unwitting inhalation of very high levels of gasoline vapors would unquestionably cause rapid loss of consciousness, followed by coma and sudden death. It all seemed to coalesce into a logical and convincing explanation.

That evening, Davis wrote up his findings with a hypothesis that the contributory cause of Moore's fatal accident at work was his prior poisoning at home from overexposure to chlorine gas. Rereading his handwritten report before handing it to his secretary for a final draft the following morning, he knew his explanation would be welcomed by the company management. The report might not exonerate the company of their safety infractions, but, at least, the unfortunate death of the young worker could now be explained as an aberrant off-work accident beyond their control.

Davis should have felt professionally gratified that his experience and scientific logic had led him to a reasonable explanation of the tragedy at the tank farm. But because he could never be absolutely certain why Denny Moore had died, he would always have some doubt. And that made him feel humble and sad.

Case **6**

No Sense of Danger

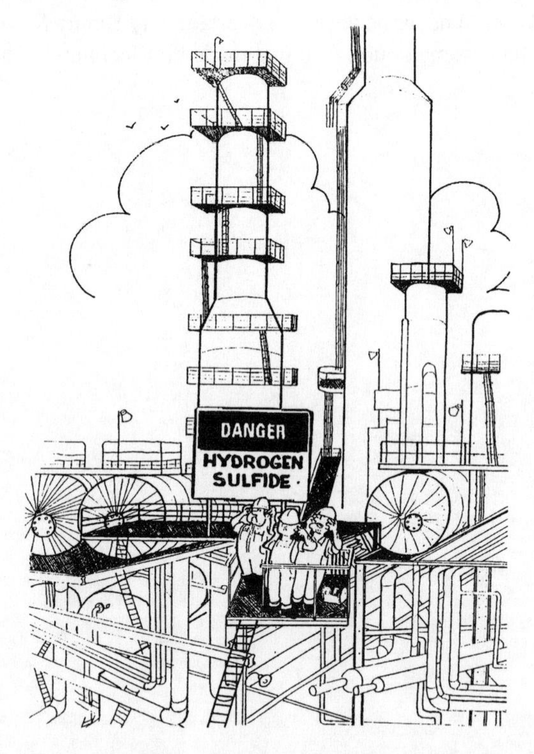

When wildcat oil prospectors hit a strike in their long-shot gamble, the sweet smell of success may be tempered by the "rotten eggs" odor of hydrogen sulfide gas indicating contamination with sulfur. With good reason, crude oils are called "sweet" when this undesirable element is practically absent and "sour" when it totals more than just a few tenths of a percent. Sulfur is trouble from the first noisome encounter with it in the oil-producing field and thereafter. It interferes with the processes which refine the petroleum products from the crude. When burned in a fuel, it produces sulfur dioxide and sulfates which pollute the air we breathe and precipitate out in the environment as major contributors to what we call "acid rain." We first try to eliminate as much of the sulfur as we can from the sour crudes, which can add up to a hefty 15 percent of the total refining costs. Where we fall short, we are often required by regulations to spend a great deal of effort and money either to prevent the formation of the pollutants or to capture them from stacks and chimneys.

We usually have good warning of very low levels of hydrogen sulfide gas, as a person with normal smell can readily detect it at less than one part in ten million parts of air. But breathing as little as fifty parts per million (ppm) of air for several minutes will make some people sick to the stomach and cause headaches. Inhalation of a single breath at a level of 1,000 ppm, or 0.10 percent, can rapidly produce a coma and death. Ironically, relying on odor detection for warning of hydrogen sulfide can be very dangerous to one's health. Breathing concentrations at about 100 ppm for an extended period causes fatigue in our sense of smell; in effect, this raises the odor detection level. Most ominously, even brief exposures at life-threatening levels can cause olfactory paralysis; thus, there would be no sensory awareness of the danger.

Small wonder that refinery workers handling sour crudes have become more accepting of, rather than warned by, these all too familiar sulfurous odors. Mercaptans, which are related organic sulfide gases in petroleum and, arguably, the most intensely foul odor commonly wafting around a refinery, have the stench of a particularly rotten cabbage at less than a tenth of the hydrogen sulfide odor threshold. The familiar smell of a "gas" leak from a gas stove or heater is actually due to miniscule amounts of ethyl mercaptan purposely added as a leak indicator. Despite the use of the best available technology to contain the hydrogen sulfide and other sulfur-containing and hydrocarbon gases, trace amounts inadvertently released during process treatments, storage, and transport help create the special aura that identifies a typical refinery.

Mike Rossi and Tom Updegrave had started work together as laborers at a refinery in the Texas gulf region a year after graduating from the same high school class. The labor pool serves as an extended rite of passage for entry-level employees who are willing to patiently endure their mindless cleanup and burdensome chores in anticipation of an assignment leading to a skilled trade or operator position. After each had served three years in the labor pool, Mike was accepted as an apprentice pipefitter and Tom became a unit operator trainee on the manufacturing units. These units sequentially process the crude oil, starting with pretreatment to remove impurities like water, salt, and sulfur compounds. The cleaned-up petroleum, which is a complex mixture of hydrocarbons, is then separated, generally, by thermal distillation into groups of hydrocarbons with similar properties and chemical composition. Finally, the larger groups are broken down or "cracked" into smaller molecular-weight constituents, or the smaller molecules may be rearranged by reforming according to their end uses. These products include heating gases and oils, automotive and aviation gasolines, kerosene and jet fuel, solvents, lubricating oils, greases, waxes, and asphalts.

The skilled tradespeople—which group Mike aspired to join—included carpenters, electricians, pipefitters, insulators, painters, among others, who perform the necessary maintenance and repairs to keep the manufacturing operations running. Refinery visitors were always incredulous of how so much product could be produced by so few workers. With this relatively low manpower requirement and little turnover in the refinery, it took almost seven years for Mike and Tom to advance to assistant pipefitter and assistant operator status.

As an assistant unit operator, Tom was qualified to make routine inspections on the units and perform simple maintenance functions. If specialized repairs were required, he would notify his supervisor who, in turn, would contact his counterpart in the maintenance and utility shop for assistance. Tom admitted that his work was usually boring in that the largely automated refinery operations were tended by smart and sensitive electronic sensors and controls, and most of the time the units operated smoothly. However unchallenged Tom may have felt, he and most of his co-workers never seriously thought about quitting the refinery. The pay and benefits were too good to give up and, deflecting the main fear of workers, they felt secure in their jobs.

The two friends regularly ate lunch together and they would occasionally discuss rumors of the infrequent openings for promotion within the refinery. However, when they heard of the company's increased activities abroad, Tom, in particular, would fancifully entertain the idea of working out of the country to help start up one of the new refineries.

"I hear that the guys who worked abroad saved a bundle with the premium pay. And you get special tax benefits, too. Now's the perfect time to make a move, Mike. Alice isn't working and the twins won't start school for a couple of years."

"Well, I may be willing but I don't think Betty would like living over there."

"It's only for two years and your family gets a free trip home once a year. Besides, when Betty finds out she can get the house she really wants with all that dough saved. . . ."

"Tom, how would you like it not knowing how the Cubs did last night, or who made it to the Super Bowl? Besides, if you ended up in Saudi, *your* wife would have to give up wearing shorts and put on a veil."

"So what's wrong with that?" They both laughed and easily reverted to their usual review of the most recent sporting event result.

Although the opportunity for an exotic overseas assignment did not arise, two years later the company announced opportunities for transfer to staff a new refinery in Illinois scheduled to be completed in early spring. Tom, for one, was more than ready for a change.

"Mike, you know we'd have to wait ten years until some of the dinosaurs around here retire for us to make first class. Why don't we bid on a transfer?" Tom implored his friend.

"The winters are so darn long and cold there. Besides, I've been to Chicago and the folks there weren't friendly like us Texans."

"Who'd want to be *your* friend?" he joshed his friend. "Heck, Mike, you know we've got nothing to lose by putting our names in."

"Okay, I'll talk it over with Betty but I'm not making any promises."

Six weeks later, they each accepted an offer to transfer to Illinois with a promotion and better chances for advancement. By early April, just before the refinery went "on stream"—that is, started up—they had bought houses in the same development and were car pooling each day as much for the companionship as to afford their wives transportation.

Later that fall on the eastern side of the country in the offices of the corporate medical department, the supervising industrial hygienist, Lazar Davis, was making up the assignments for the periodic industrial hygiene surveys of the company facilities.

"That new refinery in Illinois has been on stream for almost six months. It's about due for the initial survey," he remarked to Marge, his secretary, who was characteristically looking over his shoulder.

"Why bother now, boss? The P.R. releases said it's supposed to be a pollution-free refinery, right?"

"Maybe so, but we have to get baseline exposure measurements to see how effective their pollution controls really are. And it gives us a basis for comparison later if the controls start to show wear, or they make changes in the operations."

"Well, you might as well go now. It'll make you look good when you give them a clean bill of health for a change."

Outspoken and cynical but she's partly right again, Davis thought. When the hygienist *did* find exposure problems, the messenger and the report were often not well received by the bosses. This was particularly so when they recommended costly engineering controls which only competed with other budget expenditures and didn't contribute to the critical bottom line. Or if the findings suggested a possible employee health problem, some of the more suspicious managers felt that revealing the information to the employees only invited more complaints.

"Is a survey now at the new refinery really worth *your* time?" Marge persisted, suggesting that her boss' expertise was better spent on more demanding problems than a routine survey.

"That's *not* the reason I'm planning to go this time. I'm scheduling Randy who's been here almost a year and is ready to handle a survey on his own."

Marge, wisely, just nodded.

Davis saw analogies between his routine hygiene surveys and the periodic physical examinations of employees performed by the company physicians. Whereas the doctors were checking on the workers' health, the hygienists were evaluating their environmental health; that is, their work environments and exposures to injurious chemicals and physical agents. More often than not, both of these routine examinations revealed no major problems. The preplacement physical examination of new employees tended to select healthy workers who remained so with ongoing medical counseling and examinations. Similarly, the environmental surveys confirmed that most company workplaces were in good shape following years of periodic inspections. When the hygienists did find excessive employee exposures, they—like the physicians—would recommend action to protect the workers' health. Ideally, when either independently found unexpected illnesses, particularly, among workers similarly exposed, they would collaborate to investigate a possible workplace causation.

Later that afternoon, Davis called in Randy Barstow, a junior member in the department, who had received his master's degree in industrial hygiene the year before and was serving an extended apprenticeship under Davis before he would be assigned to a field location.

"Randy, I think you're ready to do a solo. We have an initial survey due at the Illinois refinery, which I know you can handle."

"That place is so new I shouldn't have any problems there," Randy answered, confidently, "As long as I have some help with all the monitoring. I know you want beaucoup samples."

"Sam Barsky, the safety supervisor there, is very cooperative and familiar with what we do. We trained several of Sam's people in monitoring and I'm sure he'll provide a couple of hands for the week."

"Anything special you want me to concentrate on?"

"Start by reviewing our file of refinery surveys. We're not expecting any problems so early there, but see what we found at similar operations. Listen carefully to any complaints the guys on the units make. And say hello to Peggy Brooks, the plant nurse. If there are any health problems or complaints from the workers, they'll confide in her. She'll know of problems before anyone in the employee relations department suspects anything."

"Will do. And I'll make sure to get plenty of benzene measurements."

Randy was well aware that benzene exposures were a particularly sensitive employee health issue in the petroleum industry. Following a contentious battle in the Supreme Court, the industry had won a delay of OSHA's proposal for a tenfold reduction in the allowable OSHA exposure limit. The government claimed the lower limit was necessary to prevent the risk of leukemia. The industry argued—technically correct at the time—that the existing higher level of 10 ppm had not been proved to cause leukemia in humans and, therefore, there was no cost benefit for requiring the industry at considerable expense to comply with an unproved "significant risk of harm" at the lower limit. Years later, when there was a scientific consensus that benzene exposures at 10 ppm were reasonably implicated in human leukemia, the government was successful in establishing the 1 ppm limit as a permanent standard and now all industry had to comply.

Randy spent a full week in late October performing the survey at the new refinery with the help of Sam Barsky's safety personnel. They took scores of personal breathing zone air samples of refinery employees on the manufacturing units, the shops, laboratories, and storage and transport areas, as well as in the ambient work areas. They found no unusual levels of benzene, or any of the usual other hydrocarbons. Gas tests for sulfur dioxide, ammonia, and ozone were similarly low. Even the ineluctable stench of hydrogen sulfide was moderated to levels just above its limit of detection and certainly well within the allowable exposure limit. Dust concentrations around even normally dusty units elsewhere were barely visible. The airborne asbestos fiber concentrations were later confirmed by their analytical laboratory to be at the limit of microscopic detection and well below the permissible exposure level. All their measurements of noise and vibration, ionizing radiation, temperature and humidity, and lighting levels were monotonously within acceptable levels. They approved the adequacy of the ventilation systems, the workers' use of respirators and other personal protective equipment, and the presence of warning signs, among many other items on their checklist of control measures. And although the work accident reports showed the usual number of fractures, bruises, burns, and injuries from the inevitable falls and mishaps, in the occupational illness category, no one had ever been asphyxiated or made seriously ill from a chemical overexposure or from entry into an oxygen-deficient atmosphere. None of the employees told Randy about any health complaints from their work.

At the clinic, Peggy Brooks, the plant nurse, confirmed their reports to Randy.

"The problems I hear from them don't have anything to do with their work. Compared to the old refinery where I started, I see very few with any work health problems."

"What about the usual accidents and injuries?"

"The company knew what it was doing by bringing in experienced people to run the place. Most of the problems come with the younger kids who don't know the ropes yet and aren't as careful."

"You mean you see more injuries than sickness?"

"Oh definitely, but we haven't even had any really bad accidents like fires and explosion. And, God forbid, no deaths."

When Davis reviewed the draft of Randy's report the following week, he had to agree with the conclusions that there were no evident or anticipated exposure problems. In the final report to management, he almost apologetically included some minor defects about slightly low face velocities in one chemical hood and the failure of a carpenter to wear his ear protectors in a noisy area where a warning sign required it. It was almost embarrassing to have expended so much manpower in a survey of a refinery that was so patently trouble-free. Because many of the older company facilities were having trouble keeping up with the increasingly more restrictive exposure standards, Davis considered increasing the interval between the next scheduled survey at the new refinery by six months.

If you had asked Tom or Mike then whether there were any health problems from work at the new refinery, they might seem puzzled that you even raised the question. Big as it was, their 200,000 barrels per day refinery seemed too clean to be true. This daily volume of refinery production, or throughput, is the number of barrels of crude oil processed. A small to moderate size refinery might have a throughput of about 50,000 barrels, but the economics of production has practically restricted oil refining to 200,000–300,000 barrel behemoths. The barrel unit is a hypothetical forty-two gallons, a size which cannot be found in any refinery or plant. Thus, a typical refinery in the United States daily processes over ten million gallons of product.

Tom and two fellow assistant unit operators were assigned to a multiunit crude treatment area, where they rotated principal assignments on one unit every three months. When not occupied in the control rooms or providing backup for the others, they would make at least one complete surveillance tour of their assigned unit on each shift. In the spring following Randy's survey, Tom was assigned to the desulfurization unit, which reacts hydrogen gas with the sour crude under high pressure and temperatures in the presence of catalysts to release the sulfur as hydrogen sulfide gas. Under normal operating conditions, the gas produced is captured by washing, or scrubbing, in a chemically neutralizing solution.

In the new refinery, really significant leaks from the unit were infrequent. If the airborne level of hydrogen sulfide momentarily exceeded the allowable short-term—defined then as ten minutes—exposure limit (STEL) of 20 ppm, special gas detectors would erupt with an excruciatingly piercing siren. No unauthorized person could then enter the contaminated area. Before responding to investigate the source of the leak, the unit operator had to notify his supervisor first before entering the area and then only when protected by a full-face respirator with a cylinder of compressed breathing air. Usually, the leak was minor and simply due to a loose valve or connection which the operator would tighten himself. According to the written safety procedures, only when the closure was completed and the gas in the atmosphere had been sufficiently diluted to silence the alarm was the area safe for workers to reenter. On one rare occasion when the source of the leak was persistently elusive, the horn kept on blaring. The repair crew was so unnerved while trying to finish the job, they temporarily disconnected the sensor to muzzle the alarm.

Back in their former Texas Gulf region, Tom and Mike had been accustomed to generally mild winds barely cooling the enervating sultriness that persisted through most of the year; that is, except for the occasional hurricanes in late summer and fall. But in their new midwestern home, the winds were more capricious. The wind activity or, more properly, the lack of it might cause a pocket of hydrogen sulfide to accumulate in the detector area and the alarm would go off. Moments later, the horn would be mysteriously quieted by the diluting effect of a random gust of wind. During one week, there had seemed to be an unusual spate of almost daily alarms on the desulfurization unit. Then, inexplicably, for several days Tom did not have to respond to a single hydrogen sulfide alarm.

"It was the darndest thing," Tom recalled to Mike on their ride home that week. "I feel like we had a leprechaun on the unit. Not ten minutes after the siren goes off, I start my investigation and my spot readings barely show more than a few ppm. If there's a leak, it's so low I can't find it."

"Maybe that stink gas has started to corrode away the fittings, or the gaskets, or something," Mike suggested. "I remember when I replaced the old fittings on the sulfur unit back in Texas, how the gaskets and packings were all chewed up."

"Barely a year old and you think the desulfurization unit is ready for an overhaul, Tom?"

"That's not for me to decide. That's what those high-priced boy engineers are paid to do."

"Well, those alarms can drive me nuts. I never know whether the leak's for real, or from some other unit upwind."

"Tom, do you ever worry if that gas might knock you out, or make you really sick?"

"Yeh, it can happen. But you know I'm real careful. I never go in without my respirator when the alarm goes off."

Mike reflected on the possible health effects from *his* work. He had just watched with some concern a TV program reporting on litigation brought by former asbestos workers, including pipefitters suffering from asbestosis and lung cancer more than twenty years after their exposure.

"Remember back on labor crew, when we tore out all those old asbestos pipes during the renovation? That dust was all over the place and we didn't pay it much mind."

"Well, what about it?"

"Ever worry that stuff will eat away your lungs?"

"What? That job lasted only a week or two, over five years ago. I feel fine. Besides, I never smoked and one of those doctors, or somebody, said only smokers get sick from asbestos."

"Well, I still work with the stuff every time I replace some pipe or valves and I. . . ."

Mike sensed that his friend was not really interested in discussing their impending mortality, so he dropped the subject. He tuned in to a country music station on the car radio. At the end of the day, the familiar twangy airs recounting life's sorrows and pains produced a sentimental quietude for the remainder of their ride.

Because of the report of an unusual number of gas leaks on the desulfurization unit, the preventive maintenance department began a crash program to replace the gaskets and packings in the suspect locations. The loosening of the pipe joints were expected to cause frequent and sudden releases of gas so that Mike and his fellow pipefitters and laborers assigned to the job had to breathe through cumbersome hooded respirators over full-body suits. When the weather suddenly turned unseasonably warm, their protective clothing clung to their skin like a poncho in a rain forest. The almost continuous eruption of the alarm rattled their brains and started to fray their nerves. Even the usually stoic Mike showed his irritaion.

"Can't you turn off that damn horn, Tom? I can't think straight."

"The best I can do is raise the alarm level so it don't go off so often, Mike. It'd be my rear if those safety guys found out I turned it off completely."

Tom raised the alarm threshold level from 20 ppm to 50 ppm, which was the maximum or ceiling level which could not be exceeded for any period of time for an unprotected worker. For at least the remainder of that shift, the alarm was mute. On the following morning, before they resumed their work, Tom made sure the alarm was set back to the usual 20 ppm. Later that morning when Tom was back in the control room, the alarm erupted for a barely tolerable three minutes. Then, the project was inexplicably completed with no further outburst.

The two weeks following the completion of the replacement job would end Tom's rotation at the desulfurization unit. Except for the usual residual odor of sulfide, the atmosphere on the unit was now relatively uncontaminated from leaks. It was good timing, Tom thought, to indoctrinate Ben Travis, a new unit operations trainee, who had never rotated on the desulfurization unit. With luck, they could concentrate on the process without interruption to respond to an alarm.

"I see you finished the safety training," Tom began with his young charge. "You do what they taught you and you won't get hurt."

Ben nodded.

"You know how to put on your respirator correctly?"

"Sure, Tom. I volunteer on my town emergency squad," Ben answered confidently. "I use 'em all the time."

"You know first aid, too?"

"Oh, yeh. I'm qualified in CPR, too."

Well, we got a bonus with the new man, Tom thought.

Using a schematic drawing of the desulfurization unit, Tom led Ben on a tour, explaining what was going on underneath the reactor vessels and through all the piping.

"You have to tour the unit just once a shift," Tom began. "You do the housekeeping, like making sure there's no mess or tools left behind by any maintenance or repairs. And you look out for any obvious problems, like a steam or gas leaks."

"How will I know what all to look for?"

"I'll be with you the next two weeks. Then, the unit supervisor assigns you a big brother until they think you can handle it by yourself. Most of the time you spend in the control room just making sure all the operating conditions are okay. They're all under automated control. Like the temperatures and pressures."

Ben looked puzzled. "So what can go wrong?" he asked.

"That's why we're here, kid. Sometimes, things—like leaks—just happen.

That's why I want you to have your respirator and gas detector with you every time you go on the unit."

"But you guys don't always bring 'em."

"You do it 'til you finish the trainee period under me. Okay?"

"Sure, boss. I get the message."

As promised, Tom spent the remainder of the week showing Ben exactly where on the unit there might be problems. By the following week, a more relaxed Ben had enough familiarity with the operations to serve independently as Mike's gofer. Early Thursday morning of the final week, Tom casually started the weaning process.

"Ben, I think we need a new rechargeable battery on our leak detector. Hasn't been holding the charge. Can you take it over to the instrument shop for a replacement?"

"Where do I meet you when I get done?"

"There's still a mess left by the pipefitters from that replacement job. A couple of the laborers are supposed to clean up this morning and the boss wants us around to make sure they don't screw up."

He looked at his watch. "It's ten to nine. Meet me on the unit by the scrubber about ten."

If Tom or young Ben reflected that most of their working lives might be filled with an endless repetition of similar unmemorable chores, they might have proceeded less cheerfully. Throughout their shifts, the refinery workers would regularly exchange playful gibes or gossip with their work buddies in their travels around the refinery like a slow-motion version of busy ants momentarily halting to make antenna contact. This social interaction was a palliative for their quotidian boredom. Their camaraderie would also serve to bind them together in a time of crisis.

There was no witness to Ben and Tom's rendezvous later that morning. Tom had left the control room about a quarter to ten and casually mentioned to one of the operators that if Mike Rossi called him, he'd be back by lunchtime. As usual, he put a peg opposite his name on a wall locator board. There were no unusual releases of odors and, certainly, no one heard the gas detector alarm go off. In fact, no one in or near the unit could recall anything untoward. If it were not for the labor crew's arrival on the unit—late as usual—no one would have suspected that anything was amiss.

Approaching the second landing level of the unit, one of the two laborers asked the supervisor, "Does it always stink this bad?"

"It always seems worse when you climb 'cause you're breathing in more. You get used to it."

Unconvinced, the young laborer responded with an exaggerated groan. They continued their climb at a reduced pace.

As they approached the landing above, the other laborer looking up, suddenly stopped.

"Those two guys, there," he yelled. Two men lay motionless on the ground, pressed close against the wall of the center tower and shielded from any wind.

Ben was slumped across the supine body of Tom, eerily frozen in an attempt to give mouth-to-mouth resuscitation. The black tubing from an air-supplied respirator coiled on the ground nearby. As they approached the two bodies, the supervisor grabbed the two laborers, screaming, "Get the hell out of here. I got to call for help."

He and his men withdrew to an uncontaminated area, vaguely aware that there was a deceptively sweet odor in the atmosphere they had just evacuated. The supervisor blurted out a cry for assistance over his walkie-talkie. Waiting to direct the rescue crew, they were now beginning to feel strangely light-headed.

Within minutes, a wailing siren heralded the arrival of the refinery emergency squad. Wearing total respiratory protection, they expeditiously carried the comatose victims on stretchers down to a waiting ambulance, where artificial resuscitation and oxygen administration were attempted en route to the hospital. Checking for vital signs, the experienced rescuers suspected that the younger of the two had probably expired, but the older man, with no measurable blood pressure in either arm and showing depressed respiration, still had a rapid pulse. As the rescuers feared, Ben was declared dead on arrival. Despite Tom's violent seizures and obvious severe pulmonary distress, the hospital staff kept him alive, if barely, by endotracheal intubation and oxygen administration. After lingering for almost six weeks, he died without ever regaining consciousness.

Once started up, refinery processes and operations never entirely shut down. But for days after the accident, there was such an uncommon quietude among the refinery unit operators and trades personnel, it seemed as if they were performing their work in a trance. Genuinely mourning the loss of their two young co-workers, understandably, they also reflected soberly on their own vulnerabilities from the dangers at work.

As required by law, OSHA initiated an immediate investigation and confirmed that the deaths were caused by the sudden release of an unusually high concentration of hydrogen sulfide. Because the company had, in good faith, been recently responding to the problems of leaks and, otherwise, had an excellent safety program and below average injury and illness rate for its industry category, OSHA essentially exonerated them of any serious wrongdoing. As customary, the final OSHA report implied that certain corrections were in order and cited the company only for minor noncompliances. The company responded to the OSHA suggestions with immediate new restrictions on entry and mandatory wearing of respiratory equipment in posted areas where hydrogen sulfide release could result in dangerous levels. A special task force of process safety and materials engineers was also appointed to conduct a more studied inquiry, which was, in effect, an internal soul-searching to determine what they had missed in anticipating and preventing the accident. As the report from their investigation pointed out three months later, although the company had heretofore never had a fatality from hydrogen sulfide exposures at any refinery, they were able to identify extenuating conditions. First, because of a huge oversupply of sour crudes and a greater demand for sweet crudes that year, the refinery was forced to process a significantly higher sulfur crude until prices and supplies stabilized. Thus, the hydrogen sulfide concentration from the desulfurization processes were correspondingly higher than usual. Second, the materials comprising the gaskets and packing used to effect better seals were not sufficiently resistant to the more corrosive action of the higher gas concentrations. It seemed obvious that a more rapid deterioration was responsible for the unusual number and greater intensity of gas leaks. Conferring with the research department of their gasket and packings material suppliers, they were able to identify a far more chemically resistant substitute material. Management approved a major replacement program within a year of all gaskets and packing on the desulfurization unit with the new material.

When Lazar Davis in the company medical department first learned of the deaths in a terse company bulletin, he was first shocked and, on reflection, felt some anxiety. Granted, Randy Barstow's initial industrial hygiene survey at the new refinery had found no evidence of a serious hydrogen sulfide exposure problem. But might his own participation there as a more experienced hygienist have helped identify a less than obvious failing? He was determined to learn what could have prevented the tragedy. Although he had not been invited to participate in the task force investigation, through an informal contact with a friend in the safety department, he learned of their findings and conclusions. For more detailed background information, he spoke for twenty minutes on the phone with his friend Sam Barsky, who was the safety supervisor at the Illinois refinery.

As customary, and particularly because of possible medical and toxicological implications, the refinery deaths were discussed at the weekly medical department staff meeting. Reinforced by his own sleuthing of the case, Davis briefed his colleagues on the reported findings and then answered their probing questions with the most reasonable explanations for what was not actually witnessed.

"Why did that more experienced man go on the sulfur unit without a respirator?"

"They don't usually use a respirator on a routine visit, which this was," he began. "They had just completed some repairs of some leaks and had been testing the atmosphere daily with a gas detector. The levels were considered normal, so no exposure problems were expected."

"But the first worker was overcome immediately. Could it have been a heart attack, or some kind of seizure," one of the clinic nurses suggested.

"Dr. Robertson?" Davis tactfully deferred to the medical director.

"Oh, yes, I've talked to our panel physician in Illinois. The coroner gave chemical asphyxiation from hydrogen sulfide poisoning as the primary cause of death. The victim was in his early thirties, in good physical condition, and had no prior medical history of problems."

"Then why was he overcome without any warning or awareness?" one of the paramedics posed to Davis.

"They think there was a sudden massive release of the gas from a leak they had missed during the repairs the previous week. About ten years ago, I was working at the research center and one of the technicians had filled a large reaction vessel with hydrogen sulfide gas from a pressurized cylinder. We heard an explosion, rushed in within seconds, and found the guy unconscious on the floor. We rushed him to the hospital immediately, giving him artificial respiration. They say the timing of treatment is critical, and, remarkably, he suffered no permanent effects. But when he awoke, he swore he couldn't smell the sulfide gas immediately after the explosion. In other words, at the concentration which knocked him out, his olfactory senses were paralyzed."

Nothing like a personal anecdote to make your point, Davis thought, as the group uncharacteristically listened attentively to his explanation. With a raised interest in the details of the case, they pressed him with more questions.

"They said the younger man trying to rescue his boss first had a respirator on, but he died almost instantly. Why?" Dr. Ken Snyder, the associate medical director, asked.

"He may have had the respirator on when he went in to rescue his boss, but instead of dragging him to an uncontaminated area to start artificial respiration and call for help, he ripped it off. He had to take a deep breath to begin mouth to mouth and was immediately overcome. Remember the concentration was so high you couldn't smell it."

"Then why didn't the other man succumb at the same time?" Dr. Snyder persisted.

"In an acute exposure like this, hydrogen sulfide acts mainly as an enzyme poison. Like cyanide, it inactivates the cytochrome oxidase. That's the enzyme necessary for cellular oxidation. The body can detoxify a lot of the sulfide to form harmless sulfate before it can react with the enzyme. But, it seems that there's a critical level of about 1,000 ppm of exposure which exceeds the body's capacity to detoxify. If the blood supply in the brain is anoxic even for a short period of time, the damage is irreversible. The first victim had probably stopped breathing, so his total dose inhaled was less than the younger man who died almost immediately. In any case, his dose was insufficient to cause immediate death but above the level for conscious recovery."

His colleagues seemed to be satisfied or, perhaps, had run out of questions. Dr. Robertson concluded the discussion with the dubiously mitigating reminder that notwithstanding the impact of the tragedy, the company had one of the lowest fatality records in the industry.

There were other contributory factors which had passed through Davis' mind which he did not mention, believing they were not of particular interest to the medical department. As noted, there were the higher sulfur crudes being processed which would produce unusually high levels of hydrogen sulfide, greater and more rapid corrosion of the seals, and more gas leaks. In seeking a clue to what might have been the single critical preventive measure, Davis was tantalized by other anomalies. His safety department confidant had told him something about the operator having a hydrogen sulfide detector with a bad battery. Were the unit operators getting deceptively low concentration readings which gave them no indication that the seals were failing at a higher than normal rate? Then there was, above all, the gnawing question of why the gas-sensing alarm had not gone off. Was this an instrument failure or might the exposure have been too localized to be detected by the sensors? With his attention being drawn in the following weeks to other workplace health problems on the job, Davis was unable to focus on the sulfide deaths.

Nine months later, he was invited to a refinery managers meeting held at the Illinois refinery to report the results of his group's extensive monitoring of benzene exposures that had been mandated under OSHA's more restrictive new limits. Set back a quarter of a mile from the highway in a rural area, the nearly new refinery contradicted Davis' customary sensory expectations. As he drove along the approaching road after registering at the guard station, he noted no perceptible odors or dusts in the air or oil leaks along the ground. No ditches or ponds by the approaching road soiled with multifarious wastes, or junk piles of rusting pipes and tanks, or fractured bricks and concrete blocks from units cyclically torn down and replaced by the newer technology. These silent steel and concrete constructions making up the complex refinery operations had an alien planned sense of order, cleanliness, and efficiency.

The managers, normally a tough audience to impress and not overly receptive to lectures from someone from the medical department, paid careful attention to his talk. Davis was never sure of his reception at these meetings and was pleased when Sam Barsky, the refinery safety supervisor, confirmed his success at lunch.

"Those guys actually seemed proud when you told them their operations were in compliance with the new benzene limits. Last year, when they first got wind of the proposed lowering, they were worried as hell," Sam said.

"Well, to their credit, they put in the controls we'd been recommending for years and it paid off."

After they had exchanged reminiscences of a trip they had made together to a uranium mining operation in southwestern Texas that the company considered buying, Davis segued their talk to the deaths at the desulfurization unit.

"Did you ever find anything to add to the story?" Davis asked cautiously.

Sam hesitated, before replying, "No. The management seemed satisfied that we've done everything we should."

The, he added, uncomfortably, it seemed to Davis, "We don't talk about it much, now."

Davis sensed he should not pursue the matter when Sam quietly added, "Funny you should ask now just when they're finishing the replacement of the seals with that new gasket material. But if you want to look over the unit, Lazar, I'll send one of my boys over with you."

On their walk to the desulfurization unit, Davis learned that Joe, his chatty guide, had come to safety work at the new refinery two years ago after having been a unit operator trainee at an east coast refinery of the company. Yes, he knew about the accident and the two men who were gassed on the unit. That's why he would never go there without his respirator and a gas detector that worked. Joe's recapitulation of the tragedy was not revealing.

At the unit, hazardous area signs now warned of the presence of hydrogen sulfide as an extreme health hazard. Entry required wearing of approved respiratory protection and, of course, only by authorized and trained persons. The replacement crew had almost finished their work when they arrived. Joe explained to Davis how the desulfurization unit worked and where there had been leaks.

"Do you know where the gas detector alarms are, Joe?"

"Sure, and they all work perfectly."

He located all the detectors for Davis and then seemed to take delight in demonstrating that the alarm really worked by pressing a test button which caused the siren to blast. The work crew started at the sudden noisy onslaught. When Joe playfully repeated an extended blast, one of the startled pipefitters cursed him, concluding, "That ain't funny."

Aware that he had probably gone too far, Joe apologetically said to the pipefitter, "That really bothered you, didn't it? I'm sorry."

The man nodded. "I was on the replacement job here last time and that siren drove me nuts once."

Davis who was quietly listening to the exchange, instinctively said to the pipefitter, "Really?"

"Damn right," he replied, "I turned it off that time it wouldn't stop."

Was that it? Davis thought. *They never turned that sensor back on.* Or at least, not until after the accident and those poor guys had no warning or sense of their danger.

When it was obvious from Davis' silence that he had no further questions, Joe surmised that his mission was over and suggested returning to the safety office. Before they started their descent, Joe stopped to chat with the pipefitter who appeared to be in charge of the replacement job.

"I hear you're leaving us, Mike. Where are you going?"

"I always wanted to go overseas for a spell. I got a two-year assignment as leading man to help start up that new refinery in Venezuela."

"Then you're coming back here?" Joe insisted.

"Not really. I made a deal to get me reassigned back home."

Joe pondered the pipefitter's reply for a few seconds, shrugged, and concluded, "You Texas boys never really leave home, do you?"

SECTION THREE

▪

Solving the Skin Problems

Case 7

The Girls in the Machine Shop

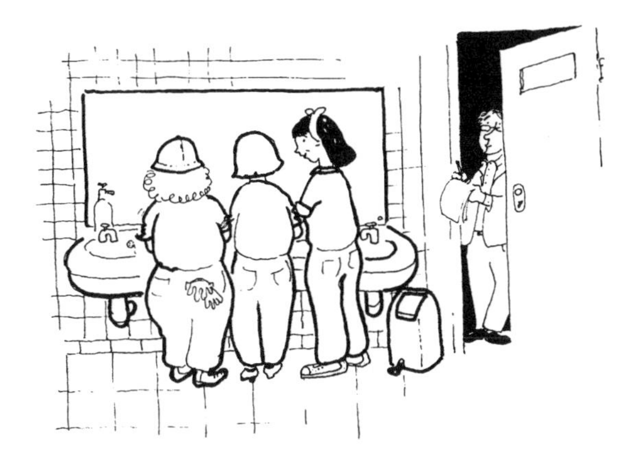

Arnold Schultz had been a highly regarded supervising chemist at the company research and development laboratory for twenty-two years when Dr. Orson Brown, the director of the laboratory, inexplicably called him into his office. Schultz, characteristically intense and unsmiling, warily entered his boss's office.

Brown greeted his visitor pleasantly but aware that reciting the social amenities only made his visitor more nervous, immediately got to the business at hand.

"Arnie, the company is concerned about all those health issues being raised about exposures to our oil products. You must have read about those skin cancer cases at the machine shop in Detroit the company just settled."

Schultz nodded, knowingly. His father, who had also worked for the company as a chemist in the refinery, had died from cancer at only fifty-three. He was certain that if he did not take extreme care in handling chemicals, he, too, would succumb to some malignancy. After once having had a suspicious looking growth removed from his lower lip, he regularly scheduled appointments with a dermatologist.

"It's bad for the company image," Dr. Brown continued. "Corporate counsel says we have to develop precautionary labels . . . to protect us. And both research and medical told the CEO we have to know more about the toxicology of our products. Maybe start some kind of testing program."

"I thought about that myself," Schultz mumbled.

"The last board meeting agreed we should develop expertise in the company to handle these health problems. They want to send an experienced employee to get a master's in some program. I think it's called industrial hygiene."

Schultz, still puzzled at the reason for the meeting, sucked on a pipe he had not lit since the year his father died.

"They're going to create a new position in medical, Arnie. You've always been interested in these health matters and you sure as hell know more about the products than anyone in the company. To put it bluntly, I want to nominate you."

Thus, well before the creation of the federal agencies regulating occupational exposures and environmental pollution and to the credit of the company's prescience, Arnold Schultz at age forty-eight was started on a new career as the first formally trained company industrial hygienist. Within the first year in his new role, he started a project to compile information sheets describing the toxicological and hazardous properties of all the company's principal blending stocks, additives, and products. Applying the newly developed information, he revised the precautionary labels on products and helped write sales literature and brochures with recommended safe handling procedures. Despite his inherent shyness and especial unease at public speaking, he frequently proselytized the pragmatic managers and marketers at company meetings about the importance to respond to environmental and occupational health hazards. After several years, Schultz's work load increased to justify acquiring an assistant and potential successor. Lazar Davis, who had recently obtained his master's degree in industrial hygiene and, like Schultz, had worked as a chemist at a research laboratory, was hired and assigned to the company medical department as Schultz's assistant.

Davis was excited at the opportunity to practice what he had recently learned in graduate school about protecting the health of workers, but he was disappointed to learn that his boss rarely performed any surveys at the company operations. Rather than dealing primarily with their own company workers, their services were more commercially directed, dealing mainly with the health problems of customers using and misusing the company products. In the marketing end of the oil business, Davis soon learned this often meant responding to skin problems. Although occupational skin disorders have been on a decline from their position as the most prevalent occupational disease, they still account for about a quarter of all such cases with an attendant large lost work time and increase in operating costs. Davis was gratified that Schultz was so smart and eager to share his knowledge, but his taciturn and almost humorless boss scarcely communicated beyond the didactics.

"Most oils and solvents aren't even very damaging or irritating on casual contact," Schultz lectured Davis early on. "You practically have to be continuously dunked in them to cause problems. You see we're protected against chemical injury to the skin by an outer layer of dead cells of the epidermis and underneath we've got glands which secrete fatty substances which help neutralize irritating chemicals. They also keep the skin pliant and moist. But the oils and solvents defat the protective fatty layer causing the skin to dry up and crack, particularly with the usual knocks and abrasions from manual labor. The bottom line is that skin problems from our products are mostly preventable."

"Then why all the problems, boss?"

"The workers," Schultz tersely concluded. "They're just slobs and don't wash up often enough, or properly. When they do wash themselves, instead of scrubbing up with a mild soap and hot water, they use those gritty abrasive powders. Worse yet, some of the grease monkeys in the garages actually clean up with gasoline or kerosene. And at the next shift, they're still wearing the same dirty oil-soaked clothing."

"So it's mainly a matter of educating the workers," Davis dutifully answered, knowing that was the message intended by his mentor.

"Right. But you're never ahead. You get new workers all the time and they don't get proper instructions. And some experienced workers think if they haven't had any problems, they're invulnerable. They slacken up on the hygiene, or won't wear the oil-proof aprons they've been issued," Schultz added. "They think they're protected by applying those perfumed barrier skin creams, but they don't last long. Then they blame us when they break out and get infected.

"I get it, but aren't some oils carcinogenic?"

"Of course. The really heavy oils—the ones that are high boiling—contain the carcinogenic hydrocarbons. They're the polynuclear aromatic hydrocarbons, or PAHs. We learned from some refining studies that treating these oils with certain solvents, like furfural, will dissolve out the PAHs. The raffinate—that's the portion of the oils that's not extracted—is then free of any carcinogens. So we only use these solvent-refined oils in products likely to involve skin contact."

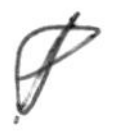

Schultz was too modest to claim that he—unquestionably influenced by his father's death from a cancer associated with handling unrefined oils—had been instrumental in convincing the company—and the petroleum industry—to adopt this practice.

In similar dialogues after dealing with actual complaints, Davis learned that the first indication of a skin outbreak due to an oil product or solvent was typically an erythema which might develop into fluid-filled blisters, pimples, ulcers, fissures, scales, or other dermal disfigurements; these might ooze, itch, irritate, burn, or cause the skin to change color. With breaks in the skin and generally unsanitary conditions in the workplace, it was common for opportunistic bacterial infections to follow. It was largely true that if the user followed Schultz's litany of exercising good skin hygiene, most skin problems from the common oil products would disappear, or at least be kept under control. Every once in a while, the

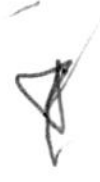

homiletic approach failed and since Schultz hated to travel, it frequently fell upon Davis to visit the ailing customer for an on-site diagnosis and remedy.

Typically, as at the Garden State Machining Company in New Jersey, even after the usual letter and phone call by Davis and visits by the district marketing representative with the appropriate product literature, the problems from the use of metal cutting oils continued or worsened. Whereas this machine shop may have experienced at any given time one or two minor skin eruptions out of an average work force of fifty workers, they recently experienced three cases almost severe enough to take the workers off the job, and several more—all in the same department of the shop—were rumored to be developing problems. The shop management was afraid if the dermatitis spread, production would be slowed down and, of course, it could give the union an opportunity to file an unsafe work practice. Insisting they had done everything they were told to do, Garden State concluded they must have been supplied with inferior or contaminated oils. When the customer threatened to turn over all of their oil product purchases to a competitor, the marketing department insisted that the company industrial hygienist visit the plant to solve the problem. Davis was then summarily dispatched to the plant to identify in a tactful manner what was expected to be a likely breakdown in their hygienic practices. Or as Arnie Schultz succinctly put it, "Look for the slobs." It worked often enough, but as Davis came to learn, the preliminary information from the field was often inaccurate or incomplete.

When he arrived at the machine shop, Bud Angelo, the obviously disquieted plant foreman at Garden State, gave him more of a complaint than a greeting.

"We got three big back orders to fill, two must-have-yesterday jobs, my kid has little league tryouts tonight, and I got to deal with those complaining dames. I told the boss a machine shop is no place for women to work."

"Your shop is integrated? I mean, well, . . . coed?"

"I guess you could call it that. A local plant shut down and some of their production girls got job retraining as lathe operators under some government program. We're expanding like crazy with all the new defense orders, so when we advertised that we had openings for trainee lathe operators, a bunch applied. The boss was afraid if we didn't hire some, we might not get any more government work."

"Are all the new hires women?"

"We also took on three guys on evening shift, but their skin's okay. Or maybe they show up a little bit like everyone who starts here, except for one pimply faced redhead. He always looks like he got something."

"Are all the bad skin cases women?"

"Right."

"Do all your new employees get instructions on how to wash up and use the protective equipment, Mr. Angelo?"

Bud Angelo looked offended.

"Of course, the girls get the same indoctrination and safety manual like everyone else."

"What about their wash facilities?"

"For the time being, they have to use the ladies' room up front for the office girls. But we got plans to add their own place with lockers back in the shop area."

"Fine, Mr. Angelo. Can I look over your operations and talk to some of them?"

"That's why you're here, right? I'll see that you talk to at least two of the girls. We just started another one this week. The new girl hasn't broke out . . . yet."

And with that, he called for "Mac" over their public address system and one of his supervisors appeared shortly. He briefly explained the reason for Davis' visit and asked Mac to accompany Davis through the plant.

"I want this problem solved before you're ready to leave, young man, or you can tell 'em to forget the next order."

Garden State Machining was both a specialty-order and production shop which precision-machined stainless-steel parts. This involved shaping the metal part by cutting, drilling, or grinding it with a fixed tool called a lathe to precise dimensions. Shaving off layers of steel with a metal cutting edge generates a tremendous amount of heat which must be removed to preserve the integrity of the metal part. The rotating parts of the drill or lathe must also be oil lubricated for heat removal and for smooth operation. Both high-boiling oils and water are excellent heat-removal agents. Thus, metal working fluids, or cutting oils, consisting of straight mineral oils, or oil in water emulsions, mixed with chemical additives like soaps, germicides, and antirusting compounds, are continuously sprayed onto the working metal part and rotating tool to provide the necessary lubrication and cooling. After impinging on the metal part and tool, the cutting fluid drains into a reservoir, or sump, where it is filtered and cooled before being recycled.

The tool operator's hands and forearms are continually wet from handling the oil-wet parts and immersing their hands and forearms in the recycling fluids. In addition to direct contact with the liquids, the rotational movement of a drill can produce an oil mist which, if not captured by an exhaust hood, settles on the workers' faces, necks, shoulders, and clothing. Davis learned pragmatically that if you can barely see the oil mist in diffuse ordinary light, the airborne concentration is lower than the allowable OSHA daily exposure limit of five milligrams of oil mist per cubic meter of air and does not present an inhalation or skin problem. Otherwise, an air sample might be required to determine the actual concentration and whether action is necessary to comply with the exposure standard.

A machine shop is not a rose garden, Davis mused, as he entered the work area. The cacophony produced by the grinding and lathe turning suggested a no-nonsense mission of busyness. Random wisps of oil mist trailed above some of the tool stations and a curious blend of odors emanated from heated and newly surfaced metals, hydrocarbons evaporating from fountains of oil, and additives—variously, pungent from sulfur and phosphorus compounds, acrid from ammonia and soaps, medicinal from germicides like phenol and formaldehyde, and unidentifiable smells from many proprietary synthetic chemicals.

The finished metal parts were neatly stacked and the housekeeping overall appeared to be equal to or better than he had seen at other shops with lesser problems. The circulating cutting oil was filtered free of the sharp metal shavings and fine-metal detritus, or swarf, that peels off from the steel parts. Most encouragingly, the metal working solutions were clean and absent the telltale malodors associated with excessive bacterial contamination from the workers' dirty hands, well-aimed squirts of tobacco juice, or equally offensive expectorations. The cutting oil emulsions contain water and organic chemicals, like natural fats in soaps, which support the growth of the bacteria and other microorganisms introduced from the air and the workers' skin. To prevent the spoilage of the product, it is necessary to add very small amounts of biocides, like slow-releasing formaldehyde and chlorinated phenols. At higher concentrations, these biocides can be skin sensitizers or irritants to some people. Thus, in a misdirected attempt to maximize the "bug" kill, workers sometimes add excessive amounts of the germicide, which can cause an allergic type of dermatitis in the susceptible individuals and which is unrelated to a purely oil-caused skin condition.

Mac, Davis' guide, was polite and answered his questions freely as they toured the facility, but he did not seem comfortable. Having heard that the union might be involved in a grievance over this matter, Mac did not want to risk being on what might be the wrong side of a controversy and protectively kept his own counsel. When Davis suggested that he might be able to continue on his own to observe the workers, Mac readily acquiesced and, pointing to his office, said he would be available there if Davis needed any help and promptly left.

Davis noted that although many of the workers' clothing had some oil stains, none was soaked or excessively wet and practically everyone wore an oil-resistant apron and safety goggles. From having worked with metals, tools, and heavy machinery, their hands were toughened and abraded by minor cuts and chafes, but he saw nothing that suggested an oil-type dermatitis. The wash-up room was clean and well lighted. The workers could choose from germicidal soap solutions, nonabrasive soap bars, and powders, or lanolin-based waterless cleaners. There were plenty of hand and nail brushes, paper towels, and ample hot water at the wash troughs and sinks. At their break time, he watched the men scrub up in nearly surgical fashion before they had their refreshments or lit up their cigarettes. And to confirm the Garden State workers' total attention to personal cleanliness, even the locker room did not have the characteristic sour aroma of unwashed clothing and towels stored in the lockers. Davis would not have been surprised had he been apprised that it was only the recent hires at the shop who developed the more severe skin problems. The unreported information that it was only new *female* workers who were afflicted was doubly unexpected. Apart from the period during the Second World War when many women worked in the usual male preserve of a machine shop, today female machinists had become an endangered species. Nonetheless, conventional wisdom held that women were, by nature, more attuned to personal cleanliness than men and, therefore, a female machinist—should there be one—would be less prone to have skin problems. Why, then, paradoxically was it only the recently hired female machinists who developed skin problems when they all used the same cutting oils?

As promised, after lunch Bud introduced Davis to two of the women at their lathes. There was little question that the sores and redness principally on their forearms were characteristic of an oil-contact dermatitis.

"Is that medicine drying it up, Bev?" Bud asked one of them.

"It stops the oozing and itching, but the doctor says it can't heal completely as long as my hands stay wet with the oil. I tried wearing one of those rubber gloves, but I couldn't hold the part steady."

"Me, too," her partner, Mary, at the adjacent lathe offered. "You can't help getting your hands wet doing this job. Just got to get used to washing up all the time."

Bud nodded impassively and led Davis to a grinder on the other side of the room to meet Lisa, the most recently hired of the female machinists.

"How's it going, Lisa?"

Lisa, smiled nervously. "Okay, I guess."

Her mentor, a patriarch among the plant machinists, answered, "She's doing great."

"Your operation looks clean to me, Mr. Angelo," Davis said. "I really don't think there's anything wrong with our cutting fluids. Do you mind if I just watch your people working and cleaning up?"

"Okay, but don't stay into the second shift or I might have to assign you to a lathe. We need all the help we can get."

Davis wandered as unobtrusively as he could around the shop area, particularly observing the work practices of the three women. At the signal for lunch, Davis guessed that Lisa would probably join the other two women at the ladies' room.

"Lisa, I'd like you to do me a favor," he tactfully began.

"What do you mean?"

"Can you show me how you clean up from the oil before you go to eat?"

"Okay. I guess the other girls won't mind."

When Davis explained to the other two women that he wanted to watch them all wash up, they eyed him strangely. When they realized this meant inside their ladies' room, they started to giggle, but, good-naturedly, they cleared the room for his entry. While he scrutinized each detail of their cleanup procedure starting with the lathering of their hands with liquid soap, they continued giggling when one of them suggested they might be party to some kinky voyeurism. They applied the lather to their forearms, more gingerly to their faces, and finished with several rinses of warm water. It appeared on casual observation that they had removed all the oil on their skin, but there was still some oil stains on their cotton sleeves and around some of their pockets. None of them applied any skin lotion, protective creams, or cosmetics before they had their beverages or smoked. They told Davis they usually waited until they got home to shower and put on any makeup, but they didn't think their work clothes got too wet with oil to change daily now, but they might in the warmer months.

It might seem that the women had performed their rites of purification in a suitable manner, but he knew otherwise from having watched many of the experienced machinists and other workers who get dirty with oil and grime. The men scrubbed themselves intensely with soap and water, sometimes applying special skin cleansers several times; otherwise, barely visible layers of the oil and grime will stubbornly adhere and accumulate. Unlike the women, the men always inspected their hands and forearms to make sure the job was done. Many of the men had either once suffered themselves, or seen others kept out of work for days and weeks with oozing and unsightly raw sores. They knew that if they didn't take the time and expend the effort to clean up, they would invite a recurrence. Most women—and notably, these novice machinists—simply did not have the experience of having worked at a grimy job which necessitated such heavy-duty personal cleaning. The women at Garden State did not even recognize that they were at risk of developing dermatitis by continuing to wear the oil-stained clothing.

Davis sensed that the apparent gender-related skin problems at Garden State would disappear if he could only convince Bud to introduce de facto coeducation. What worked for the gander would surely work for the goose.

"Are you sure the girls aren't washing up properly?" a somewhat incredulous Bud asked. "We *told* them exactly what to do and gave them plenty of stuff to read."

"You have one of the best skin hygiene programs I've seen at a machine shop, Mr. Angelo, but I don't think your women really got the message. It's got something to do with learning by doing it yourself rather than being told or reading about it."

"I guess that makes sense," Bud conceded. "But, what's this about taking Mary and Bev off the lathers 'til their skin clears up?"

"Isn't that what the doctor recommended?" Davis reminded Bud. "Besides, what did you do in the past when one of the *men* got a bad case?"

"Okay, we'll try it but if it doesn't work, we haul out all your oil."

The ploy worked. Ten days later, a grateful marketing department representative called Davis in the afternoon to report that the women's skin problems at Garden State had, indeed, cleared up and the salesman had even picked up the fuel oil account there.

Davis gleefully went in to tell his boss how his experiential hunch of poor skin hygiene had again been vindicated at the New Jersey machine shop. He waited briefly outside the office while Schultz completed the daily ritual telephone call to his wife which never varied in dialogue or time of day. If Marge Brody, their free-spoken secretary, was within earshot, she and Davis would compete with gratuitous wiseacre responses to Schultz's dependable double-barreled opener.

"Oh, are you home, dear? What are you doing?"

Davis waited a few respectful minutes after hearing the standard coda of the dialogue regarding which commuter train Schultz would take home. As he entered the office and started to make his report, Schultz barely mumbled an acknowledgment.

He was already too preoccupied with a puzzling account of a just-reported skin problem which didn't suggest any of the familiar etiologies.

Case **8**

The Dilemma of the Degreaser's Flush

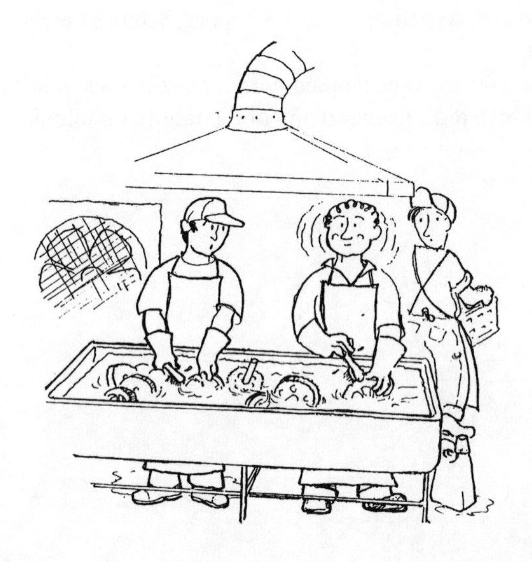

"Lazar, some little plant in Massachusetts is complaining about just one employee who started to break out with an erythema just after they switched to one of our new cutting oils," Schultz began.

"Anything different with the new product?"

"Mainly the name. They only changed the proportions of the same base oils and additives so we'd have a new product for the marketers to promote. None of their machinists there have ever had any skin problems with any of our products."

"It doesn't sound at all like a cutting-oil dermatitis. You think the guy is spending too much time in the sun?"

Schultz ignored or did not hear his assistant's question.

"The customer thinks the problem is due to the new product and wants to switch back, or go to a competitor. Marketing feels they're on the spot since they made such a strong pitch getting them and every other account to change to the new product. So they want *us* to go up there soon to solve it for them."

Davis had great respect for his boss who had taught him more practical knowledge in one month than he had learned in all of his graduate school training, but he stiffened at the possibility that he and Schultz would be in a car together for five-hour stretches to visit the plant. Arnie Schultz could just suck his pipe contemplatively while driving and comfortably not say anything that did not have to be said for several hours. Davis would feel like a garrulous fool when there was no response to repeated attempts to initiate a conversation which did not relate to work. Schultz's silence could also suspend his metabolism, so that he felt no urge to eat and was oblivious of the energy needs of others.

On previous trips when Davis would desperately suggest by mid-afternoon that they might want to get some lunch, if not breakfast, Schultz assumed a look of reenlightenment. "Oh yes, my family always had to remind me to stop to eat on the drives up to our country place."

Davis felt unabashedly relieved when Schultz announced, "I've got to give a talk on the new hearing protection regulation at the safety department meeting in Chicago this week. If you don't mind, you can arrange with the sales representative to go up yourself."

The following afternoon, Davis happily drove alone until early evening to an industrial town just north of the Berkshire Mountains region of western Massachusetts so he could be at the plant early the next morning. The facility made metal pins such as rivets and bolts and tightening nuts to exacting specifications of tolerances and performance for high-technology applications. He had learned some disarming facts from his initial telephone call with the sales representative. Apparently, the affected worker did not even work on any of the machining tools and had only minimal contact with the suspect cutting oil. His job, as degreaser, was to clean off the residual cutting oil from the finished metal parts with a chlorinated hydrocarbon solvent like trichloroethylene (TCE) or perchlorethylene. These synthetic chlorinated solvents are extremely effective in removing oil and grease, leaving a cleaned wet surface which dries quickly. Unlike the pure-petroleum-based solvents, they are not normally flammable or explosive and might be regarded more as a "safety solvent" were it not for the associated health hazards from inhaling their vapors and possible absorption through the skin from liquid and vapor contact. As an alien man-made substance, the body gets rid of some by exhalation, via the lungs, or by detoxification in the liver and excretion through the kidneys. If the dose absorbed inside the body exceeds the limit which the lungs and liver can safely handle and rid, the excess toxic solvent and its metabolites can cause permanent and life-threatening damage to the liver and kidneys. Coursing through the body, the solvent molecules can also defat the protective myelin sheath covering the nerves and impair nerve function. Exposure to excessive concentrations of the toxic vapors can be controlled by adequate ventilation or respiratory protection, but repeated and prolonged skin contact with the liquid solvent will produce a dermatitis that is usually distinguishable from that caused by oils.

The fabricating shop was on a ten-acre lot a mile outside the town in a cinder block building which had been faced with an attractive semigloss white paint, and remained so, in testimony to the unpolluted country air. Hardy red geraniums were interspersed among a dense cover of periwinkles in a border around the front of the building, and a sign identifying the company name with letters artfully formed with bolts and nuts hung from an extended wrought-iron bracket above the office entrance. Parking for employees and visitors was located unobtrusively behind the rear of the building on a tree-lined lot notably free from litter and cigarette butts. Brad Henry, the plant manager, welcomed Davis into his office as he might a visiting dignitary and graciously led him to a comfortable sectional Naugahyde sofa around a beautifully crafted oak pedestal table on which was placed a large pot of hot coffee with Vermont stoneware cups and saucers and a large plate of Mrs. Henry's oatmeal cookies.

Mr. Henry had never heard of an industrial hygienist before and seemed genuinely interested and impressed when Davis explained what he did. He also asked how Davis had got into his line of work, where he had gone to school, how many children he had, and whether he liked trout fishing. What a nice laid-back change in ambience and client, Davis thought. Most of the managers and foremen at the plants he more commonly visited in the industrialized and heavily trafficked metropolitan areas were not necessarily rude or uninterested in talking about work health problems or social exchanges; they just seemed too pressured by the pace and priorities of their work to take out time for small talk.

"This new young fellow, Billy, who just started to break out like scarlet fever almost every afternoon," Mr. Henry began, introducing the reason for Davis' visit. "He's just an apprentice, you know, and doesn't work the lathes yet. We started his rotation out at the degreasing operation. That's a two-man operation where we clean off the cutting oil and dirt from the machined parts. He's been working there for three or four months and never had any kind of skin problem until we started using your new cutting oil."

"Have your tool operators using the new cutting oil had skin problems recently?"

"Not really. You can always find somebody out there with some pimples or infected cut but nothing unusual."

"Any of the other degreasers breaking out like Billy?"

"Don't think so. Billy's very sensitive about it now. Everybody's been getting Billy's goat, if you get my drift. As I say, he usually starts to break out in the afternoon and seems like he just gets redder and redder by the end of the shift."

"Where does he break out?"

"All over his face and neck. I think he gets it on his shoulders and chest, too."

"But not on his hands or forearms?"

Mr. Henry thought a while and shook his head, no. Then, he added, "We sent him to see a doctor, but by the time he could get to the office, the redness had already faded. When Billy told the doctor what he did at work, the doctor said it was likely an irritant contact dermatitis from his working with oils and chemicals. He wouldn't give Billy any medicine unless he saw the outbreak himself, but he felt that it probably wasn't serious and told Billy to come back if it got worse."

Davis knew that a true contact dermatitis involves an outbreak specifically at the point of skin contact with the causative agent and it was not reasonable to see the skin erupt on distal areas of the body. Unless, of course, the dermatitis of an allergic, or sensitizing, nature which develops by an entirely different mechanism. Basically, our immune system responds defensively to the initial presence of certain foreign bodies or chemicals—called allergens—by producing antibodies. In the case of infectious disease agents like viruses and bacteria, the body produces a family of similar but specific antibodies called immunoglobulin. Certain atopic, or inherently allergic, individuals develop a hypersensitivity to the nonpathogenic allergens, which are harmless to virtually 80 percent of the people. Ironically, the defensive antibodies produced in these individuals can elicit all sorts of dermatological miseries, including excruciating itching, boils, hives, and welts either at the point of skin contact or elsewhere, or both, in the hapless allergic individual. Some chemical or biological agents like epoxy resins, chromates and nickel metal, poison ivy, and cashew nut oil are such potent skin sensitizers that a significant portion of the general population will react after being exposed. More accurately, they become sensitized after an incubation period of anywhere from five days to several weeks following the initial contact.

It was entirely possible that Billy had become uniquely sensitized to one or more of the additives at the concentration in the new formulation, or possibly to the solvent cleaner. You never know why someone who is not atopic mysteriously develops an allergic response to some heretofore harmless agent. Identifying this malefactor was more than Davis was professionally qualified to handle. The hygienist defers that one to a medical specialist like an occupational dermatologist, who might resort to controlled skin patch testing and blood antibody analysis for a confirmatory diagnosis. From the practical consideration of medical management and given the inability with standard industrial hygiene controls to eliminate Billy's exposure, if the dermatitis became severe or debilitating, Billy might have to be reassigned to other work.

"What other assignments does Billy have?" Davis asked.

"Trainees help out anywhere. Billy does some gofer chores. Right now he goes into town at lunchtime to deliver and pick up the mail. Maybe to the hardware store if we need something."

Davis suggested that he had enough background information and would appreciate touring the shop and, in particular, observing and interviewing Billy at the degreaser operation. Mr. Henry apologized, saying he wanted to accompany Davis himself but had a prior appointment that morning and had assigned his foreman, a man introduced as Gus, in his stead.

"I'm sure to be back before noon. You're my excuse to go out to lunch, today."

As expected from the initial impressions on his arrival, Davis found little to fault the plant in the personal hygiene and cleanliness of their operations. There was no evidence of oil spills, stains, or debris on the floor and even the tool machines looked like they were wiped down daily by their proud operators with the devotion of a teenager to his or her first car. The company provided their employees with tan-colored cotton work pants, shirts, and caps bearing the company name and logo, which were worn only at work so that they could be changed weekly, or more frequently, if soiled. The employees had to change into their own street clothes at the end of the shift and showered on site, if they wished.

Gus showed him a check-off list on a wallboard, indicating that the cutting fluid was replaced monthly with fresh charge notwithstanding that the recycled fluid was continuously filtered and personally monitored for evidence of contamination.

"It may cost us a few bucks more to replace the oil this way instead of when it starts to smell, but it's cheaper than running into trouble," Gus reported.

"You mean preventing skin problems?"

"Yes, that too. But I got this theory that like changing your car engine oil, the machining goes more smoothly with clean oil. And our parts come out looking sharper."

Gus boasted that the structural integrity of several of the successfully launched space capsules had depended on the use of their superior rivets. But for whatever reason they were changing the cutting oil, Davis could not question their success in being relatively dermatitis-free in such a problem-prone environment. Except, of course, for the singular mystery of Billy's scarlet flush.

"I'd like to look at the degreasing operation before lunch, Gus," Davis requested.

"Okay. Let's start at the beginning. Follow me."

Gus led Davis to the machining area and pointed to dollies near the workstations where the finished batches had been placed to drain off.

"When they get finished with the batch, the pair of young guys working the degreaser—that'll be Billy and Mike—will alternate wheeling these back for cleaning," Gus explained.

As if on cue, a young man sauntered up, rolling an empty dolly. Stopping momentarily to look around for a finished batch to return, he looked scared when Gus loudly called, "Billy, come here to meet our visitor."

He introduced Davis as some kind of "expert" from the oil company, who wanted to watch him do some degreasing and maybe answer a few questions. Billy nodded, barely looking up at Davis, who noticed that, at least at this time in the late morning, the cause of any reddening of the shy young man's complexion was more likely emotional then chemical. After Billy had filled his dolly with finished parts, they followed him back to the degreasing room. A rectangular metal wash tub filled with 100 gallons of TCE cleaning solvent was supported by waist-high stilts in the center of the room, directly above which was suspended an exhaust hood, appropriately called a canopy. Suspended four feet above the liquid surface to allow enough free space for the degreasers to access the bath, the vapors were exhausted by a powerful fan into the hood face and through conveying ducts to an air discharge on the roof.

Billy transferred the oil-wet parts from the dolly into a large metal bucket fashioned from a heavy low-gauge screen. He then placed a metal hand rod through the bucket handle, with which he dunked the bucket with a swirling motion several times in the bath.

"Does the solvent dip get all the oil off, Billy?" Davis asked.

"Mostly," he muttered. Then, after a nervous pause added, "Sometimes, if the parts are greasy, I have to scrub-brush 'em first on that table there."

Davis noted that there was an open quart-size can half-filled with solvent with several tooth brushes on a metal cardtable against the nearby wall. Billy then transferred the now cleaned parts onto a clean dolly and delivered them to a separate quality control room for inspection. For certain high-specification jobs requiring ultraclean surfaces, an ultrasonic cleaning bath was used to remove any miniscule particles of dirt or metal fines that might be lodged in the thread of a screw or other crevices. This high-technology bath utilizes the tiny shock waves, produced by the passage of ultrasonic waves through the bath solution, to bombard and free any stubbornly adhering particles. Because the energy imparted by the waves had been demonstrated to cause cell injury and disruption, the immersion of hands or other body parts in the bath during operation presents a hazard to the operators. Consequently, an activated bath is frequently covered or equipped with an interlock to prevent possible exposure with a precautionary sign of do's and don'ts posted. Although the ultrasonic waves are of such very high frequencies—greater than 20,000 cycles per second—that we cannot hear them, it is possible that they can affect our hearing, and the level of the bath liquid is marked to provide a sufficient volume for absorption and containment of the radiation.

Notwithstanding his assigned mission to determine the cause of a suspected contact dermatitis, Davis was now concerned with the potentially more serious health implications from Billy's likely excessive exposure to the TCE vapors and liquid.

"Has anyone ever checked out the capture velocity of this hood?" Davis asked Gus.

"You mean does it work okay?"

"Exactly."

"We paid an outside contractor enough to install it so I guess it's okay. Anyway, we kind of got used to the smell."

Davis was less certain; rather, he was fairly confident that even without having instruments to measure the capture velocity of the hood and the airborne levels of TCE, this hood did not provide sufficient exhaust to capture all the vapors, or enough of them, to prevent an unsafe exposure level in the workplace. There was also a considerable release of vapors when greasy parts were hand-scrubbed on the card table and the cleaned solvent-coated parts were allowed to dry, both outside of the hood's capture zone. As well as he could recall, neither inhalation of the vapors nor dermal contact with the liquid had been implicated in causing an ephemeral erythema. Putting a finger of suspicion on the TCE exposure as the causative agent for Billy's reported end-of-shift facial flush looked like a dermatological red herring. Surely, the plant's apparent failure to control their degreasers' exposures to the TCE vapors was the more significant health risk. As an industrial hygienist, he could not ethically fail to report his concerns, even though that was not the reason he had been called in and the customer might even resent his implied criticism of their operation and his intrusion.

"You need anything more from me?" Gus asked his guest.

"I'm just fine if you need to go back to your office. I'd like to just observe for the rest of the morning and maybe ask Billy some questions."

Davis felt more comfortable on his own with a quirky unresolved problem. It was better just to keep on observing, asking questions, and think, alone. He watched Billy and his partner, Mike, repeat their work cycle for the rest of the morning. Neither Mike nor several of the other trainees who ambled into the degreaser room to chat with their buddies had any apparent skin disorders or facial redness. Nonetheless, he became more convinced by his observations that the degreaser employees had a significant TCE overexposure in the room resulting from the open drying of the solvent-wet parts and the inadequate design of the canopy hood to capture the vapors from the tank. A pungent and characteristic chlorinated hydrocarbon solvent odor was immediately sensed on first entering the room, if any sensory confirmation of the fugitive vapors was needed.

Just before the lunch break, Billy started to clean up before going out on his assigned daily chores in the town. Davis approached him as gingerly as you might go to pick up a wounded and frightened bird.

"I hear you break out with some sort of flush on your face and body some afternoons," he began.

Billy just nodded, not looking directly at Davis.

"Do you have any idea what's causing it?"

"They say it's got something to do with the new cutting oil we're using," he answered quietly. Then with a slight rise in confidence added, "But I don't feel nothing. It just makes me look funny and it goes away quick."

"Do the TCE vapors bother you?"

"I can feel them in my throat and eyes. Sometimes I get, like, a little bit dizzy but not so's I can't work."

Davis sensed from Billy's shuffling that he was getting anxious about leaving.

"I have to pick up the mail and stuff in town, so I got to go now," Billy explained.

"Okay, thanks for your help," Davis said. Then as Billy started to leave, he asked, "Are you the only worker who goes out to eat?"

"I guess so. Everybody carries lunch pails here. See you later."

While waiting in the main office for Brad Henry to return, Davis pondered

Billy's bizarre temporal flushes which in no way squared with his apparent workplace exposures. The reaction described strangely reminded him of an incident involving Sammy Chang, a Chinese-American chemist he worked with at his first job after college at a government testing laboratory. Some of the unattached members of the laboratory formed a social nexus which would occasionally meet after work for a few beers at a bar. Perhaps in deference to Sammy's sensitivity, none of the group ever asked him why he always passed on the beer order and drank only iced tea or fruit juice. When Davis announced that he was getting married, had been awarded a master's degree fellowship in industrial hygiene, and would be leaving the laboratory shortly, his friends gave him a farewell party. In the sweep of the festivities and encouraged by Davis, Sammy good-naturedly joined the group in a celebratory champagne toast. Within the hour, Sammy's face had lit up with a brilliant scarlet flush.

"Many Chinese people react this way to alcohol. For me, just a couple of sips of wine will do it," Sammy explained to astonished friends. "I only know it's happening when people start staring. So I don't drink. Anyhow, I don't even like the taste."

This peculiar syndrome of a racial genetic trait was reinforced in Davis' mind years later when he dined out in a group with another Chinese-American colleague who, following the lead of everyone else, generously dowsed his New Orleans turtle soup with sherry wine. The poor fellow smiled nervously when all eyes at the table were mesmerized by his sudden radiance.

As Davis finished jotting down his observation Mr. Henry arrived just before noon, and indicative of the hospitality accorded guests, he took Davis out to the local country club for lunch. After they had placed their order, and finished admiring the view of the golf course, Mr. Henry pleasantly asked, "Well, young man, have you figured out what might be causing Billy's problem?"

"It's not that I doubt you, Mr. Henry, but I myself haven't seen any reaction on Billy yet," Davis started slowly, adding, "But it just doesn't appear to be like any kind of skin disorder associated with oils or chlorinated solvents. In fact, I haven't seen anything that Billy is exposed to at work which could reasonable explain it."

"But if we didn't have any problems before you brought in that new product, I'm afraid we have no other choice but to stop using it."

Davis could not refute Mr. Henry's logic, but if he did not come up with a better explanation and ultimate solution, his company might lose the business there. He told Mr. Henry that he was not minimizing their concerns with Billy's outbreaks, but he believed their employees might incur far more serious and possibly permanent health effects to their liver, kidneys, and nervous system from their failure to control the TCE at the degreaser. He described in some detail why he felt they needed an industrial hygiene engineer to evaluate the effectiveness of their canopy hood, measure the employee's daily exposures to the vapor, and institute the appropriate controls to comply with the recommended OSHA limits.

Mr. Henry listened carefully and with obvious concern to the advice, and thanking Davis, said he would certainly attend to it. He even asked Davis to recommend a consulting hygienist. When they arrived back at the plant, Davis said if Mr. Henry did not object, he would continue his observations and interviewing until the end of the shift. So assured, Davis returned to the degreaser room to find Mike, the other worker assigned there, alone.

"Hi, Mike. Is Billy still out to lunch?"

"Yeh. He probably had to wait at the post office for the mail," Mike explained.

Unlike many plant employees who are reticent and continue their work seemingly oblivious of any visitors, Mike was curious and uninhibited.

"Are you with OSHA?" he asked directly.

"No. I work for the company that supplies your metal working fluids."

"Thought you might be here because of Billy's problem. I don't think that new oil has anything to do with it," he volunteered.

"Really? Why do you think that?"

Mike paused for a few seconds, looking like he was not sure he wanted to share his secret.

"For one, by the time we get to handle the parts, most of the oil has drained off. You see how those guys at the machines bathe in the stuff? They don't break out."

And this guy didn't have to go to graduate school to figure it out, Davis thought, admiringly.

"Then what do *you* think is causing it?"

"I didn't say I knew. I just said I didn't think it was the oil."

Tantalizing fellow, Davis thought. Mike started to move toward an empty dolly for a pick-up of the finished parts, when on impulse, Davis suddenly asked, "Do you ever break out like Billy?"

Mike broke out with a sheepish grin.

"Maybe, sometimes. But never here at work.," he insisted. "Just once a while in the evening. And it's nothing bad like Billy's."

And with that for Davis to ponder, he left. Billy returned with the mail less than ten minutes later and immediately joined them at the degreaser.

"How come you're back so soon?" Mike asked his friend. "You feel okay?"

"I'm all right, I guess. Just didn't feel like eating today."

For Davis, the rest of the afternoon's work activities was a repeat of what he had already seen in the morning and almost perversely, Billy showed not a shade increase in ruddiness by quitting time. If anything, he seemed paler. At four o'clock, the two young workers left to clean up before going home.

When Davis returned to the office to say good-bye to Mr. Henry, he reported that he had nothing conclusive to add to his earlier remarks at lunch.

"Just so long as it's only Billy and thing's don't get worse, I guess we can live with it," Mr. Henry said, considerately. He thanked Davis for his effort and said if he ever came up this way again to be sure to say hello. No plant manager had ever said this to Davis before.

Since the customer had been satisfied, the marketing department would be happy and for that reason, Davis' trip was successful, but his failure to establish a clear-cut causation for the skin problem was gnawing. He had been mulling over the common and disparate factors of the case. No one who worked directly and solely with the new cutting oil was affected, whereas only workers heavily exposed to TCE reacted. Billy's flush appeared only late in the afternoon and only at work, whereas Mike's alleged lesser reaction occurred only at night and away from work. Unlike Mike and the rest of the plant who brought their lunch to work, Billy was the only worker who regularly ate outside, presumably in the town. And the capstone of this contradictory mishmash was the degreaser's flush itself. What kind of cockamamie occupational dermatitis is this that appears so unreliably on the stage like a temperamental and flashy walk-on with no real effect?

As he left the building to walk to his car on the parking lot, he spotted Mike at the entrance, dressed in a baseball uniform, obviously awaiting a ride to the ball field.

"Big game tonight?" he asked.

"No. Just regular practice. League games are on Friday."

His knowledge of the national sport was too limited to extend any meaningful conversation, but he had needed an opener with Mike to satisfy a gnawing speculation.

"Mike, would you happen to know where Billy usually goes for lunch in town?"

"I suppose he goes to The Continental. They got the best cheese steak and fries."

"Is that the local watering hole?"

"The what? Oh, I get it. Yeh, we head there after practice for a few brews."

"But Billy didn't eat lunch there today. Right?"

"You heard him," Mike confirmed. "He said he wasn't feeling so good and he skipped lunch."

Shades of Sammy Chang, Davis chuckled to himself. He vaguely recalled somewhere in his memory bank a research article he had read dealing with a temporary rash induced in college student volunteers exposed in a test chamber to some chlorinated solvent vapors shortly followed by their ingestion of some alcoholic beverages. He would later confirm on a rereading of the article back in the medical department library that the erythema was believed to be due to the production of excess acetaldehyde, a metabolite of ethyl alcohol, in the body; hence, the term, acetaldehyde syndrome. The body metabolizes alcohol by sequentially breaking it down with specific enzymes made in the liver for each stage of the way. Simply put, the alcohol is chemically converted first to acetaldehyde, then to acetone, and ultimately to carbon dioxide and water, which are exhaled or excreted. In the case of the Chinese affected, it is believed that they inherently lack sufficient acetaldehyde dehydrogenase, the enzyme needed to advance the process beyond the first stage, with the resultant accumulation of the flush-producing acetaldehyde in the blood.

In the workplace, excess exposure to chlorinated hydrocarbon vapors like TCE is believed to cause the disruption of normal liver function which produces the required acetaldehyde dehydrogenase. With just intermittent exposures within certain vapor concentration limits, the liver is probably not permanently damaged despite the unsightly rosy countenance. Davis was, understandably, more concerned about the degreasers' prolonged daily exposures above these tolerable limits which could lead more to permanent and life-threatening damage than any temporary cosmetic effect.

"Mike, I have a hunch what's causing Billy's—and your—skin problem," Davis said.

Mike looked skeptical. "It's not the new oil?" Then, defensively added, "Anyway, I never said *I* had a problem. It's Billy who breaks out like a fire truck."

"I thought you should know it probably has something to do with your exposure to the TCE solvent vapors. They're going to have someone come in to improve the ventilation over the entire operation there so you don't get overexposed. They'll probably give you some suggestions to help reduce the exposures further. Like brush cleaning and handling the solvent only under the hood and maybe, wearing special gloves."

Mike thought about this a while. "You expect me to swallow that? Look, Billy's been working with me at the degreaser for months and he never broke out 'til you brought in that new oil couple weeks back."

"Good point, Mike, but there's another player here to strike out. When did Billy start to go out for lunch?"

"He just started picking up the mail beginning last week. So what?"

"When Bill does go to The Continental for lunch, do you suppose he has a beer with his cheese steak?" Davis ventured.

The young man looked uncomfortable, as if an indiscretion had been compromised.

"Okay, Mike, I won't say anything," Davis said, in leaving. "But just ask Billy to see what happens when he switches to milk."

Case 9

Who's Itching Now?

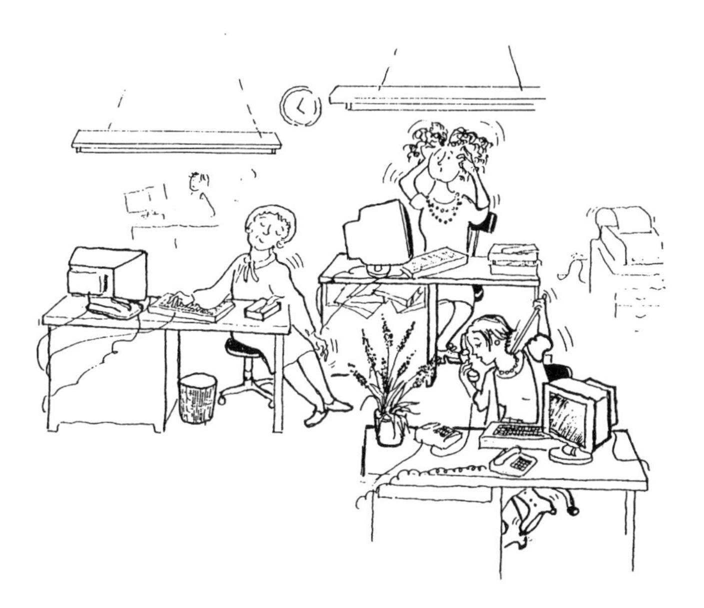

On any list of company functions in which occupational illnesses are notably endemic, the office and clerical staff might seem a surprising entry. Having grown up in a blue-collar coal-mining town and worked in many grimy summer factory jobs through college, Frank Barr, the personnel manager of the Acme Realty and Mortgage Corporation, could understand why workers got sick breathing dense clouds of rock dusts or mixing foul-smelling chemicals all day in sweaty, noisy workplaces. But why should the polyester collar workers in their sanitized air-conditioned offices inevitably attribute—in sheep-like procession—so many health ailments to their workplace? They got headaches from the smell of painting of the hallways or from a co-worker's perfume, or from reading under lighting subjectively reported as being too bright and too dim. Their uncommon colds developed from a dichotomous atmosphere concurrently hot and cold, drafty and stuffy, and humid and dry. And absent a physical causation for their illnesses, there was, reliably, the emotional and psychological stress of the job to account for all, and more, of the above.

Just before getting ready to leave for his biweekly Lions Club luncheon meeting, Barr was understandably apprehensive when he was stopped at the door by an ominous-looking Myrtle Fink, his billing office supervisor. Myrtle had the unsettling effect on Barr of seeming to deliver every report of ill tidings with an I-told-you-so air of triumph.

"Yesterday morning Barbra broke out at her desk with itches on certain unmentionable parts of her body."

"So?"

"In the afternoon, Mary Beth says she started scratching her arm where there were—like, you know—little mosquito bites, only redder."

"It's December, Ms. Fink. We don't have mosquitoes now."

"That yellow hibiscus plant that's on Barbra's desk. . . ." she said, cryptically.

"The what?" he questioned, trying not to sound too dense at failing to divine the obvious.

"The hibiscus, Mr. Barr. Barbra saw little creatures crawling all around the leaves and flowers."

"Well, did Barbra get rid of the plant?"

"Of course, she threw it out last night. Barbra's grandmother said the hibiscus was infested with plant lice."

"Good. So the problem's solved now."

"We're not sure, Mr. Barr. Just this morning, Linda, whose desk is on the other side of Barbra's, says her legs have been itching. She thinks it has something to do with the carpet cleaning."

"But that was last weekend. Well, has anyone else. . . ."

"That's all . . . so far."

"All right. We'll try to find out what's been bugging the girls when I get back from lunch." He eagerly left the stone-faced Ms. Fink for his regular Lions Club lunch meeting where he could forget the problem, or, at worst, feel free to complain about it to sympathetic ears.

"I could understand their sore eyes and neck pains from sitting at that computer screen all day . . . even with all their breaks," he conceded to an associate at his table. "So we paid some expert to install ergonomic chairs and show them how to adjust the lighting on the screen to reduce the glare. That problem was solved and everybody's happy. But, it's these pesky off-the-wall complaints which drive me bats."

"You'd think they'd be happy just to have a decent paying job these days," his friend whispered, just as the Lions Club president called for order to introduce their luncheon speaker, a retired physician and professor of public health. The doctor had just returned from setting up an immunization program at an impoverished Indian village in Central America funded by the Lions. Barr, who never missed a National Geographic special on public television, was vicariously transported by the doctor's spectacular video camera capture of the life of the Indians, who find revelation in their mythological religion with the mind-freeing peyote drug derived from a cactus. He felt he could use some peyote when he found Ms. Fink stalking him when he returned to the office.

"We think the insects from the plant are still around. Now Mary Beth says she feels itchy. She thinks she definitely felt something crawling but hasn't seen anything."

"Anybody else . . . ?"

"Ted Rogers' left foot has been itching all morning, but he hasn't seen any bugs. And Rhonda who sits in front of Barbra has three tiny red marks on her leg that just started to itch."

"But Ted's desk is on the opposite window side of the room nowhere near Mary Beth's desk."

"That's why some people think we ought to call in an exterminator. But of course, we'd have to have them come in on a weekend because Susan and Meredith are allergic to insecticides."

This is getting out of hand, he thought. We don't even know if we have a real problem, let alone, what might be causing it and they're ready to call in a bomb squad.

"I think we need some professional help, Ms. Fink, before we. . . ."

"Of course," she agreed, condescendingly.

On several previous occasions regarding claims of damage, Barr had learned that their company insurance carrier used a consulting company with a staff of all kinds of technical experts. He called their agent who referred him to their consulting company, who, in turn, said that their expert in health problems at work was a professor of industrial hygiene at a local university.

After having completed over twenty years of service as a supervising industrial hygienist with a major oil company, Lazar Davis was fortunate to achieve what most people yearn for but rarely attain: a second career that was a first choice. As a newly appointed professor, he started a graduate program in industrial hygiene at a well-known urban university and, like his highly qualified and experienced engineering and scientific colleagues, also served as a private consultant.

Barr sounded apologetic reporting the current skin-irritation problem to Davis after recounting the many unsubstantiated employee health complaints in the same office.

"An outbreak of dermatitis in an office from a house plant?" Davis dubiously asked himself. Given the myriad of chemical products commonly used or generated in the modern office, somebody was destined to have some kind of contact dermatitis. The ammonia solutions from some wet-process duplicating machines, solvent cleaners for office machinery, carbonless copy papers, and ozone discharges from poorly ventilated and inadequately filtered photocopiers have all been implicated in offices. Indirectly, airborne dusts raised by drilling into a cement floor or from damaged glass fiber insulation, or vapors from certain recently treated textiles have occasionally been cited as causes for skin disorders among office personnel. Because some air-conditioned offices are overheated with excessively low relative humidities, the drying atmosphere has elicited erythema, scaling of the skin, and the severe itching of a pruritus condition. The proliferation of video display terminals (VDT), photocopiers, and electronic facsimile machines into the modern office might seem to be a less than obvious dermatological hazard. Nonetheless, Davis had read reports attributing skin rashes, tingling sensations, and, occasionally, papular eruptions usually on the face and chin of the VDT operators despite the absence of any contacting chemical or clearly identifiable causative agent. In fact, he had once been called in to investigate complaints at a police department van of upper respiratory irritation, burning of the eyes, and, to a lesser degree, itching of the fingers from the recipients of electronically relayed crime reports.

None of these factors were apparently associated with the problem of his caller, who was understandably more concerned with the cure than the cause.

"Professor, to be honest with you, I think their complaints of itching from the plants or the bugs or whatever are, well, . . . more in their heads. I want an expert to tell me whether their problem is really work related."

"That's my job, but I can understand your skepticism, sir," Davis commiserated. "When I interview them—which I'd like to do soon—I assume that their complaints are real."

He quickly added that although he thought he could help Barr, he had to admit he had had no prior experience with plants or insects that *proved* to be the cause of a dermatitis in an office.

"Okay, but how soon can you get out here?"

"Let me look at my calendar." Then, adding the kind of silly gratuitous remark that undermined his commitment, "Sometimes, these problems just disappear as mysteriously as they appear."

"Maybe so, professor, but I can't count on that. I hope you can get out here soon."

"Oh, I didn't mean that," he sputtered, with mild embarrassment. "I can be there first thing in the morning."

Davis had only once been involved with a purported occupational dermatitis that was not associated with any of the commonly associated causes of skin problems at an office. That was at a large suburban hospital which called him to investigate the source of skin irritation complaints from several of their billing clerks in a basement office alleged to be caused by the "paper-eaters" in a damp claustrophobic file room. Having recently acquired a daughter-in-law who had majored in entomology, Davis was now able to supplement his admittedly limited knowledge of the habitat and diet of literary insects, both fiction and nonfiction. He was apprised that the little creature popularly classified as a "paper-eater," along with "paper fleas" and "book lice," is a real insect, misleadingly named "silverfish." It feeds indiscriminately on the bindings of books and paper sizing but is otherwise harmless to man. The scientific evidence notwithstanding, some phobic people believe that any crawling or flying arthropod is a threat to their health.

On investigation, Davis learned that the three hospital clerks complaining of mild irritation were far less specific about what was responsible for their discomfort. While an expansion in the hospital was being undertaken, a previously unoccupied and dust-accumulated basement area with a scant six-and-a-half-foot ceiling had been converted into offices for their department. They were uniformly convinced, however, that they only started to feel "dirty and itchy" since having been relocated into the dank and somber subterranean offices. When Davis toured their new location, it was hard to fault them for their discomfort and sense of incarceration. His measurements of the air quality and ventilation indicated that the building engineers had not provided sufficient fresh makeup air, so that the air was indeed stale, humid, and smelled of mold. If air filters had been installed, they were ineffectual in preventing the deposition of a fine black dust on their desk tops and papers. Although Davis did not specifically state that the work environment caused the health complaints, the hospital management readily inferred from his report that they had made a tactical error in creating such an insalubrious and crowded work environment. When they moved the filing clerks back above ground with windows to the world, the complaints subsided along with the retreat of the "paper-eaters."

Based on the sketchy preliminary information, the reports of itching imprecisely attributed to plant lice, or more accurately, aphids, at Acme Realty and Mortgage did not seem to be much more substantial than the book lice at the hospital. When Davis arrived at the personnel manager's office to begin his survey the next morning, Frank Barr was impatiently awaiting his arrival.

"Good morning, professor. I'll take you around the office first for a quick see, but believe me, there's not much out there to cause real problems. I already scheduled your interviews like you said. You can use this back office," he said, explaining, "It's better if you talk to each employee privately without letting everybody here know what's going on."

Davis nodded agreeably, convinced that every clerk on the floor would know exactly what had been revealed and learned well before they left work.

He had to agree that Barr's allusion to an essentially healthful albeit unesthetic workplace appeared to be on target. There was a computer screen, a telephone, and piles of paper on each of the three dozen desks evenly spaced in three rows in the center of the large room, a bank of file cabinets along the inside wall, and not much else. At least, there were no equipment or activities in this essentially functional and unremarkable office to suggest a likely cause of skin irritation.

His goal in interviewing the complainants was first to determine if they all really experienced a common health effect and, second, to figure out what specific agent(s) and conditions in that environment were known, or suspected, to cause that kind of problem. Once the suspect causes were identified, he then had to confirm whether they were present and under the propitious conditions. With most occupational exposures to chemicals or physical agents, propitious also means exposure at sufficient concentration, or dose, known to cause the effect to the average healthy worker. For example, just being exposed to very low levels of carbon monoxide, as might exist in a room with an occasional cigarette smoker, is not likely to cause carbon-monoxide-induced headaches. The exposure has to be above a certain concentration or for a period of time to deliver a sufficient dose. With the "nonaverage" allergic or highly susceptible individual, this dose may be considerably lower.

Davis applied the classical epidemiological approach in determining the disease causation by identifying which of the trinity of interrelated components (namely, the Host, or the victim, the Environment, or where the exposure occurred, and the causative Agent) was the critical factor. Sometimes, an intermediate or Vector was necessary to deliver the agent to the host. When it is not apparent why only certain people in the same environment become victims (i.e., the hosts) while others similarly exposed remain unscathed, we attribute the causation to their particular susceptibility or possibly their lesser exposure. Thus, not all asbestos insulation workers in the same plant succumb to asbestosis or mesothelioma any more than everyone develops flu during an epidemic. The first two factors in the current situation—the itchers and their common environmental workplace—were fairly evident, but the specific agent causing the problem was less than obvious.

Barr updated Davis with the news that there were now three complainants to be interviewed out of a total office staff of thirty-four. The others had been eliminated when Linda's doctor confirmed that her skin reaction was caused by her inadvertent wearing of wool socks to which she was known to be allergic and Ted Rogers realized that his problem was a flare-up of a prior condition of athlete's foot.

None of the women interviewed indicated exposure to any of the items on Davis' checklist of the various chemical products and activities reported to cause dermatitis in offices or professed to have any history of skin or other type of allergy. Each of the women interviewed agreed that they had felt their itches initially and most strongly while at work, and Barbra, in particular, maintained that she still felt itching at work and usually in the morning. When asked what they thought was causing the problem, they parted company. Barbra, who was the first employee to report a problem was firmly convinced that she had been bitten by small bugs that were now resident in the office. In fact, she claimed to have seen a tiny black beetlelike insect about an eighth of an inch long jump from her arm after she had been bitten, but she didn't catch one then or since. In a separate audience, Linda, Barbra's desk neighbor, having seen no insect other than the aphids on the hibiscus and not having been bitten since the plant was thrown out, was less convinced that she still had a problem and implied that her appearance was to provide credence to Barbra's claim that all was not well within the environs. Rhonda, who sat in front of Barbra, was as firmly assured as Barbra that the itching on her legs had been caused by a resident insect which she, too, had observed in flight after being bitten. She claimed her assailant was definitely a reddish-brown winged bug about a half an inch long that resembled a fruit fly, but she, too, had not caught the culprit. With such conflicting eyewitness reports, it was impossible to support what Davis had begun to suspect was the most likely insect candidate; namely, the fleas from domestic animals.

Davis' daughter-in-law had explained to him that these common fleas feed preferably on the blood of their animal hosts, with man generally a second choice. Several years previously, Davis had had an excruciating demonstration of the fleas' compromising feeding predilection when he agreed to help rent and oversee the vacated house of a friend who was now living abroad. Apprehensive of possible property damage from rambunctious children and their irresponsible parents, the absentee landlord had been delighted to learn that his first tenants were a childless working couple with a "few" cats. The couple never specified the exact number in that they never knew how many cats they had accrued with their ongoing feeding and addition of wayward felines. With the rent several months in arrears, the couple absconded—fortunately, with all the cats—to the relief of their neighbors who had been complaining to Davis of their unsightly yard with an overpowering stench of cat urine. When Davis and his wife entered the empty locked-up house a week or two later to arrange for a cleanup, they were overwhelmed in less than a minute by multiple itches all over their bodies and were forced to rush outside, slamming the door behind them. Apparently, when starved, adult fleas denied their customary cat blood and hungry pupae emerging with no prior taste cultivation will attack human hosts with a vengeance.

When Davis asked the women the obvious question about pets at home, only Linda reported having a dog, which she claimed never had fleas or, at least, no one in their family had ever been bitten by one. Without the recovery of a live or dead insect from the hosts or their environment, Davis knew he could not attribute the reported itches to an insect or, indeed, anything else at this point. He said as much when Barr joined him at the conclusion of the final interview.

"We need a writ of habeas corpus for this one, Mr. Barr."

"You mean a dead bug?"

"Live or dead. Otherwise, I don't see anything here at work which can be implicated."

"That's fine with me."

It was not exactly satisfying with Davis who felt that he had missed something which could explain the clerks' mysterious itches.

"Sorry, I can't give you a more definitive answer on this one, but that's the way it goes sometimes," Davis said, as he left.

"I'll be sure to remind the girls to catch the next bug they find crawling on them here," Barr laughed.

Davis had just about filed the case in his mind when he received a call from Barr just two days after his visit.

"Barbra just brought me in a squashed bug which she caught biting her leg this morning," Barr reported. "I can get it wrapped carefully and delivered to your office."

"Fine. Send it right over."

Davis knew that the state university maintained a local cooperative agricultural extension office, where a Dr. Brown was the part-time consulting entomologist. He promptly called to make an appointment to have the insect identified. When he arrived at the extension office and carefully explained the reason for his request, Dr. Brown nodded confidently, as if the story was monotonously familiar. Davis wondered how the entomologist could possibly identify an insect from the partly disjointed and crushed body parts hidden under a swath of absorbent cotton inside the polyethylene plastic bag that Barr had sent him. Dr. Brown delicately transferred the reconstructed insect parts onto a glass slide for viewing under a low-power microscope and within seconds of focusing tersely announced, "cat flea."

"The kind that also bites people?"

"Oh, sure, they don't discriminate too much. For some reason, the so-called cat fleas are more likely to jump on a person than the dog fleas."

"I can believe that," Davis said and recounted his experience at his friend's rented house.

Dr. Brown had heard variations of that story, too. Davis thanked him and then called Barr to tell him of the breakthrough.

"Could you find out if any of the women have been in contact with a cat?" he asked Barr.

"I thought only Linda had a dog and the other didn't . . . ," Barr accurately recalled.

"Right. None of them said they had a cat at their *home* but I'd like to know if they've been anywhere near a cat recently. Or a dog for that matter."

"Okay. I'll call you back as soon as I find out," Barr replied pleasantly.

Davis was not surprised when Barr called a few days later to state that Barbra had been recently taking care of an elderly neighbor's cats while the neighbor was in Florida.

"She says she's gotten so attached to them she gets up early every morning just to feed and pet them before leaving for work," Barr added.

"It's obvious Barbra's been both the victim and the vector in the case."

"Well, then, if Barbra brought the fleas in from outside, we can't blame the employer for the problem. So the case of the mysterious itches is solved. Right, professor?"

Whatever does blame have to do with the case, Davis wanted to ask but he thought otherwise, answering, "Right, Mr. Barr. The cat's out of the bag."

SECTION FOUR

▪

Metal Poisonings

Case 10

Our Son's Just Not the Same

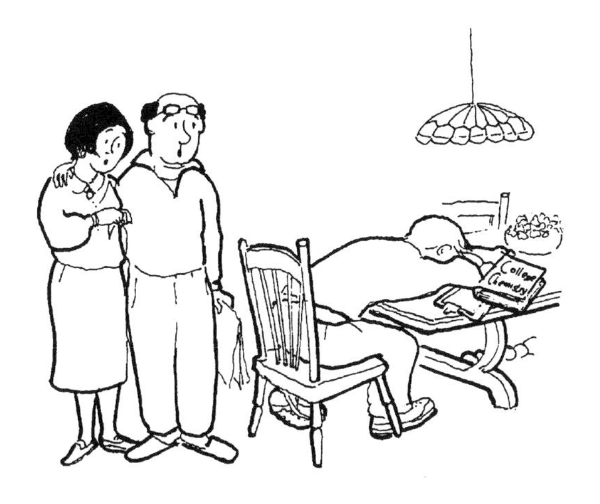

Terry Dugan, an eighteen-year-old part-time college student in business administration, rarely asked questions in class or had time to participate in the extracurricular activities and campus hoopla, so his fellow students and faculty had only a vague awareness of his presence. Commuting to school from a family of modest means, he worked part-time at a restaurant to help pay for his tuition. From the time he was a young teenager, he loved to experiment with chemicals in the unfinished family basement which was staked out as his private retreat. He thought of becoming a chemist, but his high school counselor tactfully convinced him that his science grades might not be strong enough for him to get acceptance into a rigorous college chemistry program. When a summer position as a clerk in the chemical storeroom of the chemistry department at the university became vacant, he applied and was selected by default when none of the preferred chemistry majors applied. That he was contented satisfying his interest in chemicals with the surrogate part-time job could only be surmised by his pleasant demeanor because he did not talk very much at work either.

After over thirty years of neglect and abuse from faculty and graduate students, the chemical storeroom had become a disorganized repository for hundreds of misplaced reagents, laboratory equipment, and abandoned and unmarked chemical containers. Because OSHA had recently been investigating chemical exposure hazards and safety violations in the heretofore sacrosanct laboratories of academic research, the university administration was fearful that failure to clean up their chemical junkyard might jeopardize their federal research grant program. Consequently, when school resumed in September, Terry was offered and happily accepted the opportunity to continue to work part-time on the high-priority project to reorganize and clean up the storeroom.

Adjustment to college for a diffident and untested young man like Terry had gone well. He had a girlfriend and though barely a middling student, he had kept his head above the academic waters and was praised for his diligence on the job. Unaccustomed to having an undergraduate assistant working in the storeroom mess without having to be constantly told what to do, his boss insisted that Terry continue on the job part-time when school resumed in early September and offered him the unusual option to work a few extra hours each week.

When Terry started to talk more volubly and excitedly at home, his mother at first attributed it to an awakening of confidence in her normally taciturn son. Certainly, there had been no indication that anything was amiss is his apparently unstressed life, but by late October, he uncharacteristically began to start arguments with his two brothers or a friend often claiming that they had made fun of him behind his back. When he fought and broke up with his girlfriend after accusing her of two-timing, his parents assumed that he did so not knowing how to terminate his involvement in a relationship which had cooled. They were less certain of his behavior when he began to show irritation and often anger at any harmless remark made during the ordinary banter at the dinner table from which he would stalk away claiming he no longer had any appetite. At school, he accused the graduate students of stealing equipment when he could not remember where he had put it, and he angrily argued with the teaching assistants and instructors when he was reprimanded for forgetting to deliver orders despite repeated reminders. The assistant department head who tried to talk to him about the reports of his forgetfulness and his antagonistic and uncooperative behavior was nonplused when Terry screamed and cursed that everyone had been lying about him. When Terry continued his behavior, unrepentant, his boss regretfully had to fire him.

Shortly after the mid-term examinations, Terry had received warning of failing performance in his courses, which he did not disclose to his parents. They had been told that college gets progressively more difficult, but they were startled when their son suddenly announced just before Christmas that he was quitting school and refused to talk about it, or see a counselor. He complained of stomachaches, was not sleeping well, and seemed more irritable and tense. His father suspected that he had gotten involved with drugs at school, which was vehemently denied in what developed into a continuing series of disturbing confrontations. The parents wanted to believe that college and working had proved to be too stressful for their son and that he would come around to his former self if he just took it easy for a few months. In early January, he inexplicably disappeared, and the next day a policeman called from Norfolk, Virginia reporting that Terry had been picked up wandering the deserted streets in the middle of the night and did not know how or why he had come there. With the untutored wisdom acquired from handling all kinds of personal crises, the veteran policeman advised the desperate parents to take their son to a doctor. The day following Terry's safe retrieval, they importuned him to see Dr. Baron, their family physician who had treated him since he was a toddler.

Noting that Terry had lost weight and seemed nervous and agitated, the doctor asked gently, "What seems to be the trouble, Terry?"

"Nothing wrong with me," he snapped.

"How's school going?" the doctor asked, casually.

Terry looked away and said nothing. His mother looked pained and on the verge of tears.

Then answering elliptically, Terry said, "It was those assholes at school. I couldn't take all their lying about me."

"Of all my boys, Terry was always the quiet one," Mrs. Dugan interjected, adding between sobs, "He'd never say anything bad about anyone, and now. . . ."

Mr. Dugan, who had said nothing from the time they entered the office, put his arm around his wife and said plaintively, "Our son's just not the same."

Stone-faced, Terry stared into space as if he did not belong in the same room.

"Terry, why don't you just step into my examining room," Dr. Baron said, gently, indicating that the parents should wait in the lobby.

Dr. Baron could easily recognize the broad-shouldered young man before him as a mature version of the shy cherubic boy with curly brown hair he had first seen as a toddler, but he was taken aback by his personality turnabout. Less then six months had passed since he had performed the required physical examination for Terry to enter college and noted that the young man was slightly overweight though otherwise healthy and was still as low keyed and compliant as he had ever been. This time he seemed tense and appeared to have a slight tremor, which could be attributed to his understandable nervousness in view of the high-tension dramatics going on in the office. The doctor noted the abnormality and performed the standard physical examination of the vital functions, which is not designed to provide clues to account for a change of personality. Like Terry's father, the doctor suspected that the young man might have gotten involved with drugs at college, but there were no obvious signs. Acknowledging that he could not come up with a diagnosis, he recommended to the parents that Terry should see a specialist in internal medicine and possibly a neurologist for a more complete workup and examination. The internist who subsequently examined Terry noted during a test to determine manual dexterity that he had some difficulty in coordination and had a slight tremor in his hands. The patient, he recorded, sweated profusely, protested that there was no reason for his being there, and was barely cooperative. When neither the internist nor any of the half-dozen or so other medical specialists and consultants reviewing the case during the next several months was able to agree on a physical causation to explain Terry's symptoms, a psychiatric evaluation was proposed, although there was no family history of mental disease or apparent predisposing stresses. The jargon-laden report on the psychiatric examination confirmed what everyone already knew—Terry Dugan manifested paranoia, antisocial behavior, and erethism, which is a nervous irritability—and provided no reasons to explain how or why they suddenly developed.

Not one of all the examining and consulting physicians had bothered to follow a simple recommendation of a seventeenth-century Italian physician that might have put them on the right track. Bernardino Ramazzini, who published his monumental study *The Diseases of Workers* (*De Morbis Artificum Diatriba*) in 1700, suggested that an examining physician should simply ask the ailing patient his or her occupation—that is, where do you or did you work and what did you do there—for indications of a possible work-related causation. Fortuitously, although months later, one of the stymied physicians mentioned the case to a colleague who suggested to his friend that the young man might have been exposed to some chemicals like pesticides at work. It was early June when this doctor referred Terry to an occupational health physician on the staff of a labor-sponsored organization that dealt with the health and safety problems of workers.

The sole faculty member on campus who was an expert on the health effects of occupational exposures and could have helped solve Terry's mysterious personality change was totally oblivious of the student's existence. Professor Davis dealt entirely with graduate students in industrial hygiene and only encountered the undergraduates on his forays across the campus where they gathered in good weather to toss frisbies, schmoose against the background of booming rock music, or in the library if they needed to have more confidential conversations. Despite their avowed mission of promoting and exchanging knowledge, the university administration feared adverse publicity might result from news of Terry's behavior and dismissal and, therefore, imprudently put a lid on any disclosures. Had Professor Davis been advised of Terry's symptoms and work in a chemical storeroom, he would have strongly suspected chronic mercury poisoning.

Mercury, first mentioned by Aristotle, is unique among the heavy metals in that it is a silvery liquid at room temperature; hence, the common designation of "quicksilver." It evaporates slowly, producing toxic vapors in the breathing atmosphere with no warning properties. The liquid metal and the vapors, to a lesser extent, can also be absorbed through the skin so that someone handling mercury at close range is at double jeopardy of exposure. It was also found to be easily recovered by simple heat retorting of cinnabar, its principal ore source, which chemically is mercuric sulfide (HgS). The ancient Romans had learned that mercury can readily alloy with gold at room temperatures, and by the fifteenth century, it was found that this amalgamation also worked for silver and many other metals such as copper and tin. It soon became extremely useful in extracting these valuable metals from their ores, or for their purification. An amalgam with tin is used to deposit the reflective silver coating on a clear glass plate that creates a mirror. The fascination with the many properties of this "mercurial" metal exists among children who delight in magically transmuting a copper penny into a silvery coin by rubbing it in the liquid.

Unhampered by modern bureaucratic requirements for proof of efficacy and harmlessness, Paracelsus in the sixteenth century (whose contributions to medicine and science have been described by Herbert and Lou Henry Hoover as " . . . the unparalleled egotistical ravings of this half-genius, half-alchemist") prescribed mercury as a chemical therapeutic treatment for syphilis. It is purported that even today some males of certain Mexican and Central American Indian tribes inject globules of the metal into their blood to enhance their mettle. The Romans, at least, were aware that breathing the vapors and dusts from mining, extracting, and handling mercury could cause debilitating illness. Pliny the Elder, a Roman scholar in the first century, reported that workers processing cinnabar to make vermilion, a widely used mercuric red dye and pigment, wore the pervious lining of an animal bladder as a protective breathing mask.

Dentists and their technicians routinely prepare amalgams of silver to fill the cavities in our teeth, sometimes using their unprotected hands to prepare the mixture in poorly ventilated offices. Although the mercury is believed to be largely bound up in the amalgam such that it is essentially inert, low levels of mercury vapor can be detected above the restored teeth and mercury ions may be released from the galvanic action of the other metals present. Thus, it was inevitable that health concerns would be raised both about the ambient exposures to the personnel working in the dental offices and those internally to the patients with the amalgamated fillings. Once when Lazar Davis had a talking moment in the dentist's chair while getting a filling, he asked the dentist if he were concerned about his possible exposure to mercury. The dentist looked askance at the suggestion, claiming that they were very careful in handling mercury and, besides, they had never experienced any ill effects. Davis pointed to the globules of loose mercury which had spilled out on the amalgam mixing table beside him and observed that it was likely that some of the mercury had probably fallen onto the carpeted floor, where it lay hidden under the pile and would be an ongoing exposure source. To prove his supposition and with the dentists's permission, he returned on his follow-up visit with a direct-reading instrument which determines the airborne concentration of mercury based on the strong absorption of ultraviolet light by the mercury vapor. The dentist was obviously unsettled watching the instrument dial sweep up the scale, indicating that mercury vapors were indeed emanating from his carpet. Confirmation of the prediction might have looked like black magic to the dentist, but Davis had had sufficient prior monitoring experience at a large research laboratory to know that invariably portions of the elusive liquid escape Houdini-like from open manometers, broken thermometers, and pressure devices which incorporate mercury as a seal. The fugitive mercury collects unobtrusively in and under floors, in drawers, and in sink traps.

Trying to clean up a spill of the elusive mercury is tricky. It has long been well known among chemists that powdered sulfur sprinkled on and mixed with mercury would form a nonvolatile chemical complex, which could then be harmlessly swept up for disposal, or for recovery. Later, commercial preparations of metal chelating agents, like the versenes used for treating severely lead-poisoned patients, became available to swab a mercury-contaminated area. The ideal tool in large laboratories or workplaces where mercury spills are fairly common is a special vacuum cleaner equipped with a charcoal filter on the air exhaust to capture the mercury vapors. Unfortunately, many dentists, chemists, and other users of small quantities of mercury are not fastidious about the cleanup of their spills or tend to ignore them.

Although exposures that may occur in the dental offices have not been demonstrated to be of sufficient magnitude to elicit any of the classic symptoms of mercury poisoning of the practitioners, that has not stopped controversial speculation that subtle and insidious effects—particularly, on the central nervous system which controls thinking and voluntary movements—may still warrant our concern. The American Dental Association claims that widespread studies have proved that the very low levels from the internal exposures from the amalgam fillings do not cause health problems, but there are several dissenters among their ranks who have stopped using the amalgams and some even recommend their removal. Consequently, some frustrated patients desperate for relief from various undiagnosed ailments have targeted mercury as the cause of their bane and had all their amalgam fillings removed and replaced with permanent but costly gold or silver alloys, or less durable and sometimes troublesome plastic resins.

The fairly common ailments of fatigue, headaches, weight loss, sleeplessness, and headaches which can arise from many causes are often seen in early chronic mercury poisoning, but there are several less common conditions which often develop later and are more distinctive of the illness. First, there are the tremors and indications of possible nerve and muscle damage. Unlike the involuntary and almost continuous movements seen in some neurologically impaired people, there was the slight hand quivering—called an intention tremor—which Terry showed only while trying to perform some voluntary action like the coordination test in the doctor's office. Second, there are psychological and behavioral manifestations, such as a Jekyll to Hyde personality transformation, paranoia, argumentativeness, and irritability. The expression "mad as a hatter" is alleged to refer to the hat makers' mad—meaning "crazy" rather than "angry"—behavior, which in this context could be attributed to their former use of mercury compounds to depilate animal furs to make felt. Third, although Terry was not seen by a dentist during this period, gingivitis, or a diseased condition of the gums, invariably shows up with advanced chronic poisoning and suspiciously so in the absence of any prior gum or dental problems. Another associative symptom which could hardly have gone unnoticed had it developed in Terry would have been excessive salivation, called ptyalism. Finally, mercury taken in the body at excessive levels will be excreted in the urine at concentrations above the normal background level, accumulate at above normal levels in the hair, and will show up in the perspiration.

Urine sampling and, to some extent, analysis of the sweat can serve to establish that an individual has recently been exposed to and absorbed mercury in the body. The cumulative storage of certain other toxic metals in the hair, most notably including arsenic and mercury, has provided forensic experts and historians with a tool for investigating suspected toxic exposures in victims long since expired. Not only is our hair fairly resistant to decomposition but in preference to the collection of teeth and bones, which also serve as long-lived repositories of past exposures, locks of hair from the departed—particularly, of the famous—are made available for evidential purposes. Napoleon, for example, was suspected of being poisoned by arsenic during his exile at Elba and analysis of a hair sample from the great general's head was purported to have been high, which, in turn, spawned a spate of theories about the possible sources and significance of the findings.

Sir Isaac Newton, regarded as one of the supreme mathematical and scientific geniuses of all time, became chronically ill in 1693, complaining of sleeplessness and fatigue with an aversion to eating. During the succeeding three-year period, he inexplicably became reclusive, argued and broke off relations with friends, expressed paranoid thoughts, and reported imaginary conversations. Biographers have variously suggested explanations that depression and fatigue had set in during an intellectual slump following his monumental achievements, or that the dependent bachelor suffered an inordinately lengthy melancholia following his mother's death. Based on indications that during this period Newton was carelessly performing experiments with mercury at elevated temperatures at home, P.E. Spargo and C.A. Pounds hypothesized in a report in the journal *Science* in 1981 that Newton was manifesting classical mercury poisoning. Their analysis of a lock of his hair indicated an abnormally high mercury content of 197 parts per million (ppm) and other elevated toxic metal levels. Although Dr. Leonard J. Goldwater, a respected mercury expert, dissented, claiming that Newton's handwriting should have reflected the characteristic intention tremors to clinch the diagnosis, the implication of poisoning associated with such extremely high mercury in hair levels—assuming validity for the sample and the analysis—is compelling, considering that a normal average mercury value in hair is only 5 ppm. In a case closer in time to Terry Dugan, a family was poisoned when a student spilled 200 grams of filched mercury at home and the mother attempted to clean up the mess with an ordinary vacuum cleaner. All four family members hallucinated, developed tremors, and had mercury levels in their hair ranging from well above normal to a maximum of 17.5 ppm in the son.

By the time Terry was referred to Dr. Harold Berry, the occupational health physician with the labor safety and health group, he no longer was hostile or expressed paranoid suspicions, but he still complained of not feeling right and at times, appeared withdrawn.

Dr. Berry's cluttered and unprepossessing office was appropriately located in a less advantaged area of the city that is euphemistically tagged as a working-class neighborhood by more advantaged people who live and work elsewhere.

"I hear you worked part-time for the chemistry department at college," Dr. Berry began pleasantly in an effort to engage his visitor.

Terry looking sullen, barely nodded.

"Well, can you tell me what you did there?"

"I gave out all the chemicals and equipment."

"You didn't work in the labs? Like helping with the experiments?"

"They wouldn't let me help with the research."

"Did you have any exposure to chemicals? Like from cleaning up spills?"

"I didn't spill anything, but I sometimes cleaned up after anybody who did."

"Terry, did you ever do any experiments with the chemicals yourself?"

"Why do you want to know that?" Terry asked, defensively.

"I heard you were interested in chemistry and I thought you might have been exposed to some chemical."

The young man shook his head and stared at the floor.

"Terry, I'd like to get samples of your blood and urine. I think it might really help us figure out what might be causing your problem."

Unexpectedly, Terry agreed to provide the samples and Dr. Berry sent them to an industrial hygiene laboratory which specialized in the analysis of biological specimens for toxic metals and chemicals. Based on all the symptoms, Dr. Berry strongly suspected that the young man had been exposed to the one uncombined chemical element that is ubiquitous in chemical laboratories and storerooms worldwide.

From 8000 to 10,000 tons of mercury have been used annually worldwide for the past twenty or so years, and concerns about toxicity and pollution notwithstanding, the projections are for continued and possibly greater demand due to industrial expansion. As a weighty measure of distinction, mercury use and production are often uniquely reported in units of "flasks," which represents the 76.5 pounds of mercury that had historically been marketed in an iron bottle. The use of mercury most evident to the average person is probably as the silvery liquid enclosed in the bulb and graduated column of a glass thermometer, which indicates the temperature reading by expanding or contracting in response to the fluctuations of the environmental heat. Aware of the toxicity of mercury, a parent might have understandably panicked if a child accidentally bit off and swallowed the end of an oral thermometer, only to be informed by a poison control center at a hospital, or other knowledgeable source, to feed the kid plenty of bread, mashed potatoes, or other bulky food of his or her preference and report any blood in the child's stool. Since metallic or elemental mercury is insoluble, virtually unabsorbed, and nontoxic when ingested, it is is excreted fairly quickly in the feces. A greater hazard than the mercury toxicity might arise from internal bleeding caused by the sharp edge of a similarly insoluble and nontoxic glass shard caught up in the inner lining of the body in its exit journey; hence, the advice to facilitate a bowel movement with protective bulk. Besides thermometers, liquid mercury is extensively used in laboratories and technical operations in mechanical measuring devices and instrumentation like barometers and manometers to measure pressure or to produce vacuum seals.

One of the major volume uses for mercury today is in batteries, electrical switches, and instruments, which does not present a likely exposure during use but is of considerable concern as an environmental pollutant when they are ultimately disposed of, usually by land burial, as potentially hazardous waste products. The greatest tonnage use for mercury has been in the chemical industry for manufacturing mercury compounds, or mercurials, such as pigments in paints and ceramics, preservatives, germicides, antifouling agents, antimildew compounds, pharmaceuticals and pesticides, and as process catalysts. Its specific use as a catalyst in the electrolytic process for making chlorine and alkali from brine in the chlor-alkali process has been projected to be the greatest single use for mercury. Until pollution-control measures were imposed, large amounts of mercury were routinely discharged in the huge aqueous wastes from these processes, which led to extensive and disastrous pollution problems.

Mercury is also often found *in situ* with fossil-fuel sources, so that the mining and burning of coal and the drilling, refining, and combustion of oils and natural gas annually contribute as much as 5000 tons into the environment.

It may seem contradictory that we are overly concerned about environmental pollution from the release of mercury from anthropogenic sources and uses, which has been estimated to be derived from about 10,000 tons produced worldwide annually, when the contribution from natural sources evaporating from the land, oceans, and rivers has been estimated to be from two and a half to ten times as much, annually. A similar analogy can be made with carbon monoxide, arguably the most commonly produced toxic chemical on the planet, whereby the natural contribution from plant and animal life also readily exceeds what man generates from industry and transportation. Apart from the possibility of being downwind from a forest fire, no human or animal in the woods need worry about getting overcome from the biogenic carbon monoxide. In a reprise of Paracelsus' dictum that it is the amount (i.e., the dose and concentration of the substance) which determines whether it's a poison, carbon monoxide from natural sources is slowly and continuously being released and diluted throughout the entire world, whereas man gregariously tends to huddle in his habitat and produce his pollution locally in concentrated spurts of activity. Furthermore, the carbon monoxide is chemically converted to relatively harmless carbon dioxide by plants as part of the life-supporting cycle of photosynthesis, so that the toxic carbon monoxide never accumulates above barely detectable, let alone toxic, levels. The inorganic mercury from wastes, on the other hand, that might escape into the water table of a residential area from an unsealed land fill or what is dumped into a local river or bay from an industrial process waste always remains as some form of toxic mercury. The effects of mercury pollution at sea is particularly insidious in that the mercury is taken up by microscopic plant and animal organisms known as plankton, which are subsequently ingested by tiny fishes, and then by their successively larger marine diners which progressively concentrates the mercury in the diets and bodies of the marine animals with the largest appetites. The biggest food fishes such as tuna and swordfish which live and eat for a long time might then be expected to store up the mercury to the highest levels for man, the ultimate consumer. Whether that part per million level of accumulation is an actual human health hazard may be debatable, but the potential risk has been sufficient for the EPA, the FDA, and other government watchdogs to propose acceptable levels for human consumption.

The toxic nature of metal compounds varies according to their chemical makeup and properties including, among others, valence, or chemical combining power, solubility, whether the substance is a gas, a liquid, or a solid, and how it is subdivided or mixed, and whether it is an inorganic or organic compound. Thus, changes from one chemical form of mercury to another may have significant effects on the toxicity and route of entry of the mercury compound. For example, mercur*ous* chloride ($HgCl$), known as calomel, had been medicinally used in small amounts as a laxative, but if the same chemical constituency were given in the higher valence form as highly toxic mercur*ic* chloride ($HgCl_2$)—which, atomically speaking, only involves the loss of a single electron—the dose might be the patient's final purge. The organic mercury compounds, in common with the organic forms of other metals, are not only more readily absorbed through the skin than the inorganic compounds but they also often cause distinctive and severe neurotoxic effects.

The tragic consequences resulting from uncontrolled industrial mercury pollution were not immediately apparent when a mysterious debilitating disease was first seen in 1961 among the villagers living near Minimata Bay in Japan. Early symptoms of the victims appeared as numbness and tingling, then in difficulties with their walking, swallowing, speaking, and thinking, and in the extreme cases, tremors, spasticity, coma, and death. Because the human fetus is particularly vulnerable to the uptake of the mercury, their infants seemingly normal at birth later evinced seizures and impaired physical and intellectual development. The waste sludges and effluent discharged into the Minimata bay from a nearby chemical plant manufacturing acetaldehyde were known to contain elemental mercury used as a catalyst in the process. Consequently, mercury pollution was suspected by the public health officials and physicians investigating the cause for a mysterious disease outbreak, but they could not reconcile the apparent symptoms with those associated with metallic or inorganic mercury poisoning. Rather, the symptoms suggested the toxicity of the organic form. Indeed, the mechanism for a biotransformation of inorganic to organic mercury was cleverly deduced to suggest the nexus of causation. The metallic mercury submerged in the sediment of the bay was anaerobically converted by microorganisms in the sediment of the bay, and apparently, also when taken up internally by some fish, into organic methyl mercury. Thus, a concentrating chain of transfer was begun, leading to the fish making up a large portion of the villagers' diet. Other human poisoning cases involving organic mercury products have been more readily identified but no less tragic in consequences. Perhaps the worst epidemic in a series of incidents involving ingestion of organic mercury occurred in 1971–1972 in Iraq when 459 deaths were reported from more than 6500 hospitalized victims who had eaten grains recently treated with methylmercury pesticide.

Terry's symptoms clearly implicated exposure to the inorganic form of mercury, and if the laboratory storeroom and chemical laboratories were the venue, the exposure was most likely to be liquid mercury, simply because more of it, by far, is used and released there through spills and carelessness than any other mercury compound. To help determine whether Terry might be suffering from mercury poisoning incurred at work six months after his last exposure, Dr. Berry knew it would be telling first to demonstrate that there were abnormal levels of mercury in his body. Second, it would be incumbent to establish by an industrial hygiene survey—even after the fact—whether Terry could have been exposed to mercury levels in his work at the university that could cause illness consistent with his symptoms.

Dr. Berry's concern was that although the concentration of mercury found in the urine and blood samples does not necessarily correlate with the extent of the exposure, time is of the essence for confirmation. Since the body tends to excrete some, although not all, of the absorbed mercury, the likelihood of finding a level significantly above the normal background range diminishes with time since exposure. Not unexpectedly, the laboratory now equivocally reported that the mercury level in Terry's urine sample could be interpreted as being ". . . somewhat elevated but at the upper range of normal values for unexposed individuals."

Dr. Berry hit upon a novel way to confirm that Terry might be continuing to express mercury in a way not shown by people with normal background levels. Although mercury is also excreted in the perspiration of exposed people, it rarely shows up in the unexposed. By collecting the perspiration of a heat-stressed subject on a sterile absorbent cotton pad and analyzing for the mercury content with a correction run on a blank sample as a control, it might be possible to confirm that Terry was expressing telltale traces of the metal. Dr. Berry was afraid he would have a hard time convincing the young man to come down to his office to undergo the sweat testing without revealing specifically what he was looking for, but Terry willingly appeared. A week or so later when he received the laboratory results indicating that the sweat pad samples were unambiguously positive for mercury, he felt the time was right to raise the question of exposure directly with Terry.

"Terry, did you happen to handle any mercury at the university?" he asked, casually.

"Of course, we kept mercury in the storeroom and everybody used some in the labs. So what?"

"Did you ever help out in the labs using it?"

"They wouldn't let me work in the labs."

"Well, did you ever have to clean up a spill?"

"They broke thermometers sometimes and I might of cleaned it up if it was in the storeroom."

"Do you have any idea where you might have been exposed to lots of mercury, anywhere besides work? At home?"

The sullen young man looked away and said nothing. Dr. Berry could not tell if the body language indicated hostility or hesitancy.

"Okay, Terry, maybe you were exposed and didn't know it. My organization feels the likelihood of a work-related exposure is high. You've heard of OSHA?"

Terry nodded.

"If a worker believes he got sick from work, he can file a complaint to OSHA. Then the government has to investigate. Legally, I guess it's to find out if the employer has been complying with the health and safety regulations and, if not, to get the situation corrected."

"So, you want me to file a complaint?" Terry asked, then thoughtfully added, "Suppose they they find lots of mercury there. Do you think I can sue the bastards?"

"I don't know about that. Right now we have no proof of your exposure, but regardless of where you picked up the mercury, we think it's important to help your body get rid of the mercury."

Terry agreed to undergo treatment to facilitate the naturopathic elimination of the mercury from his body by sweating it out in the steam baths at a Y.M.C.A. gymnasium. He also readily agreed to sign a complaint to OSHA.

Less than a week after OSHA formally received the signed complaint, the university received their notice that a compliance officer from the agency would perform an inspection of their facilities with respect to the specific alleged violation.

Betty Brentano, the twenty-six-year-old compliance officer assigned to the case, had been with OSHA less than two years and already had a reputation for being thorough, smart, somewhat abrasive, and would have been labeled a "feminist" had the term existed then. Dr. Cyrus Walters, the fifty-two-year-old head of the chemistry department, had been on the faculty of the university twenty-six years and was known nationally as an expert in x-ray spectroscopy and, locally on campus, as a no-nonsense administrator to the faculty and a tough marker to his students. In current vogue, Brentano would have dubbed *him* a "sexist." At their opening conference, Dr. Walters virtually preempted his visitor's explanation for her inspection by smugly stating that the limited and controlled uses of mercury in his domain precluded the likelihood of any significant exposures.

"Young lady, our safety committee inspects the labs and storerooms regularly and except for some broken thermometers and an occasional blowout from a manometer, they're never reported any. . . ."

"Maybe so, Dr. Walters, but I'm here to survey the area where the complainant worked, as required by the law," she said, while showing him her credentials.

"Are you a chemist, Miss . . . ?"

"No, sir. I think I had enough chemistry courses at college to be familiar with the labs and chemical storerooms, but I'll need someone representing the university to guide me around. You know the complainant is also entitled to have a representative of his union or employee group accompany me during the survey," she added.

"He didn't belong to any union or employees' group here. So that's not a problem." Dr. Walters answered, adding, "Not a chemist? I'll have my assistant department head, Dr. Brodsky, take you around and answer your questions. I'm sure you'll have many. By the way, how many mercury surveys have you done at universities?"

"This is my first."

"Really? And how many mercury surveys have you done in industry?" he pressed.

"I've done some checks for mercury in a quality control lab, but I guess this is my first complete survey."

Dr. Walters half closed his eyes, smiling ever so faintly.

"I'll give you a full report of my findings in an exit interview, Dr. Walters, when I'm finished and I'll be happy to answer any of *your* questions," she answered.

Dr. Stuart Brodsky, the assistant department head and her guide for the inspection, had arrived and was introduced by Dr. Walters. Brentano very pointedly explained the purpose of her visit and the applicable OSHA standards at issue and then they started the tour and inspection.

Despite her lack of prior experience evaluating mercury exposures in workplaces, Brentano knew exactly where and how to measure for the airborne levels of the metallic mercury vapor once Dr. Brodsky had identified all the places in the department where the mercury was used and stored. If electronic survey instruments can be personified, the mercury detector available at that time was not very sensitive, temperamental, and required an understanding operator for obtaining reasonably reliable results. With some judicious adjustments and interpretation, Brentano was reasonably certain from her readings that all the airborne concentrations were below 0.05 milligrams per cubic meter of air, as an eight-hour time-weighted daily average. She spent the entire morning scrupulously looking for evidence of spills in all the areas of mercury usage and storage, and measuring the ambient atmospheres with particular focus on the levels in the likely breathing zones. There was some indication of mercury vapors above some of the sink drains and some questionable instrument quivers just above the floor joints from some of the lab tops. Brentano questioned several of the graduate assistants and instructors, the storeroom clerk who had replaced Terry, and even one of the janitors about their experiences and observations of spilled mercury. Apart from cleaning up the debris from some broken thermometers and an occasional blowout of mercury from an open-ended manometer, no one could recall any appreciable amounts of fugitive mercury or confirm that Terry had had any particular involvement with it. She also reviewed all the minutes of the safety committee for the past five years and found nothing substantive noted about mercury exposures.

There were always some infractions of the myriad OSHA regulations that any inspector could find at any workplace—a frayed electric cord, an unsecured compressed gas cylinder, a lab technician failing to wear safety glasses—and are often so noted in the inspection report as if to justify the visit. But in the paramount concern, Brentano had to conclude that there was no evidence of any appreciable mercury exposures in the chemistry department that could account for the recent chronic mercury poisoning.

Usually an exit interview in which a federal compliance officer reports that there are no serious infractions, or noncompliances, elicits a noticeable sigh of relief from an employer, similar to a taxpayer being given a clean bill of health by an I.R.S. auditor. Dr. Walters accepted the findings with such aplomb that Brentano felt that their roles had been reversed and it was she and her agency that had been cleared.

"Young lady, our students have been handling toxic materials without incident for years. I presume you observed how very strict we are with them in observing safe laboratory practices and. . . ."

"I'm sure you do a fine job, Dr. Walters, but OSHA is legally responsible for protecting the workers so that. . . ."

"Not interested in our safety program? Sounds like a typical bureaucratic response," Dr. Walters riposted.

She smiled and wisely bit her lip.

"Will you send me a statement indicating that we have had no mercury problem here?" Dr. Walters asked.

"An official of the university will have to request that in writing to the director of my office for a decision, sir," Brentano answered bureaucratically, and when Dr. Walters coldly indicated that he had no further questions, she left.

The findings and conclusion of the OSHA inspection may have exonerated the university, but they were baffling to Dr. Berry and his associates at the labor safety and health organization. They had been convinced that Terry had frank chronic mercury poisoning—presumably from exposures at work. If neither the inspection nor the observations from Terry's close co-workers and faculty could uncover significant mercury exposures in the chemistry department, where else then might the young man have possibly been exposed?

No longer appearing angry or acting irrationally, Terry now insisted that he had been poisoned by mercury when he had had to clean up "all those broken thermometers at school." Claiming that his symptoms rendered him incapacitated to work, he testified in hearings before government agencies proposing regulations for the emerging "right-to-know" regulations to protect the worker and the public from toxic and hazardous chemicals. He became a cause célèbre for the labor health and safety group when a newspaper article highlighted the mystifying circumstances of his alleged occupational illness. He described his symptoms using the terminology of medical references such as "loss of motor skills, severe memory loss, full body tremors, degenerative gum disease, full or partial paralysis and heavy chest pains," and having incurred permanent heart, brain, and nerve damage; he claimed that he suffered from severe mental anguish and physical pain.

Distraught at the prospect that her son might be permanently incapacitated, Mrs. Dugan became his relentless advocate in a legal suit claiming toxic tort damages from the suppliers of the mercury. It was rumored that a large settlement had been made, notwithstanding a failure to unearth the source for his exposure.

Few members of the faculty, staff, or administration at the university were aware of the Terry Dugan incident until the newspaper article appeared and even that, coming as it did at the time of a threatened strike by the physical plant workers, was given only passing discussion. At the table in the faculty dining room where the presumably more knowledgeable and interested members of the chemistry department regularly congregated, Dr. Stuart Brodsky, who had accompanied Brentano during the inspection, was asked his opinion of the former student's claim.

"We really didn't see much mercury around and nobody ever saw him cleaning up any spills or fooling around with it," he answered, carefully.

"We've all been working around mercury at one time or another and nobody ever got poisoned by it," one of the professors asserted.

"I heard this Dugan kid had his health problems before he ever came to work. The boss suspects he was just setting us up," an instructor added.

"I don't know," Dr. Brodsky said, adding reflectively, "they say it's very unusual to have mercury in your perspiration, so it had to come from somewhere, right?"

Most of the group nodded, but curiously not one of the scientists at the table seemed sufficiently informed or interested to offer a possible explanation, and the conversation turned to more practical considerations of how they would cope with a breakdown in the utilities for the laboratories if the physical plant workers carried out their strike threat.

At the opposite end of the dining room, Lazar Davis was having lunch with Dr. Jack Miller from the civil engineering department, who shared his distaste for the frequent discussions of campus politics at the larger tables, so they often chose a table for two. Miller had just read the newspaper article and thoughtfully posed a similar question to his friend as that logically raised by Dr. Brodsky.

"If that student has a confirmed case of mercury poisoning, where else could he have been exposed if not here?"

"I only know what I read in the papers," Davis quipped.

"When has that ever stopped you from offering an opinion?"

"Of course I thought about it and I have a possible explanation," Davis admitted. "When I worked at the oil company, the security guards would to do random inspections of the workers' lunch pails whenever too many hand tools started disappearing. They caught this guy filching a flask of mercury. There's not a big market for the resale of mercury, so what do you think was his reason?"

"He brought it home for his kid to play with?" Miller suggested, only half in jest.

"Not far off, but it was the kid in him. You know there has always been some kind of mystique about mercury to some people. The worker was intrigued with the stuff and claimed he wanted to experiment with it making some jewelry, or whatever."

"So you're suggesting that this Dugan kid was also pilfering mercury for home entertainment?"

"Getting to the bottom of this, I heard he had a basement lab at home. He could have been working with it close to the heater. There's probably no ventilation there. I would certainly have investigated it."

"Whatever gave you that idea?" Miller asked.

"When I was a kid I loved to fool around with mercury in what we called the cellar. I've been thinking about that recently."

Case 11

The Plastic Maker's Infirmity

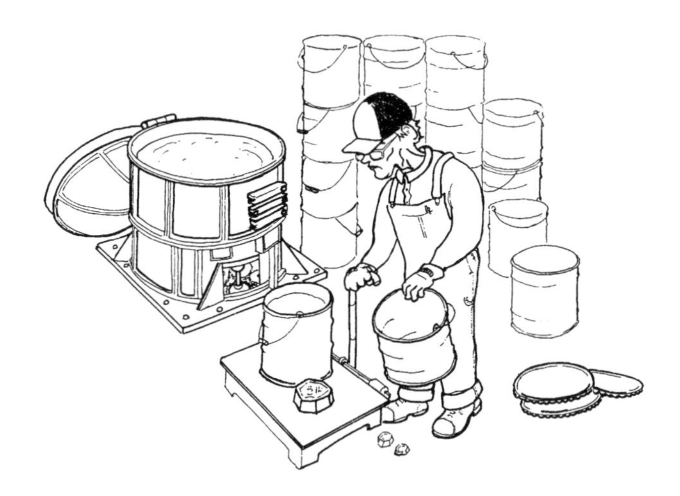

Lazar Davis had no clues what chemical exposures at the Superior Technology Company plant could possibly have caused the claimant to be permanently and physically disabled. The work force there simply assembled and installed the components of various electronic instruments inside the instrument case. Apart from occasional repair soldering with a nonleaded compound and very small quantities of acids and solvents used for cleaning, they did not even have any industrial chemicals on site. But Davis had learned from premature accounts of other unlikely cases of work-related illnesses, in accord with Yogi Berra's admonition, there's no early call on the game.

His initial skepticism was reinforced, but for different reasons, when Jim Crane, the employer's insurance agent, called to explain the nature of the alleged chemical exposure.

"They use all different kinds of plastic gaskets in their assembly work, so they set up their own custom-making unit to stamp out the exact forms they need. Roger Bean—that's the guy claiming the disability—worked all alone making the plastic sheets."

"What kind of plastic, Jim?"

"It's PVC. That's polyvinyl chloride, right?"

"Right, but there's no chemical exposure with the polymer. PVC is virtually inert."

"Maybe so, Lazar, but Bean's doctor said the cause of the disability was exposure to vinyl chloride."

The doctor's association of life-threatening damage with vinyl chloride *gas* exposure was reasonable, but his knowledge of the chemistry and hazards of polyvinyl chloride was flawed or, at least, outdated. Davis hesitated about giving the technical explanation to Jim that PVC *poly*mers are complex compounds made up of thousands of the same simple molecule called *mono*mers linked together in long chains. The monomer making up the polymer, vinyl chloride, is a highly reactive chemical both with itself and sometimes adversely with vital human organs. Once formed as a polymer, PVC is essentially stable and unreactive and does not break down readily to form toxic materials, including the vinyl chloride monomer.

"From what I know about finished PVC, I can't see how the man could have been exposed to VC gas. Something else there may be causing the man's problem but. . . ."

"Okay, Lazar, but we'd like you to evaluate the situation there. In over twenty years of operation there, the company has never had any serious worker health problems. They're running scared."

Recognizing and evaluating the hazards of working with vinyl chloride depended on when the question was raised. During the 1950s, if you worked in a plastics plant synthesizing or forming PVC from the highly flammable vinyl chloride (VC) gas, you were told that the main workplace hazard could arise if the VC vapor level approached the lower explosive limit of about 40,000 ppm or 4 percent by volume in air. At that enormously high concentration, a spark from an electric tool or from static electricity could easily set off an explosion and fire. Human toxic effects were not then regarded as significant, so the earliest workplace exposure standards in the United States in 1945 recommended a value for VC as high as 1000 ppm, indicating more concern for inducing sleepiness in workers from its narcotic effect than from any observed damage to a vital organ. In fact, VC was regarded as so innocuous to human health that there were even suggestions from anesthesiologists that it might be appropriate for use in the operating room. Even when the daily occupational exposure limit was lowered to 500 ppm, and then lower, the plastics industry was able to comply and it was assumed that any risk to the workers' health was virtually nil.

Understandably, the industry was shocked by successive reports in the early 1970s of the deaths of PVC manufacturing workers from a very rare mixed tumor in the liver called angiosarcoma. OSHA issued a temporary emergency standard immediately limiting the daily average exposure limit to 50 ppm. When the same type of tumors were produced by animal studies in mice and rats exposed to VC, industry had reason to panic. OSHA responded to the confirmatory animal results shortly thereafter with a permanent standard of only 1 ppm. A jeremiad from industry protested that compliance with such a restrictive limit was unattainable and would effectively shut them down. Their fears could be appreciated, since the process of making the PVC polymer from VC monomer always resulted in an excess of unreacted VC, which as a gas readily escapes from the reactor and the finished resin. Even minuscule leaks of VC gas would quickly produce workroom air concentrations well in excess of the daily average eight-hour limit of 1 ppm and only 5 ppm for any fifteen-minute period.

With hindsight, it may seem that industry protested too much and the government overprotected. The polymerization reaction was optimally controlled by the manufacturers to minimize the excess VC gas in the finished PVC powder. By also applying well-established control technology to contain the release of the VC gas from the reactors, industry painlessly achieved compliance with the 1 ppm workplace limit in a remarkably short time. On the other hand, when the occupational cancer deaths attributed to VC were examined, it appeared that the only afflicted workers were those whose activities had involved excessively high exposures of several hundred parts per million or more, such as the tank cleaners of the reaction vessels *and* who had had an average exposure period of about twenty years. Because actual VC exposure levels had already been on a downward trend since the initial cases were reported, angiosarcoma and other serious health effects associated with occupation exposure to VC have virtually disappeared.

When Lazar Davis, by chance, met Roger Bean in the office, just before starting his investigation of working conditions and exposures at the Superior Technology plant, he felt that he might have been mistakenly introduced to a pensioner returning for a nostalgic visit with his former co-workers. This asthenic, hunched, and sallow man was shaking slightly and required a cane to walk. Davis had been told that Bean was forty-four years old.

George King, the plant foreman, led Davis to the one-man PVC forming operation where Bean had worked for the past several years in a small room adjoining, but totally separate from, the main instrument assembly area. A young man in his twenties and apparently Bean's successor at the operation was cleaning out equipment with an air blower when they entered the area. Clouds of dust rose like miniature tornadoes where the airstream from the blower impacted the layers of dust which had settled throughout the area.

"Yes," King agreed with Davis, "all that weighing out and mixing of powders makes it pretty dusty here."

He reached for an opened drum of one of the additives and grabbed a handful of the powder just to show Davis how fine the dust was. When he allowed the raised mass of powder to fall back into the container, a very fine cloud erupted like a puff of smoke which very slowly and gracefully dispersed. The individual dust particles were actually less than six microns in diameter, or below our visual detection limit of about forty microns, and only because some of the particles are clumped into larger masses are we able to see the suspended material.

Davis recognized a ball mill which is used to mix the uncompounded PVC powder thoroughly with various powdered additives, principally stabilizers to prevent degradation, and plasticizers and lubricants. He watched while the worker added the entire contents of several one-hundred-pound bags of the uncompounded PVC powder into the steel ball mill. Like a cook following a recipe, the worker checked off the entries on a formula sheet and carefully measured out on a small balance the much smaller quantities of additives required. When all the materials were added and enclosed within the mill, a roar erupted within the small room from the rotating steel balls when the worker activated the mixer with a preset timer. King motioned to Davis to escape the din outside for the several minutes it took to homogenize the mixture.

They reentered the room as the worker was transferring the mixture to the enclosed heating unit in which it was fused into a plastic mass after about twenty minutes. This material was introduced between critically separated heated rollers—a process called calendering—where it was form into a sheet with subsequent cooling.

In preparation for his visit, Davis had read several review articles on the industrial hygiene aspects of compounding and forming the finished PVC and none of the experts noted any special hazards of toxic exposures but did mention possible pulmonary irritation from the plastic dust. Although the young worker was not wearing a dust mask—or any special protective equipment apart from safety glasses—the mask would have served primarily to prevent the subjective effects of a nuisance dust. Otherwise, Davis could not identify any exposure at the operation which could be reasonably implicated in Bean's illness.

As a routing matter and for completeness of his evaluation, he asked King if he could provide him with some background information including a list of the materials and amounts used to make up a PVC batch and the Material Safety Data Sheets (MSDS) from the suppliers, detailing what was in the additives and their properties.

"I guess I can get you that information back in the office, sir," King answered, "but I'm sorry I can't tell you too much about this plastic-making operation. This was Roger's thing, you know, and the rest of us just didn't. . . ."

"That's okay, Mr. King. I'll appreciate whatever you can get."

"I'll have to get all that stuff out of files," King apologized, "but I'll be sure to get you copies of everything by next week."

Davis called Jim Crane at the insurance office that afternoon to report his preliminary findings that he found nothing there to account for Bean's disability, but he needed to review the additional material on the additives that he had requested from the company before sending in a report. When the information containing the MSDSs on the additives arrived the following week, as promised, he was startled to learn that the stabilizer additives, which amounted to as much as

6 percent of the total product, were largely *lead* compounds such as dibasic lead phthalate, carbonates, chlorosilicates, and silicate sulfates. Amazingly, nobody at the plant had ever said anything to him about lead compounds being used in the process, or recognized that its use even as a minor additive in an isolated process in the plant was hazardous. For Davis, it was the immediate and obvious suspect to account for Bean's infirmity.

It did not take long to get biochemical confirmation from Bean's blood level that he had been chronically poisoned from overexposure at work to the finely divided lead stabilizer dusts which he had been handling almost daily for the past five years. Bean was, indeed, permanently and totally disabled from a classical occupational disease that was oddly not even under suspicion at any time during his exposure. He was the first and only case of severe lead poisoning that Davis had personally seen.

This tragic anomaly may be better understood given the prescient observations of Dr. Robert A. Kehoe written in the early 1960s on the direction of occupational lead poisoning. Despite great progress in reducing *serious* occupational lead poisoning due to greater awareness in industry of the hazards, Kehoe expected a gradual increase in cases from innovative industrial uses for lead, particularly in workplaces with no prior experience with its hazards. The observation attributed to George Santayana that those failing to learn from reading history are doomed to repeat their mistakes is no less true with occupational diseases.

At least, that's what the case of Roger Bean's lead poisoning seems to say.

Case 12

The Workers' Right to Know

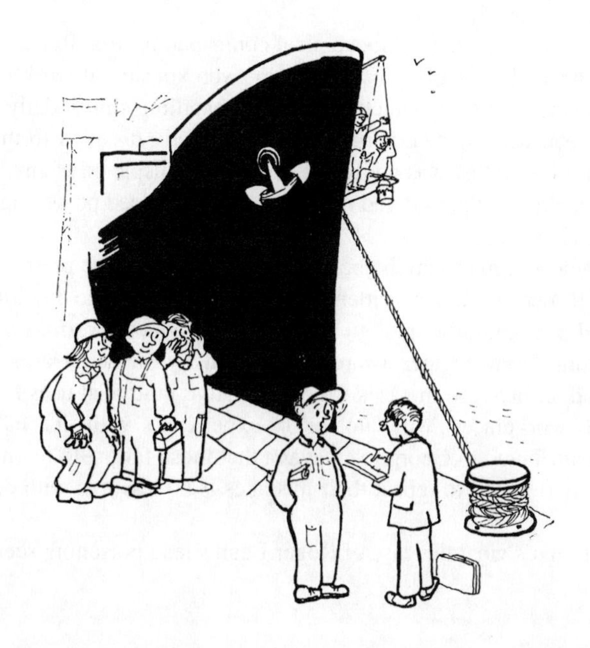

In over twenty-five years of industrial hygiene experience in industry and government where lead metal and its products were used, Professor Lazar Davis had encountered only one occupational lead poisoning case and with reason. The industrial hygiene control measures and medical surveillance for preventing excessive employee exposures were well established and effective. If properly implemented and enforced, as they were in his experiences, it was arguable that lead poisoning from work was totally preventable.

As a young analytical chemist working at a government shipyard laboratory, Davis was responsible for performing the routine but tedious colorimetric analyses of the painters' urine for the excreted lead as an index of their exposure from applying and removing lead-containing paints. Lead serves no biological use, so the body tends to get rid of it, but a minute residual amount normally remains in the body without apparent adverse effect at an equilibrium level between what goes in and what gets excreted—in effect, a "background" body burden of lead. The input is derived from the small amounts of lead in our daily food and water intake from natural sources (i.e. lead in the soils) as well as from man-made sources from food processing and containers; for example, lead solder had been widely used to seal canned foods. It has been suggested that when the lead intake exceeds the amount normally excreted, the lead is then biologically available to cause toxic effects.

Although most of the shipyard painters' urine results were only slightly higher than what you might find in controls from nonoccupationally exposed people, Davis was mystified why George Kinderman—Davis actually got to know his subjects—invariably had lead levels at least two or three times higher than his peers. The men all did essentially the same work in the same area with the same paints, and when Davis stopped by the painters shop before lunch one day to ask the foreman if there was anything different about George's work, he got a quizzical stare. When the painters returned to eat and heard that George was running higher urine values, they erupted in uncontrollable laughter in a game of sophomoric taunts having to do with "getting the lead out" of George. With open season on George, the men continued with more giddy cracks when George ate his daily lunch of those smelly Portuguese sardines. Davis later was to learn that lead solder was still used particularly in the imported sardine cans and was the probable source of George's elevated values.

Rarely, if one of the painters' urinary levels was particularly high, Davis might be requested by the shipyard doctor to analyze the worker's blood as a more reliable measure of the lead burden in the body. The laboratory measurement of lead in blood then required an all-day and fetid procedure of decomposing the samples by boiling with acids to dryness over a hot plate under a laboratory hood. Because of the trace amounts of lead being measured, all the glassware, chemical reagents, and distilled water had to be scrupulously free of lead contamination and the analysis was performed in an isolated lead-free laboratory. Aware of the government laboratory's expertise analyzing biological samples for lead, a local hospital had urgently requested analysis of a blood sample, which was delivered to Davis. The dependency on lengthy wet chemical methods has long since been obviated by the advances in instrumentation. All analytical and most hospital clinical laboratories have their own atomic absorption instruments which accurately and directly measure lead and other metals in biological samples without the messy preparations and handling.

Davis had never seen such a high result as that in the exogenous blood sample. He assumed he had made an error or the sample was contaminated until he learned that the blood was drawn from a colicky inner-city toddler who had been nibbling away for many weeks at the peeling lead-containing paint from the woodwork in an old house. This inexplicable and highly injurious craving of children and others to ingest nonfood substances has been termed "pica," the Latin word for magpie, presumably for the bird's nondiscriminating eating habits. The lead pigments in the dried paint chips are not water soluble, but the lead, which often comprises more than half of the total weight, is dissolved out by the hydrochloric acid in the stomach and absorbed through the intestinal wall into the blood which will distribute it throughout the body. Low levels of lead may be in household dust and garden soils contaminated with the accumulated deposits of automotive and industrial emissions of lead, so that the hand-in-mouth habits of young kids further contributes to their lead intake. Although low-level lead poisoning of children does not often cause symptoms initially, several studies suggest subtle and adverse effects on normal growth, hearing acuity, and possibly, a decrement in cognitive skills. With repeated and higher dosages of lead, the child may become irritable or show signs of gastrointestinal pains and, continued unabated, may result in anemia, kidney damage, irreversible cerebral impairment, and death.

The lead which does not get taken up by the soft tissues in the body and is not immediately excreted can be inertly stored in the bones as a villainous substitute for the essential calcium. This is particularly damaging to growing and poorly nourished children because even if the child stopped ingesting the leaded paint, the banked lead gradually leaches out into the blood to exacerbate the toxic effects. Many pediatricians and health researchers believe that young children are so sensitive to lead that subtle and damaging effects can result at blood lead levels in excess of only ten micrograms per deciliter, a value which has long been considered to be within normal background range of asymptomatic urban adults. There are indications that the developing fetus may also be particularly sensitive to very low levels of lead; thus, the mother's lead intake during the pregnancy period should be kept even lower than the normally recommended limits for adults. With estimates that over half of the housing in the United States has leaded paints and many drinking water supplies contaminated from lead-containing household plumbing exceeding the U.S. Public Health Service recommended limit of fifteen parts per billion (ppb), lead poisoning has become a national public health concern.

A nonoccupational case some years later involved a not uncommon expo-

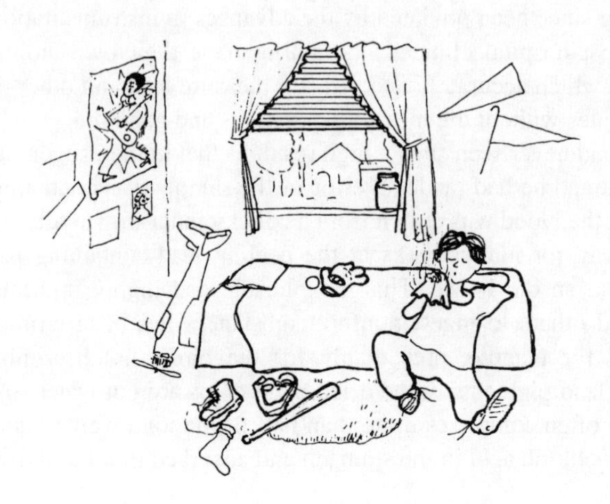

sure to a lead-containing product but with an unexpected and rather bizarre consequence. Having been referred to an oil company industrial hygienist purported to be knowledgeable in the health effects of petroleum products, an inquiring physician had momentarily disarmed Davis.

"Can you develop lead poisoning after getting high from sniffing gasoline?" the doctor wanted to know.

Davis was momentarily tempted to ask jocularly whether the patient was using high test or regular gasoline.

"No, doctor," a composed Davis politely answered. "All the studies have indicated that inhaling leaded gasoline doesn't cause. . . ."

The doctor's association of lead exposure with gasoline was understandable to Davis, but lead exposure by inhalation of gasoline vapors had not been shown to be significant by measurement of blood lead levels in workers exposed in gasoline manufacturing or with gasoline station attendants. There was far greater public health concern then for the increasing airborne lead concentrations that had resulted from the enormous daily emissions from automotive traffic burning leaded fuels.

About three to four milliliters of organic lead liquid compounds, equivalent on average to one gram of lead per liter, had been regularly added to gasoline to increase the octane rating of the fuel and prevent the engine "knock" from uneven combustion. When burned, these lead alkyl compounds—mainly, tetraethyl lead (TEL) and tetramethyl lead (TML)—are converted to inorganic lead particulates which are largely discharged into the atmosphere with the exhaust gases. Because lead aerosols had been regarded as major air pollutant and were designated as a national ambient air quality standard under the amended Clean Air Act, the U.S. Environmental Protection agency required the gradual phaseout of alkyl leads in gasoline beginning in 1975.

The pure alkyl lead compounds are extremely potent neurotoxins to man and, as highly volatile organic liquids, they can deliver their toxic effects by both the inhalation of the vapors and by permeation of the liquid through the skin. Direct and unattended skin contact with the concentrated liquids can rapidly cause disorientation, hallucinations, and psychiatriclike manifestations erupting into violent convulsions, maniacal behavior, coma, and death. When leaded gasolines have been stored for long in the same vessel, organic sludges often collect in the tank bottoms and eventually have to be manually cleaned out. Because the lead alkyl compounds are often concentrated in the sludge, the tank cleaner has to be totally protected against all contact with the sludge and the vapors. During the 1960s, a gasoline tank cleaner in Greece, despite wearing respiratory protection inside the tank, died from acute organic lead poisoning while wearing permeable cotton work clothes and gloves heavily soiled with the leaded sludge.

However, handling commercial gasolines at typically low concentrations of less than 0.1 percent lead alkyls has been shown to produce little skin absorption or inhalation of the lead. To be sure, handling leaded gasolines presents real fire and explosion hazards and possible dizziness and headaches from excessive inhalation of the vapors but not a lead toxicity problem.

The conventional wisdom notwithstanding, the doctor's response had a sobering effect.

"I have a teenaged patient who's been sniffing the stuff for several weeks. His blood lead level is slightly elevated, but his urinary lead is almost 100 micrograms."

"Hm. That's very interesting," Davis mumbled, stumped for an explanation.

Getting a "high," or feeling euphoric from the acute inhalation of organic solvents like gasoline, was a fairly well-known experience among some adolescents, principally male. Some painters or employees using organic solvents have been known to seek escape similarly from their tedium at work. Occasionally, a surreptitious teenaged sniffer may become addicted to the faster-acting and less irritating vapors of toluene in a bottle of hobby glue, long-term dosing of which can result in severe but reversible kidney and liver injury.

"How and . . . where was he doing it?" Davis finally asked. "Gasoline is such a giveaway, I wonder how he got away with it in the house."

"He kept a pint-sized mayonnaise jar stuffed with cotton gauze on his bedroom window sill. He would just sniff the soaked cotton by the window until he got high."

"How long was this going on?"

"Maybe a couple of weeks. It stopped when his Dad thought there was a gas leak in the house. He traced it to the bedroom when the kid forgot to close the window."

"Does he have any other signs of lead intoxication, doctor?"

"Not really. He seems like your ordinary lethargic teenager, so it's hard to tell."

Davis meekly offered to think about it and call the doctor back. The patient was healthy otherwise and seemed to have no complications. The doctor admitted he was more intrigued by the reason for the elevated urinary lead than the prognosis, since the sniffing had been snuffed.

When Davis reflected a little more about the routes of entry for the lead from the gasoline, he realized that the teenager had been repeatedly holding a wetted cloth in his hands for several minutes, day after day, and that his skin had probably remained wet with gasoline until it evaporated. But the jar containing the gasoline had been practically open to the atmosphere on the window sill and was significantly reduced in volume by the evaporation of the more volatile gasoline components. The lead alkyl compounds are less volatile than the ordinary gasoline hydrocarbons, and would tend to be concentrated, as they are in gasoline tank sludges. Skin absorption from the fortified lead in this gasoline was then not only possible but likely.

Davis never heard any other concerns raised about lead poisoning from inhaling gasoline vapors thereafter. By eliminating lead alkyl from most gasolines, the EPA had made that question moot. A metal-free organic liquid, methyl tertiary-butyl ether (MTBE), has largely replaced the lead alkyls as the octane booster in gasoline. Whether MTBE enhances or lowers the euphoric effects of sniffing gasoline has not been raised yet.

Many years later, these earlier tangential experiences had not conditioned the then Professor Davis to expect a telephone request for his help with serious occupational lead poisonings at a time when the classic disease was assumed to be well understood and under control. He could only identify the final surname in the secretary's crescendo announcing the roster of law partners of the firm but that wasn't his caller. She said, simply, "Mr. Roman is ready for you, Professor."

Anthony Roman was forthright.

"Professor, I got your name as an expert in occupational exposures from an associate you helped out once. I'm representing several workers at a metal recovery plant in the city who are probably dying from lead poisoning. We think the defendants never told them that they were being overexposed. Are you interested in helping us with the case?"

Dr. Robert A. Kehoe, one of the foremost experts in occupational lead poisoning, had noted a quarter of a century earlier that the more severe forms of lead poisoning had largely been brought under control and, consequently, there were very few cases of *severe* lead poisoning, let alone deaths. For the rarity alone, Davis might be interested.

"I'll be happy to serve as a consultant for you, but whether I can help with your advocacy in the case depends on. . . ."

"Sure. Sure," Roman interrupted, "I know how you academics hedge, but when you review the records on this one, you won't have any doubts."

"You may be right, Mr. Roman, but I'll need to review the records. A description of the operations, any industrial hygiene survey reports, OSHA inspections, their blood lead values. . . ."

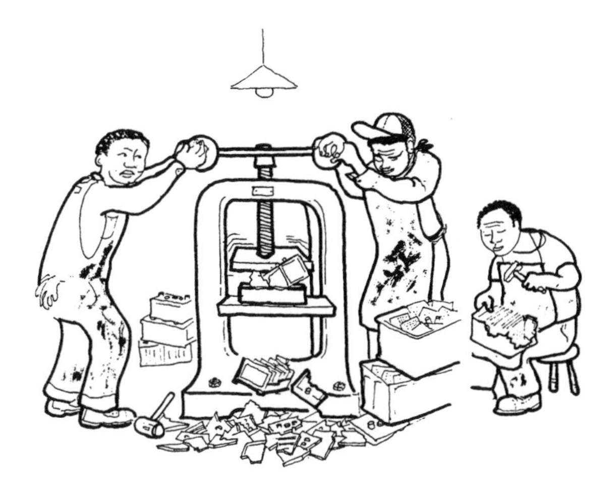

"Of course. We've just started to take depositions and we're waiting for replies from the defendants to our interrogatories. My assistant's Lisa Taylor. She'll send you what you need as soon as we get it assembled. Then you can come in and tell us what you think. And call me Tony."

Davis said that sounded reasonable with the implicit understanding that Roman was free to accept or reject his independent opinion. The following morning a large manila envelope was delivered to his office. He learned that the original lead recovery company and employer of the plaintiffs was founded by Harry Porter, a metallurgical engineer and businessman who ran the operations for five years. Porter then sold the business to Automotive Energy, a major storage battery manufacturing company in the area, which recognized the advantage of owning a subsidiary as a local lead supplier.

The parent company had a part-time medical director who assumed responsibility for the medical surveillance of the lead recovery workers and a health and safety manager, who provided some guidance on employee health and safety. The recovery operation remained a subsidiary under Automotive Energy for twenty years before the business was finally sold to a conglomerate, also engaged in battery manufacture. After only one year, the new owners decided that to meet the air-pollution control requirements of the city and the health and safety requirements of the new OSHA lead standard, operation of the recovery business at that site was no longer cost-effective and within a year the plant was dismantled and the property was vacated and put up for sale.

The surviving five members of the original recovery plant employees, who were eligible for a modest early retirement, were now uniformly in poor or failing health. Because the men had been assured over the years by their employers and company doctor that their occupational exposures were under control, none of them attributed their malaise and disabilities to their work. When one of them was taken to the emergency room of a hospital with evidence of kidney failure, the examining physician reviewing the occupational history suspected of possible complication from lead poisoning. The wives of two of the men were instrumental in getting their reluctant husbands to talk to an attorney.

Davis called Roman's office to confirm that he was willing to serve as their industrial hygiene consultant on the case because it clearly involved occupational lead exposures with probable adverse employee health effects. Several days later, he received another large package containing a copy of the case file. In keeping with personal injury custom, the Roman firm named all the owners past and present as defendants.

From the depositions of some of the former owners and plant foreman, the essential facts of the work histories and exposure of the men to lead and other toxic metals were uncontested. They all agreed the work was dusty and the lead exposures were probably high, but they had been operating that way for years and without serious illness. An inspector from their insurance company performed semiannual workplace surveys and they had implemented recommendations of providing dust masks, personal protective equipment, and even workplace change of clothing and showers for the workers. The limited air-monitoring results of the workplace exposures indicated to Davis that the operations routinely produced airborne concentrations of lead dust that exceeded the then-current recommended exposure limits.

Although blood lead testing was the standard measure of the workers' exposure, no records of the results were provided. In one report, the company medical director equivocally reported that ". . . the blood values were elevated but not excessive for that kind of occupational lead exposures." During this pre-OSHA period, lead poisoning was a required reportable occupational disease in the state, but the diagnosis of condition was a medical judgment; consequently, no reports of cases at the plant had ever been filed.

There were many visits from city agencies dealing with building inspections, licenses and permits, fire prevention, and air pollution, but none dealing with employee health or exposures. In later years, the plant had only been inspected once by OSHA and that was largely in response to an explosion of molten metal which resulted in half a dozen workers requiring treatment for burns at a hospital. With no opportunity to confirm the exposure conditions at a now defunct plant and an incomplete paper trail of unverifiable records, Davis would be hard pressed to provide Roman with a professional opinion that would answer the lawyer's critical questions. Did the management and their medical and safety advisers, largely during a pre-OSHA period, properly evaluate their workers' exposure to lead and act responsibly to prevent harmful injury? To be fair to the value system of the times, you would have to consider to what extent the company could have reasonably been expected to reduce the exposures to safe levels, given the costs involved and their claimed slim profit margin of operation.

As a successful personal injury attorney and senior partner, Anthony Roman had become bored and emotionally uninvolved as the firm point man handling the indistinguishable pedestrian claims of car accident victims for whiplash and back injury. He had leaned of the workers' claim of lead poisoning, variously termed "plumbism" or "saturnism," while having lunch with one of the partners who normally handled workplace injuries and illnesses but who knew nothing about metal poisoning. Seeking a change with a challenge, Roman offered to take on the case. For reasons which his fellow attorneys could not fathom, he became so drawn to the cause of the dying lead workers that the case evolved into an evangelical call for righting an injustice. It was not difficult to commiserate with the five plaintiffs, none of whom had advanced beyond the sixth grade but were hard-working, soft-spoken, and uncommonly polite black men who, having been laid off at textile plant in North Carolina in 1959, sought work in the industrial North.

Roman admitted that his prior knowledge of lead had been limited to his childhood experiences casting toy soldiers with the molten metal. Nevertheless, his penetrating and accusatory interrogation of the past owners and foremen in the depositions impressed Davis. The lawyer had clearly done his homework, having become rapidly conversant with the history of lead, the secondary lead recovery business, and the causes and medical effects of lead poisoning. If a defendant expressed ignorance of the employees' symptoms of chronic lead poisoning, Roman might mockingly point out that Hippocrates had described lead poisoning way back in the fifth century B.C.

Depending on which historian you cite, man began to mine and use this soft, easily melted, heavy, and highly toxic metal to make art work and useful objects over five thousand years ago in Asia Minor. Galena, or lead sulfide, is the principal ore processed from over 200 lead-containing minerals, many of which contain valuable amounts of other metals, including copper, gold, silver, and platinum. When the Romans in the second century B.C. extended the use of the metal into their plumbing and in food containers and utensils, the potential for toxic absorption of lead was tremendously increased. (Note: Plumbum is the Latin name and derivation for its chemical symbol, Pb.) One can fancifully speculate on the contribution of endemic lead poisoning to the decline and fall of Rome from daily binges with acidic Italian reds stored and drunk in leaded vessels.

Today, about six million metric tons are used annually worldwide, 60 percent of which is provided by the primary smelting of the ore and the balance from recovered scrap. The primary smelting treatment commonly consists of roasting the crushed galena ore in air to convert the sulfide to lead oxide, which is then reduced with coke in a blast furnace to form molten lead, the by-product metals, and lots of slag. It is a hot, dusty, and dirty process and it might be anticipated that the smelter workers would be at high risk of lead intoxication. The availability of lead, or indeed any compound, to exert its toxic effects is dependent to a large degree on its solubility in the body. Since the coarse smelting dusts of lead sulfide, oxides, and the pure metal are virtually insoluble in water and dissolve only in strong acids and alkalies, the primary smelter workers are generally at lower risk of developing severe lead poisoning.

Long before the environment-conscious program to recycle plastics, paper, glass, and aluminum cans, the recovery or "secondary smelting" of lead from used lead products and scrap as at the original recovery plant has always provided a significant portion of the lead used in the manufacture of storage batteries. It would appear that the work exposures and hazards here should mirror those at the primary smelting of the ore when, in fact, there are notable differences. The breakup of scrap and used materials for meltdown and recovery is not only considerably dustier than from the raw ores but the dust produced is much finer and, therefore, more readily inhaled, ingested, and absorbed by the workers. Pound for pound, the small-diameter scrap dust not only creates a much larger surface area for absorption and solubility than that of the coarse ore dust but some of the lead in the manufactured scrap has been converted to water-soluble lead compounds. Furthermore, the scrap dust likely involves concurrent exposure to other highly toxic components, namely, cadmium and arsenic, which have been overshadowed by the primary focus on lead.

Of the approximately 1.3 million metric tons of lead consumed annually in the United States, its use in the manufacture of storage batteries accounts for over 80 percent of the total. Far behind, the second major current use, which has supplanted the moribund lead alkyl industry, is in ammunition, followed by paints, glass, ceramics, and chemicals. Much lesser quantities are used in cable covering, sheet lead, solder, casting metals, pipes, brass, and bronze and other alloys. The miscellany of lead in domestic and imported products includes the foil around the cork of the champagne bottle, the crystal glass decanter storing the brandy, fishing sinkers and plumb bobs, some purportedly "nontoxic" crayons and toys, pesticides applied on imported fruit, and the darkening agent in hair lotions and creams used to hide the tattle-tale grey of maturity. Almost perversely, the worst recent industrial exposures to lead have not involved the manufacture or current use of any of these products; rather, the removal by abrasive blasting of lead-bearing paints and ongoing repair and repainting at bridges has produced worker exposures of several hundred times the allowable OSHA limits and multimillion dollar fines.

Two weeks later after having reviewed the case file and a library search of the pertinent references, Davis arranged to meet with Roman alone at his center city office. The cheery dark-eyed receptionist greeted him by name, said Mr. Roman would be with him shortly, and, in a first time ever at a law office, offered him a cup of espresso while he waited. Roman, dressed in the conservative navy blue pinstripe of his profession, took Davis completely off guard by the fervor and directness of his approach.

"Don't you think those bastards knew their men were being poisoned and never told them?"

"I don't know if I can say that," Davis demurred, adding, "But, if you mean the airborne lead level were excessive and they didn't. . . ."

Roman reached for an overstuffed manila folder, which he thrust at Davis.

"There's more to the story. We just got hold of twenty years of blood test results at Automotive Energy stashed away in the old company doctor's office. They were ready to be chucked out when they got our discovery request for disclosure. Read it and I'll be back in a couple of minutes."

Dr. Wallace Cannon, the retired former medical director of Automotive Energy, was considered to be an expert in occupational lead poisoning although he had never published in the literature or had any academic appointment at a medical school. Davis recalled occasionally seeing him at joint local meetings of their respective professional societies, but they had never met. It was rumored that Cannon had been a neighborhood general practitioner when, at a businessmen's luncheon, the plant manager of the local battery plant asked him if he would be interested in serving as their medical examiner and advisor. At a time when few physicians were interested in working in industry and fewer had any professional training in occupational medicine or industrial hygiene, Cannon accepted the offer and flourished in his newfound specialty and work. Sociable and avuncular, he relished his unchallenged status as the medical expert with the corporate executives and the protector of the lowly plant workers' health.

It did not take long for Davis to scan the blood test results and get a sense of the workers' exposure histories. For many years before OSHA and the existence of an occupational lead standard, a level of 80 micrograms of lead per 100 grams of whole blood was considered to be an upper acceptable limit. Although the recovery workers' peak values considerably exceeded 100 micrograms, the *average* values in the individual records ranged between 60 and 80 micrograms. The high points were followed by somewhat sharp drops to the lower levels, increasing and retreating gradually in an undulating fashion. Now under OSHA, lead workers would have to be removed from further exposure and not allowed to return to the lead activity until their blood levels fall below forty micrograms, Davis knew that, judged historically, the results might have been viewed then by some as less health threatening. Roman was less accepting of that discretionary view.

"Now, don't you think the doctors and owners knew those poor guys were being overexposed?" he challenged Davis.

"Looking at the results today, they were probably overexposed, but I can't say that they knew *then*."

Roman was clearly irritated that Davis was not willing to accept his assumption.

"Okay, if that's what you believe, that's what you believe. Meanwhile, I've scheduled the retired company doctor for deposition next week, so I'll need some education from you now."

They withdrew to the conference room joined by Roman's young assistant, Lisa Taylor, a young woman recently graduated from law school who had worked for EPA for two years and was now clerking at the firm until she passed the bar examination. Drew dominated the questioning while occasionally glancing at Lisa to confirm that the point he made had been recorded in her notes. The free-wheeling session lasted for over an hour and Davis, usually unflappable and relaxed in consultations with attorneys, felt at times as if he had mistakenly ended up in the opposing lawyers quarters. It was all perfectly clear to Roman that the defendants knew exactly what they were doing and was irked whenever Davis qualified *his* interpretation of the facts and just could not understand Davis's refusal to ascribe purposeful deception to them.

"Oh, by the way. Here's a deposition from one of the workers," he said matter-of-factly, handing Davis a folder when his questioning ended.

He barely nodded good-bye and left hurriedly, asking Lisa to see their visitor out. Davis chatted awkwardly with Lisa about her experiences with the EPA and learned, not too surprisingly, that she had worked with one of his former students. The quasi-contentious meeting with Roman had left him with unsettled discomfort in the role of a hired professional witness. There should be a better system to present scientific evidence and opinions in a court free from the pressure of advocacy, he reflected, as he headed back to his university office. Still discomfited on his arrival, he placed the unread deposition of the worker in the file labeled "Lead Case" and peacefully withdrew to the academic chore of preparing a mid-term examination.

Two weeks later, when he received the package with Dr. Cannon's deposition, he defensively put it at the bottom of his mail pile, reserving it for a reading on the train ride home that evening. Depositions read like play scripts without stage directions and the not-so-subtle messages from the actors' pauses and raised voices, their sneers, smiles, and poker faces. Sometimes, the opposing attorneys perform a ritualistic play within the play in which they challenge each other's integrity, claim their witness is being badgered, threaten to halt the proceedings to get a ruling from a judge, and, otherwise act like two snarling young toughs in a turf war standoff. At one of his depositions in Los Angeles, virtually ignored and unable to answer any of the questions above the shouts of the lawyers, Davis was certain the two adversaries would square off in mortal combat. When the deposition was finally concluded, Davis was flabbergasted when the two men, like actors casting off their roles on leaving the stage, calmly discussed recent acquisitions to their wine cellars and invited Davis to join them for a drink.

Davis expected that in keeping with a common strategy of treating professional witnesses deferentially rather than alienating them, Roman would tactfully elicit admissions from Dr. Cannon that would later prove to be culpable. Rather, he could hear Roman's inquisitorial voice in the deposition with the now familiar intonations and skepticism and visualize the elderly Dr. Cannon, smiling benevolently, at times, evasive and unfazed by hostile questions.

Q. Doctor, did you review the plant air lead results?

A. I guess I would see them along with a lot of other reports.

Q. Well, sir, would you please look at this document titled Plant Air Sampling Results labeled as Exhibit A? Tell us what they say about the levels of employee exposure to lead.

A. Oh, the exposures are what you would expect at a lead recovery operation.

Q. I see many concentrations of over 200 micrograms per cubic meter of air. Would you say that they were excessive?

A. The hygienists are the folks who can tell us what the dust levels should be. I suppose we would have liked to see them lower.

Q. At that time, wasn't the recommended limit 150 micrograms?

A. Recommended, yes, but the plant engineers said it was the best we could do. That's why we gave the men dust masks, had them change work clothes, and shower. But I can't say that in my medical opinion, the exposures were excessive.

Q. Let me see if I understand you correctly, doctor. These men were breathing in and covered with lead dust every working day, for what? Twenty or more years? And you, sir, state that was not excessive?

A. As I explained. . . .

Q. Well, what about their blood levels? Didn't they tell you the men were overexposed?

A. Their blood levels were elevated as expected with workers exposed to that much lead. But we managed to keep the average value within limits.

Q. You mean under eighty micrograms?

A. Right. Oh, they might jump up a bit from time to time. Then we'd make sure they were doing what they were supposed to. Like, using their masks and taking showers. The values would always come down to the acceptable range.

Q. But you weren't concerned, doctor, that they were getting too much lead in their system?

A. No. I did their physical exams and they didn't have any more problems than you see with any aging plant worker. You know, the usual emphysema, hypertension. They all smoke and don't eat properly.

Q. Did you try to counsel them about their health?

A. They're good workers and nice gentlemen, but they're country boys. Not educated. Oh yes, I did try to get them to drink milk when I read some article. Claimed the calcium helps to rid the body of the lead but it did no good.

Q. You mean they refused?

A. They said that older black folks can't drink milk because they get stomach ache and gas. How's that for an excuse?

Maybe Dr. Cannon could not believe their explanation, but Davis could. He, too, was deficient in lactase, the enzyme which completely breaks down the milk sugar and that is a common genetic problem among people of African descent. The undigested fermenting milk results in excess acid and the production of uncomfortable stomach gas. But that was hardly a factor that would allow him to support Roman's contention of willful intent to harm. The doctor could have been sincere, dumb like a fox, naive, or just plain lying, but a case could be made that for that period Dr. Cannon was following—perhaps less, than more—standard industry practice for lead surveillance. Davis was certainly not privy to the doctor's mind to attribute malice to his action or inaction.

He called Roman's office to give him his preliminary opinion that based on the limited information available, the exposures were probably excessive and that more effective industrial hygiene controls to reduce worker exposures probably could have been instituted. He tactfully deflected any request for an opinion about Dr. Cannon's handling of the workers' blood lead levels by claiming that it was a medical judgment beyond his expertise. Roman listened quietly and said, somewhat icily, "That's what I thought you would say."

"Would you like me to prepare a written report, or . . . ?" Davis asked.

"Not now. I'll call you if I need any more *help*," Roman answered brusquely and hung up.

When Davis place a brief notation about the conversation in the case file, he ashamedly realized that with all the focus on the defendant's depositions, he had neglected to read the only testimony from a plaintiff. Lying there almost apologetically was the unsealed deposition of Albert Johnson, a retired plant worker.

It often seemed to Davis that the first third of many depositions had nothing to do with the case. Mr. Johnson patiently recounted his family necrology, the ages, birthplaces, occupations, and health histories of his parents, his eight siblings, and his four children. Before leaving his native North Carolina at the age of twenty-four, he had worked as a farm laborer and a factory hand from the time he left school in the sixth grade. He described his twenty-six-year work history starting as a laborer at the original lead recovery plant in a cant that frequently required a phonetic transcription of the work processes by the stenotypist. When Johnson was asked to define the arcane processes associated with the scrap handling and smelting, the attorneys would supplement his halting, though understandable, explanations with their own muddled interpretations. Mr. Johnson seemed too polite to contradict or correct them. Davis quickly got to the questions dealing with the workplace exposures and practices, which were carefully phrased by Roman in language uncharacteristically simple and direct for an attorney.

Q. Was your work very dusty and dirty?
A. Yes, sir.
Q. Did the bosses tell you that breathing the lead dust was bad for your health?
A. Sure, we knowed you get sick if you get too much in you.
Q. What did they do to prevent your breathing too much dust?
A. They give us dust masks.
Q. Did they show you how to use them properly?
A. I suppose so. Don't rightly remember.
Q. Well, were you required to wear the dust masks?
A. Maybe we was. Lots of times, they plug up so bad with all that dust, we couldn't breathe. So we just took 'em off.
Q. Did the company do anything else to protect you from the lead?
A. They give us work clothes. Put in showers so we can clean up good.
Q. Did they always provide your work clothes and have showers at work?
A. Oh, no sir. Was just a couple of years fore we shut down.
Q. Were there any exhaust fans inside the buildings to pull out the dust?
A. No, sir. We didn't have no fans like that.
Q. What about medical exams? Did you get regular checkups to see if you were healthy?

A. Sometime we go to his office and he checks us out. Dr. Cannon is a real gentleman. When he see us in the plant, he always ask how we feel.

Q. What was your health like then?

A. Since I live up North it seem like I get lots of colds. I never did feel exactly right.

Q. Did you ever tell him about not feeling good?

A. I tell him sometime my stomach hurt something awful. Don't feel like eating nothing.

Q. Anything else?

A. Once I tell him I feel real tired lots of times. Can't sleep good.

Q. Did you have any sickness that you didn't tell him about?

A. I figure everybody get bad headaches from work. I don't say nothing about that.

Q. Did he give you any advice for your health?

A. Yes, sir, he tell us to eat good food and drink milk.

Q. Did he give you any medicine at work?

A. Yes, sir. He give me something for my bad stomach.

Q. Anything else?

A. Let me see.

Q. Take your time, Mr. Johnson. I see you're getting tired. We'll take a break soon.

A. Yes sir. Sometime every month they give us some big white pills right there at work. I guess they be vitamin pills to make us strong.

Q. Did they tell you the results of your medical examination?

A. No, sir. I suppose if we be real sick, Dr. Cannon tell us.

Q. What about blood tests for lead?

A. Yes. sir. We get them regular.

Q. Did they tell you the results of these tests? Like were they low or too high or just right?

A. We figure they's okay because they never say nothing.

The deposition recorded they took a 15-minute break.

Davis felt that the subsequent questioning of Mr. Johnson contributing an additional forty pages of testimony did not reveal anything that would materially alter his position. He was prepared to give Roman his professional opinion supported by specific examples that the company's program to protect the employees was inadequate given what was commonly known and practiced in the lead industries for that time. The workers' high blood lead levels and the classic symptoms of lead poisoning, which were ignored or minimized, indicated that the company efforts were ineffectual. Beyond that, he and Roman were at an impasse when they later met.

"Can't you see that the defendants damn well knew the workers were being overexposed, Professor? That's willful," he fairly screamed at Davis.

Davis answered firmly, "Even if I could read their minds, I'd be compromising my professional ethics to . . . ."

"Now, that's bull," Roman interrupted, "Don't employers have the responsibility to inform their workers of the hazards? Protect them instead of looking the other way? Right?"

Davis nodded.

"They even deceived those poor guys into thinking they were safe," Roman continued, his voice raised in anger.

Davis just listened and said nothing.

"And you hygienists are supposed to be the experts in worker protection? Well, as far as I'm concerned, their failure to protect was . . . *criminal.* And you ought to be able to recognize it."

Davis started to protest, "You don't practice industrial hygiene and I don't . . . ," when he felt he was mouthing one of those absurd lines of comic genius in a classic Marx Brothers movie. Groucho playing a shyster lawyer is challenged by a human-fly circus performer to follow her up on the ceiling. He declines saying he has an agreement with the house flies that they don't practice law and he doesn't walk on the ceiling.

Half-smiling and more composed, he quietly concluded, "Tony, when you start talking willful and criminal, that's out of my area. You're looking for a prosecutor, not a hygienist."

Indeed, Davis had been dealt a wild card, for up to that time, even a repeated or willful workplace exposure—however, serious the outcome—had not been regarded as the basis for a criminal charge. Years later, company executives and supervisors would be tried in criminal court on charges involving the workplace deaths and serious injuries of their employees attributable to their knowing failure to protect the workers. Smart and perceptive, Roman realized that perhaps he had misconstrued the independent role of his scientific consultant—and unfairly so.

"Okay, we've been around this barn enough times. So we'll just agree to disagree. No hard feelings, right?"

Roman was actually gracious as he escorted Davis out, thanked him for his time and tactfully indicated that his involvement on the case had been concluded with a request for an invoice for his services. Davis left feeling uneasy with a gnawing sense that Roman may well have been justified in raising suspicions. The matter would be settled through notoriously slow litigation by a trial, or a more likely out-of-court settlement. Back at his office, he turned his attention to more satisfying academic duties.

About a month later while searching in a drug store for a particular multivitamin pill recommended by his physician, the efficacy of which he questioned, Davis recalled how he reacted with similar skepticism during the deposition of Mr. Johnson who alluded to vitamin pills being prescribed for the lead workers' health. He, Davis, was in excellent health and Mr. Johnson, ill with a body overburdened by lead, would probably succumb to its ravaging effects. The vitamin therapy seemed irrelevant for both of them. Unable to visualize the particular vitamin among the multifarious offerings in the brown glass bottles, he suddenly remembered that Johnson had referred to a "big *white* pill" and every multivitamin pill he had ever seen had a color of oil—tan/amber/brown, whatever—but definitely off-white. Johnson had also said something about getting the pill "sometime every month" implying that, unlike the usual one-, or more, a-day vitamin regimen, the workers got the pills only at some prescribed time at work. If the lead workers were not being given daily vitamins, what were the sometime big white pills?

He asked an obliging pharmacist on duty behind the rear counter for her copy of the PDR (*Physicians' Desk Reference*), then sat down in the customer waiting area with the large blue covered book. As the title implies, the PDR provides a doctor with a readily available source of information containing all that needs to be known about a prescription drug or medication from the manufacturers. It covers in great detail the indicated usages, recommended dosages, side and long-term effects, contraindications, and often includes identifying color photographs. Reinforced by the information in the PDR, Davis went back to his office, reviewed the medical surveillance and treatment for lead poisoning, and then mulled over the implications of what he had learned.

As a general rule, workers who have been demonstrably overexposed to cumulative injurious chemical agents like lead and mercury, or certain physical agents like x-rays and repetitive motion, are removed from further exposure. Medical treatment depends on the particular case as evaluated by a knowledgeable treating physician who also often makes the call on when the worker can safely return to work. Lead presents a special treatment problem. Apart from any immediate therapy, there is a time bomb with lead workers or children who have had excessive exposures. As noted, the majority of the total lead taken in their bodies is stored inertly in the bones and will continue to spill out into the blood even if they are removed from further exposure. For such chronically poisoned individuals, the released lead may tip the scales to cause irreversible and life-threatening effects; most dramatically, kidney failure and encephalopathy, a neuronal degeneration of the brain. In such cases, getting the lead out of the body promptly may be critical to the patient's survival.

Chelation is a type of chemical bonding in which a metal ion is tied up by a complexing agent in a soluble form so that when administered in the body, a toxic metal is rendered less biologically available and can be readily excreted. The word is derived graphically and etymologically from the Greek word meaning "crab's claw." Unfortunately, the chelation of metals in the body is not specific and an essential element like calcium or zinc can be removed along with the target toxic heavy metal like lead or mercury. The calcium disodium salt of ethylene diamine tetraacetic acid, usually referred to as EDTA, is the drug of choice for lead, but due to its poor absorption in the stomach, it has to be injected intravenously or intramuscularly. In common with many chemicals not natural to the body, EDTA may also have some toxic effects of its own, so that the therapeutic treatment has to be carefully monitored by a physician in a hospital or clinic. The usual adult dosage involves an infusion of a pint solution containing one gram of EDTA daily for three to five days so that it would be a rather agonizing treatment for a two-year-old.

A low toxicity derivative of penicillin called penicillamine (chemically, 3 mercapto *d*-valine) is regularly used in the treatment of Wilson's disease to remove copper, which accumulates to toxic levels in the liver, brain, and kidneys and produces a telltale golden brown ring around the pupils. Copper happens to be an essential micronutrient normally present in our diet, but the victim has a deficiency of the protein, ceruloplasmin, which binds the copper in a useful form; the unaffiliated copper is responsible for the toxicity. Penicillamine will also tie up lead, and being absorbed efficiently in the intestinal tract, it has the distinct advantage of oral administration and has been used to treat children with moderate body lead burdens. But there was another less noble aspect of the deleading treatment of which Davis was aware.

Subsequent to Automotive Energy's stewardship of the recovery plant, OSHA had specifically banned "prophylactic chelation" of any lead worker, which refers to the routine use of chelating drugs ". . . to *routinely* lower blood levels to predesignated levels believed to be 'safe'. . . ." After chelation, the measurement of lead in the blood will indeed appear lower, but the true measure of lead availability and levels inside the tissues and vital organs are masked. Judged to be "safe," the worker's body burden of lead may, in fact, continue to be increased.

Is that what the Automotive Energy had been doing all those years to keep their workers blood levels within the then acceptable range? Although the exposure levels were known to be high and little was done to reduce the workers' exposures by effective control measures, their average blood levels contrarily appeared to stay within the then acceptable levels. If the PDR had not identified the penicillamine as white pills, Davis might have been able to shrug off his initial suspicion but there were too many loose ends. Lacking definite proof, it was still only conjecture and he agonized whether he should apprise Roman of his thoughts regarding the mysterious white pills. Now illegal by specific regulation, it is highly unlikely that anyone would employ prophylactic chelation today, so what useful purpose would be served? So conflicted, he did not call Roman. When he received a message at work to return a call from Roman's office, he still was unresolved and uncomfortable as to what he would say.

Uncharacteristically, he put off calling Roman for several days, only to learn that Roman was in court that day and messages would be taken by Roman's assistant, Lisa Taylor.

"I guess you heard the news, Professor," Lisa said, anticipating a reason for his call.

"What news?"

"Didn't Mr. Roman tell you we settled the lead workers' case?"

"That's good news," he said. Then, after a slight hesitation, "I suppose Tony is satisfied at the outcome."

"I think so, professor. He said the most important thing is for those poor men to be fairly compensated and . . . ." Her voice trailed off noncommittally. She was aware that the out-of-court settlement was confidential and there was no point for further comment.

"Is there any message for Mr. Roman?" she asked.

"No, Lisa, if the case is settled, then I guess there's no need for any further comment from me."

He reflected how unfair it was that as far as the law and justice were concerned, the matter could be filed in the books as a closed case; for Davis and his fellow hygienists, the concerns and problems were always there.

PART 3 The Risk Assumers

■ *This last section deals with an odd couple of occupations: cosmetologists (largely comprised of hairdressers) and firefighters, both of whose members share a status distinctive in the work force. They each face unusual and persistent health or safety hazards daily in their work, but their love of and dedication to their professions makes them willing to "assume the risks." It may be recalled that in the era before workers compensation for injuries or disabilities incurred on the job, any worker who was engaged in a work activity that was commonly known to be inherently dangerous to one's health and safety was legally prevented from obtaining financial compensation from their employer because of the common-law principle called Assumption of Risk. It is unusual today that workers would knowingly and willingly assume serious workplace risks—irrespective of their rights to compensation for their workplace disabilities, and for that alone, the two occupationally exposed groups are worthy of special coverage. The description of these unusually dedicated risk-takers also includes another aspect of the investigational aspects of industrial hygiene practice.*

The industrial hygienist in the case stories of Part 2 investigated mysterious reports of illness at work that were in one sense unique to the particular event and location. Lazar Davis applied his knowledge and the methods of his trade to solve the problem. That body of knowledge and know-how is the collective result of a broader type of investigational activity to which many industrial hygienists and occupational health professionals contribute; namely, the research and statistical analysis of occupational health studies as reported in the literature and scientific meetings. This investigative role of the research hygienist and statistician may not have the panache of a sleuth at work, but it is indispensable for understanding and advancing the science of the profession and putting the true hazards of the job into meaningful perspective.

Chapter 1

The Cosmetologists

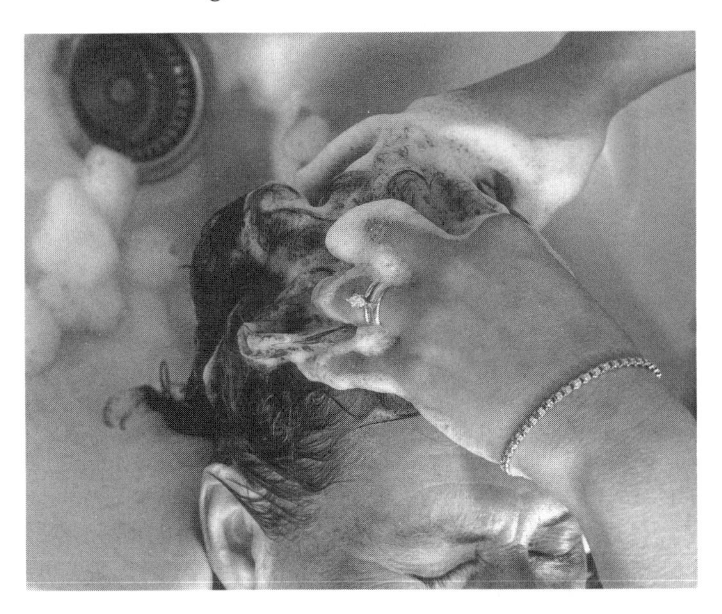

The hands of hairdressers are repeatedly exposed to the drying action of the soaps and detergents in the hair shampoos and rinses, which render their skin more susceptible to skin irritation and disorders. Most hairdressers refuse to wear protective gloves, claiming they impede the shampooing treatment and shaping of the hair.

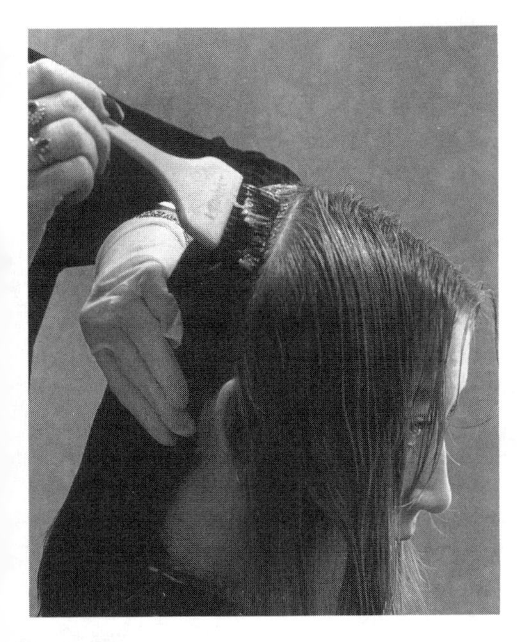

Once highly suspect of causing long-term health effects, the chemicals in hair dyes used today have been more extensively tested for safety. In this brush application of a dye, the hairdresser wears protective gloves for esthetic purposes, to prevent the staining of *her* hands.

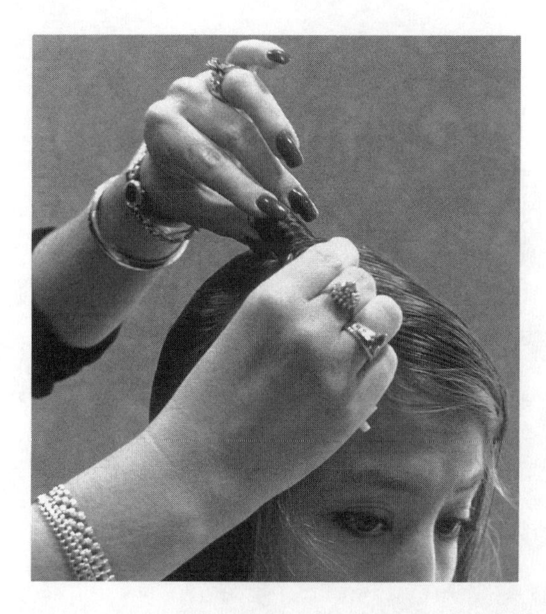

Repetitive-motion injury of the type associated with carpal tunnel syndrome has been attributed to hairdressers' extensive application of hair curlers and hair brushing.

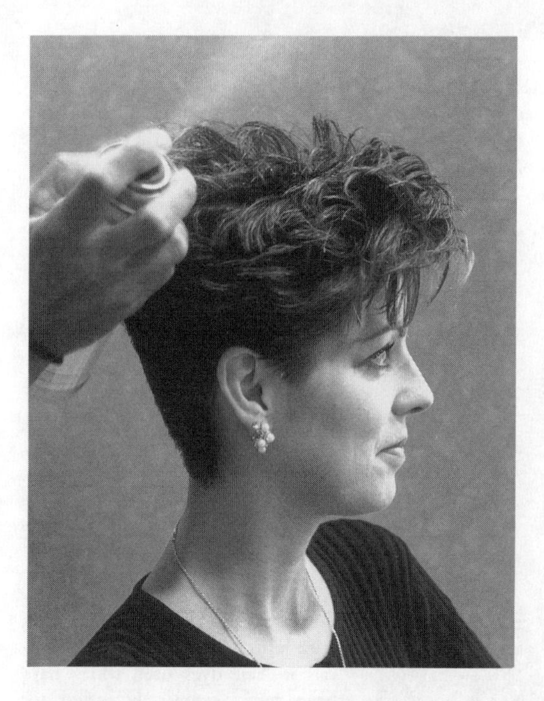

Although generally not a health problem, the indiscriminate use of aerosol hair sprays in poorly ventilated and crowded salons has led to some respiratory and subjective complaints. Some highly asthmatic subjects may incur problems and occasionally an allergic dermatological reaction occurs among sensitized or atopic individuals.

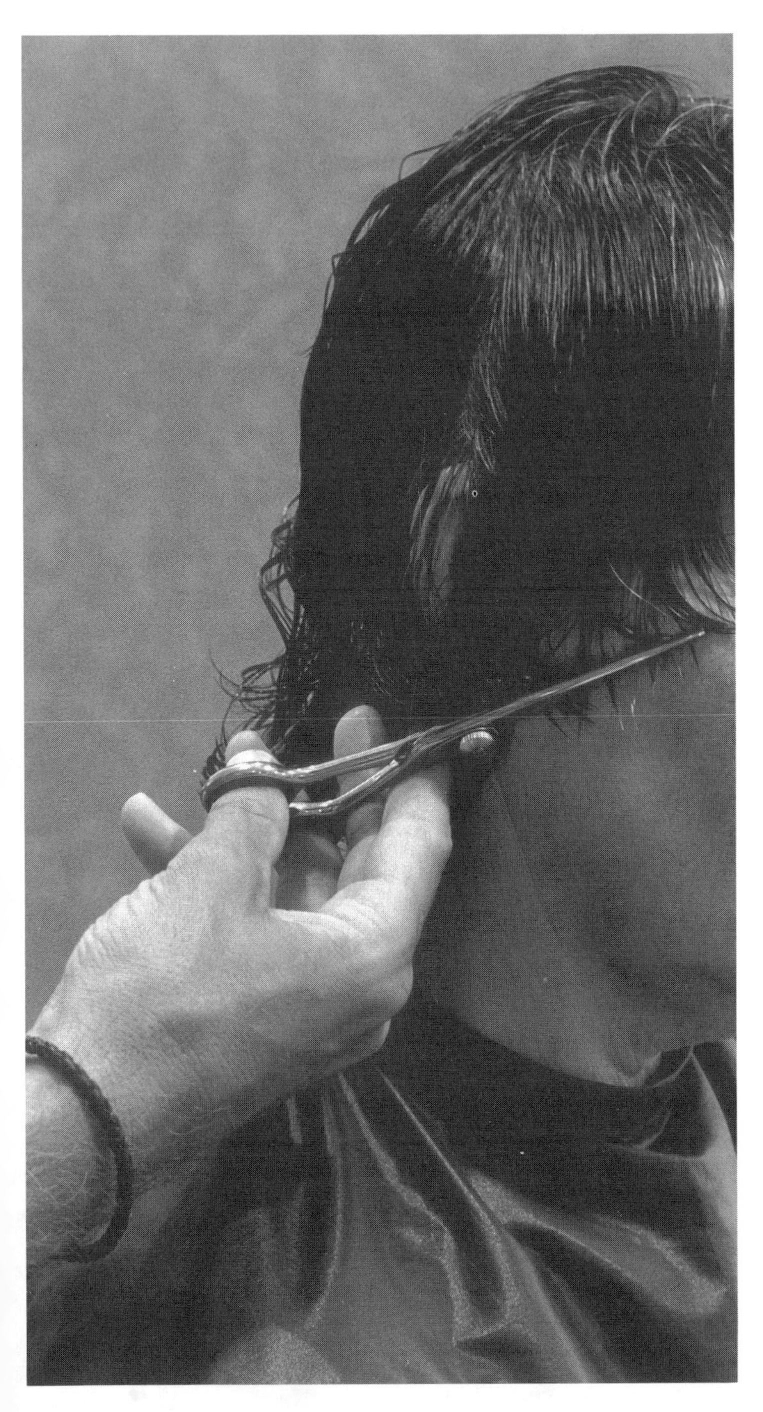

The most potent and common skin allergen affecting cosmetologists has been nickel metal. Problems can arise due to contact with the nickel present in steel scissors, other metal tools, and even costume jewelry.

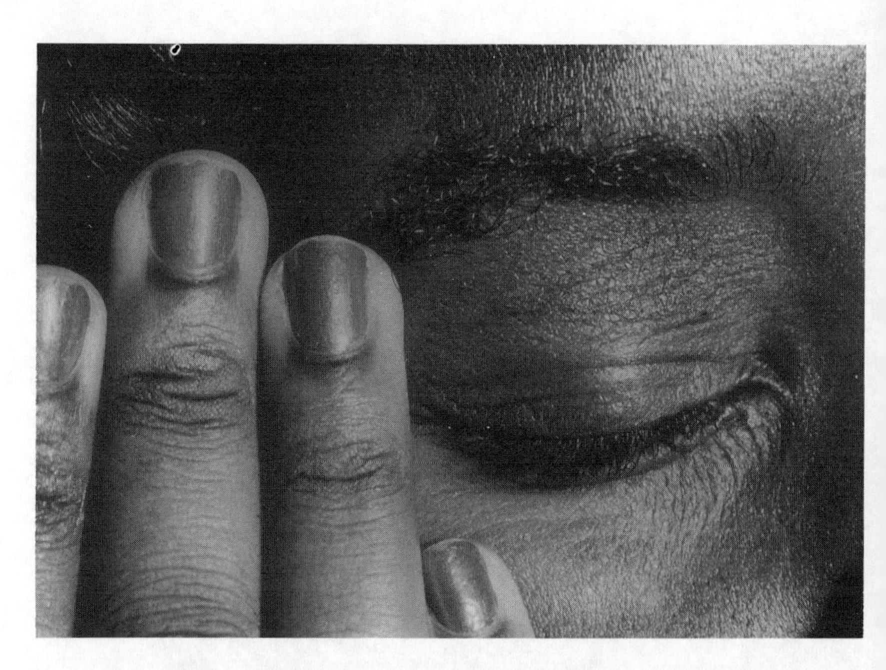

The potent nickel sensitizer is not commonly present in the chemical products used by the cosmetologist. However, a finger nail polish containing the metal elicited this allergic response in this patient's fingers.

Credits (first five photos): New York Hair Company, Yardley, PA
Photographer: Philip Taylor
(last photo): Department of Dermatology, Medical College of Pennsylvania and Hahnemann University

Chapter *1*

The Cosmetologists

Working to make people look beautiful is a relatively recent way to make a living although vanity in personal appearance probably predates the discovery of a mirror. Beauty care had largely been a personal and family activity during antiquity, with the possible exception of the grooming services provided by servants and slaves. By the eighteenth century, there were specialists in the beautifying treatment of our skin, hair, eyes, and nails to provide their services professionally to the upper class, who for good reason have since been dubbed the "beautiful people." Following the Industrial Revolution in the nineteenth century, an expanding economy entitled the nascent middle class to the same indulgences, and self-employed hairdressers began to provide their services directly into the homes of their clients. Before the end of the century, a public facility offering more extensive cosmetic services and equipment was established and was common enough by 1901 to be called a beauty shop. House calls continued to be available in the United States until the mid-1920s. About the same time, many of the beauticians, perhaps because of children at home, other family obligations, or personal preference, set up neighborhood businesses in their homes. That a parlor is a room in a private dwelling which is intended for conversation may explain the origin of the "beauty parlor." Partly because of zoning restrictions, strict licensing, and inspection requirements and more lately, liability, these home establishments have dwindled and largely been displaced by what are now more glamorously called beauty salons and unisex hair styling shops on Main Street, the shopping malls, and department stores. The large salons employ fifteen or more full- and part-time hairdressers and cosmetologists, but the majority of shops will have less than five. Whatever the size, an array of beauty-enhancing services are offered there in a spiffy, well-lit, and commodious environment by experts who personally know what their clients want or, as the case may be, *should* want.

Occupational Perspective

If the way we spend our disposable income in both good and bad times is any guide to fears about job security, the professionals providing beauty care can rest assured. For most customers of the beauty salons and barber shops, the benefits from their regular attendance justify the costs, which they treat as a non-negotiable item in the budget. For their part, the highly skilled and dedicated professionals—formerly "beauticians," now "cosmetologists"—respond like Pygmalion to each devoted customer. They love what they do and do it with pride, a strong sense of personal identity, and perhaps, most importantly, with appreciation. Instant and mutual gratification follow whenever a client beams approvingly at the daring new hair style in the mirror, or at perfectly shaped and tinted toenails.

In 1992, there were 746,000 beauty care professionals in the United States, 90 percent of whom were cosmetologists and hairdressers, with a female/male ratio of seven to one. Whereas male hair cutting had been exclusively a male-dominated profession a generation or two ago, slightly more than a third of barbers today are women. Most cosmetologists and barbers work full time, which is variably reported as meaning 40–48 hours per week including Saturday and evenings, but at least one-third only log in part-time. Both groups reflect a somewhat independent streak in that at least half of the cosmetologists and four out of five barbers are self-employed. This does not necessarily mean that they have their own shops since many work on a straight commission basis at the prestigious larger shops. Most employees get paid a straight salary with commissions usually of 40–50 percent, but all derive a considerable portion of their income from tips. Consequently, it is difficult to get accurate representations of total income based on the median weekly salaries reported annually by the Bureau of Labor Statistics, but all agree that despite relatively low beginning salaries, an experienced cosmetologist, particularly at the more exclusive salons, can comfortably qualify as a member of what a Gilbert and Sullivan of today might call the "lower upper middle class."

All states require professional licensing by a state board which usually specifies that the eligible applicants must be at least sixteen years old, pass a physical examination, and, most distinctively, be a graduate of a state-licensed school. There are almost four thousand public vocational and private schools with programs in cosmetology, comprising a satellite industry that warrants a National Association of Accredited Cosmetology Schools. The formal training consists of a minimum of a thousand hours of both practical and classroom instruction over six months, but some states require as much as twenty-five hundred hours lasting fifteen months. Students receive elementary instruction in anatomy, physiology, applied chemistry, and electricity, and with an emphasis on sanitation and health, they are attuned to recognize infections and disorders of the scalp, nails, and skin. To be licensed, the graduates must pass written and practical examinations and some are even subjected to oral examinations, or required to work a year first in a junior status before being eligible to take and pass an examination as a senior cosmetologist. It is still possible to get licensed alternatively in a few states by serving a one- to two-year apprenticeship, but the likelihood of receiving reciprocity to practice in other states with more demanding formal education is unlikely. Not only do the cosmetology schools have little trouble placing their qualified graduates, but it was estimated by the Association for the Advancement of Cosmetology that forty thousand hair-dressing jobs were unfilled in 1993. The Bureau of Labor Statistics projected that the job growth in the field will remain above the average of all occupations well into the new century.

The barber shop Figaro might well have been impressed by the current formal training and professionalism required by the largely distaff members of the business but puzzled by their limited services. As early as the seventeenth century, barbers doubled as surgeons specializing in bleeding and purging without ever having gone to a barber college or a medical school. In the well-known eighteenth-century picaresque novel *Gil Blas of Santillaine* by Le Sage, the medical procedures, principally phlebotomy, of the barber-surgeon are satirically described when the hero serves an apprenticeship to a Dr. Sangrado, introduced as "this learned forerunner of the undertaker."

Although beauty salons are attractive workplaces with the apparent sociability of a genteel androgynous locker room, the hairdressers often work standing for most of their eight- and ten-hour shifts. In addition to the physical demands of the work, they must continue to appear to be pleasant, even-tempered, attentive, and solicitous to each customer. There are many challenges to maintaining their smiles and equanimity. On the tightly scheduled and quick-paced peak weekend shifts, clients arrive late for appointments or make last-minute appointments and emergency requests. Many clients are not gracious about being kept waiting, so the frenzied hairdressers frequently have to skip lunch and keep smiling.

An unusual sense of loyalty often evolves between the cosmetologist and client that ironically leads to stresses in the business. Although in a sense the hairdresser is an employee of the salon, he and she come to regard the client as *their* customer, which tends to strain the relationship between the owner and the more ambitious and independent employees. There is a more tangible consequence of the loyalty. One long-term male hairdresser claimed that every time he had free-lanced to a new salon, 80 percent of his customers followed him and he suggested, reinforced from his own experiences as a sometime owner, that the subsequent loss of business was a principal reason for the failure of many small salons.

In addition to the loyalty between client and cosmetologist, interpersonal relationships develop, almost unique among professional personal services. According to one study, hairdressers will engage in one-on-one conversation for twenty-five minutes with each of an average of fifty-five customers a week. In about one-third of that time, customers will confide their most personal problems, most notably with their marriage, health, children, anxiety, and depression. In an actual quote from a salon that might have appeared in a New Yorker cartoon, one woman prefacing her revelations announced, "Honey, I'm telling you things I haven't even told my analyst." When a highly accomplished male hairdresser who had been practicing for forty-five years was asked why he believed his profession engendered this special relationship, he said, "I think it has a lot to do with the hands-on aspect of our work. People really have to trust you to allow you to touch them as we do."

An interview study on their role in interpersonal involvements found that most cosmetologists perceived it as an integral part of the job. Many enjoyed listening while lathering and were even flattered by their status as confidants, but they often felt inadequate to offer advice where professional help may be needed and wisely responded with sympathy, lightheartedness, or tactfully deflected the topic. For some, it was just another form of stress of the job. However, there are far more prevalent and evident risks to their well-being and health for their beauty-making.

Work Health Hazards

In surveys of reported or actual occupational health problems associated with specific occupations, cosmetologists virtually head the list on contact and allergic dermatitis and with certain types of cancer. There has been some concern expressed about adverse reproductive effects, asthma, increased mortality rates, and inflammatory bowel disease, among others, but the associations are ambiguously reported by the investigators as "negative," "weak," or "possible," with the standard caveat that further study is indicated.

The substantive and proven health effects from the work do, however, have a common etiology. Every cosmetologist is in daily and continual contact with hundreds of potentially hazardous chemicals, comprising the scores of specialized cosmetic products found in the modern beauty salon or barber shop (Table 1).

Adding injuries to the chemical insults to the body in the beauty salons are, in part, the heat, noise, and dryness from the hair dryers, cuts from scissors, breathing air blended with tobacco smoke and hair spray, the burns from curling irons, the repetitive motion injury from vigorous hair brushing, and the stress of the aforementioned nonstop dialogue with the customers. By far, the most prevalent and discomforting ailment of being a cosmetologist today is occupational dermatitis, which, at least for the professionals, belies the adage that beauty is

Table 1. Chemical Products Used by Cosmetologists

After-shave lotions
Hair: dressing, dyes, frosting
Bath: fragrance, oils, salts
Bleach: lotions, powder, cream
Bleach powders
Bubble bath
Cleansing creams
Cold waves
Colognes
Conditioners: hair, skin
Body lotions
Cream makeup
Cuticle remover
Deodorants: aerosol, cream, roll-on, stick
Depilatories: cream, powder, wax
Dusting powder
Eye makeup: pigments, remover
Eye-wrinkle cream
Eyebrow: pencil, plucking cream
Eyelash: cream, oil
Face: conditioners, packs
Fingernail: acrylic, cuticle remover, hardener, polish, polish remover
Hair: dressing, dyes, frosting, lightener, permanent wave, rinse, setting lotion, spray, straightener, tonics, pomade
Lipstick
Makeup: liquid, powder
Mascara
Massage lotion
Neutralizer: permanent wave
Perfumes
Powders: face, compact
Preshave lotion
Rouge
Sachet
Shampoo
Shaving cream: brushless, lather, aerosol
Skin: freshener, softener
Suntan lotion
Sunscreen
Tanning agent
Vanishing cream
Vitamin cream
Wavesets

only skin deep. The incidence among female hairdressers is reported to be higher than the males, but few are completely immune from an occasional disturbance. For some hairdressers, the skin problems are so discomforting and persistent that they either are endured stoically as the hair shirt price for doing what they love or may become the reason for quitting the profession. These skin and other health problems can best be understood from the historical development and use of cosmetics and new techniques of beautification.

Cosmetics

Because primping and sexually attractive odors, or pheromones, have been part of the animal courting scene since creation, it is not farfetched to assume that early man and woman were employing naturally occurring cosmetics for similar purposes. The practice of manufacturing cosmetics for enhancing appearance or personal attractiveness can be traced to the Egyptians over thirty-five hundred years ago. The Egyptian word *kemait*, referring to the aromatic herbs from which oils and oozing plant liquids were derived for skin applications, appears as *kommi* in Greek, *gommi* in Latin, *gomme* in French, and ultimately *gum* in English. Essential oils derived from plants and fats from animals were often blended with sweet-smelling scents such as those from cinnamon, peppermint, rosemary, and sandalwood, and then used as balms for wounds, rubbing ointments, and for religious purposes, as in anointing. Olive oil, in particular, was regarded as having particular purity and sanctity for anointing purposes and according to the Old Testament, failure to follow the precepts of the Lord would cut off the supply because the transgressors' trees would not bear the fruit.

When coloring was needed for the face, eyes, and lips, harmless vegetable dyes from berries, nuts, roots, and other plant parts were first used happily and safely. Earth pigments containing innocuous iron oxides mixed or appropriately fired with clay or sand provided a red bloom to the Egyptian's cheeks and lips or the golden cast preferred by the Sumerians. Sometime later in Egypt and the Eastern world of antiquity, minerals containing antimony, lead, or copper were ground up in the eye makeup to protect against the endemic eye diseases. The use of these toxic metal pigments and minerals might have produced some insidious health effects, but they were neither detected nor suspected then. A water-based paste called *kohl* made with ground antimony, soot, or galena, a common ore of lead, was commonly used in response of the fashionable predilection of the Eastern women to darken their lashes and eye brows. To this day, the eyes of millions of women, men, children, and even infants in parts of Africa, the Middle East, and Asia are coated with a formulation of *kohl* comprising 40–50 percent lead sulfide. In addition to the cosmetic and protective reasons, application is even encouraged by the Sunna, the behavioral guidelines of Islam. Although this inorganic form of toxic lead is not absorbed through the skin and does not penetrate the cornea, the makeup can cause a slight burning sensation and tearing. Young children, who are most susceptible to the toxic effects, are likely to wipe their eyes with fingers that inevitably end up in the mouth. Notwithstanding the FDA proscription against using toxic constituents such as lead and mercury in cosmetics, a Somali graduate student of industrial hygiene in the United States recently brought into class a kit containing *kohl* and applicators that were being marketed in an immigrant neighborhood close to the campus.

The ancients also developed perfumes and incense from resins, the inhalation of which was considered to be purifying and, by implication, beautifying. There probably were preparations for the teeth, shaving, and toilet, although there are no recorded recipes or remnants sufficient for analysis, but in Mesopotamia, pumice was reported to be employed as possibly the first depilatory.

Detergents and soaps which constitute the active ingredient in probably the most widely used modern hairdressing product—hair shampoos—were not developed and commercialized until many years later. We do not know just when soaps were discovered, but there are indications that the Babylonians almost five thousand years ago, and later the ancient Egyptians and Romans were believed to have made some crude soaps from animal fats and wood ashes for washing and treating skin diseases, but it was not until the eighth century that commercial soap makers started to appear in Italy and about five hundred years later in England. Whether the products were too coarse, too expensive, or the demand was not there, no one seemed to have been in a hurry to start up an industry until the late 1700s when Nicholas Leblanc in France discovered a cheap and reliable source of lye from table salt. Soaps are made by heating the animal fats or vegetable oils with a strong alkali, like lye (sodium hydroxide) or caustic and regular potash (potassium hydroxide and potassium carbonate). The chemical reaction, called saponification, forms a creamy, smelly, caustic soap which is essentially a two-part molecule made up of a water-attracting and a water-repelling—or oil-attracting—moiety. The detergent or soap decreases the surface tension of water so that the cleaning action is begun by first wetting the dirty surface, then by separating the oily dirt particle from the surface to which it is adhered, and then removing the dirt by suspending or emulsifying it in the rinse water. Hair was largely cleaned by brushing until less irritating detergents and soaps were available as attractive liquid shampoos enhanced with perfumes, preservatives, stabilizers, and dyes.

Occupational Skin Problems

As described in the skin case stories of Part 2, our natural body defenses against chemical and environmental assaults to our outer shell are highly effective unless the exposures are excessive or involve a particularly irritating or sensitizing (i.e., allergenic) component. The outer skin has a tough coating of dead skin which acts like a physical shield, perspiration provides some measure of washing and dirt removal, and the normal excretions of skin oils and fats keep the skin buffered against chemical attack, resilient, and pliant. Shampoo treatments of the hair are usually harmless to the scalp and hands even when performed once or twice daily as Mary Martin did washing that man right out of her hair at every evening and matinee performance in the long-running Broadway stage production of *South Pacific*. In addition to the purposeful cleansing action of removing grease, dirt, and debris from the hair, the detergents and soaps in the shampoos with repeated and prolonged applications will also soften the outer protective skin layer, remove the natural oils and fats, and leave a dry chapped skin that is particularly susceptible to more serious skin problems. The cold and dryness of the winters in the temperate countries exacerbate this condition, which explains a higher seasonal incidence.

After the shampoo, the follow-up rinse treatment softens and makes the wet hair more manageable, adds luster, and reduces static and snarling when combed out. The rinses also are comprised mainly of a detergent quaternary ammonium compound as the active agent, so that the already defatted skin gets further assaulted by this process.

Getting a shampoo is standard practice before cutting and coloring the hair, so most hairdressers will have their hands immersed in hot soapy mixes and rinses for more than an hour each day. Being low on the totem pole and needing the experience, trainees and junior cosmetologists may be particularly at risk of developing an irritant contact dermatitis from giving most of the shampoos in the shop, but one veteran hairdresser reported doing as many as forty to fifty a day. Shampoos are understandably and inevitably the most frequent and persistent cause of contact dermatitis among cosmetologists.

Studies of occupational contact dermatitis of cosmetologists in such diverse countries as Australia, Bulgaria, Benin, Japan, Sweden, and the United States reveal a fairly consistent experience. On the average, 50 percent of all hairdressers reported having experienced some form of dermatitis—most often an eczema of the hands—with the majority attributing it directly to the shampoos, wavesets, and bleaches. Either the Japanese are more sensitive or observant, indicating in one study of 306 female hairdressers that their prevalence rate of skin lesions on the hands and arms, or the percent of cases at a *given* time, was an alarmingly high 49 percent. Their lesions were described as dryness, roughness, hyperkeratosis (thickening), redness, and desquamation (scaliness). If you were to enter a beauty salon at random and ask the personnel if they were experiencing any skin problems, it is odds on that at least one of the attendants will show you an active condition and the rest will relate their past or most recent bouts.

A statistical multifactor analysis and interviews covering the medical histories of over four hundred cosmetologists in the United States in 1982 indicated that slightly more than half reported having had significant skin problems which they attributed to their work. About half of the cases lasted days or weeks and about a third suffered for months or were for all practical purposes ongoing. Particularly revealing was that the odds of a beauty care worker developing work-related skin problems were extremely high ($p<.001$) with *any* prior history of a medically confirmed allergy including such disparate but common allergens as ragweed, household dust, foods—of all kinds, detergents, drugs, animal hair, and, of course, beauty care products. More esoteric but no less potent to their victims were oven cleaners, insect sprays, adhesive tape, newspapers, and tobacco. One might suspect that the hapless lot of cosmetologists branded with atopy, or the inherited predisposition to develop a hypersensitivity to substances to which four out of five people are immune, are the major victims. Most, yes; but still about 40 percent of cosmetologists with no prior history develop a skin problem.

Protective gloves, of which the latex-type appears to provide the highest resistance to chemical permeation, are generally worn by the hairdressers when tinting or bleaching but are considered by most to be too restrictive for effective shampooing. Other methods of control include the use of protective and emollient skin creams and the avoidance of using products known to be more irritating than others. Although contact dermatitis from shampoos may be minimal or acceptable for most cosmetologists, there are more serious and less tolerable dermatological problems in the business.

Allergic contact dermatitis is not believed to be caused appreciably by the detergents in the shampoos, but serious skin problems of sensitization among cosmetologists have been caused by allergenic components of the shampoos, such as formaldehyde (as a germicide) and perfumes, in the scores of other cosmetic products used daily, or from the tools and the environment. Unlike the contact dermatitis caused by detergents and soaps which require continued and excessive exposures, minuscule amounts of the allergen of short duration can elicit a severe and debilitating reaction once a person has been sensitized by an initial exposure. Fortunately, not all allergens are sufficiently potent to elicit a reaction with most people and many people seem to be relatively immune. The highly susceptible "atopic" individuals, who are fated genetically by familial history to break out with no prior exposures or apparent cause, invariably predominate among the afflicted. It might seem an easy solution just to eliminate the allergens in the cosmetic products and the beauty shop to solve the allergy problems, but there are practical limitations to a complete exclusion, as there would be in trying to provide a germ-free environment.

Consider the most potent and common allergen affecting female hairdressers and women in general. Consistently, about 40 percent of all hairdressers develop contact allergic dermatitis from contact with the metal *nickel*, which, with the exception of nail polish, is not usually a constituent of any of the chemical products but is present in the metal alloys making up the scissors, clips, pins, and rods, and often in the costume jewelry worn, most notably pierced earrings and bracelets. Although the amount of nickel that is leached out of a nickel hairpin or from an earring is barely detectable by the most sophisticated analytical techniques, it is sufficient to cause a skin reaction in the sensitized hairdresser. The jewelry problem may be solved by switching to 14-carat gold or all-plastic adornments, but it may not be so easy to obtain nickel-free metal tools, pins, and the like, including the coin of the realm. As might be expected with the hundreds of synthetic chemicals comprising the permanent wave preparations, hair dyes, bleaches, and other cosmetic products in near daily use in the beauty salon, some are fairly potent skin irritants, some are allergic sensitizers, and some may be both.

In many cases, the price of countering nature to produce or enhance a desired beautifying effect for the client is at the expense of the cosmetologist's skin. Our hair is naturally made up of helical chains of protein, called keratin, which are linked by disulfide bonds that strengthen and shape the hair. Unfortunately, the shape is more often naturally straight than naturally curly. In order to reorder the structure of hair so that the hair fibers will follow the desired curlicue direction, the hair bonds were first primitively broken down by an alkali and heat from a curling iron. A second step involves using a chemical oxidizing agent to rebuild the bonds into a "permanent" wave.

In the 1940s, a cold chemical process was introduced as an alkaline perm using a chemical, ammonium thioglycolate (ATG), to break the bonds. Although dermal sensitization does not appear to be a problem, applying the alkaline ATG is not innocuous since it can cause an irritant dermatitis if it is left on the skin too long. By the 1970s, a related chemical called glyceryl monothioglocolate (GMTG) largely displaced the ATG as a so-called acid perm. For whatever benefits the GMTG brought to the hair styling it did so at the cost of dermally sensitizing about 20 percent of the hair stylists based on patch testing studies. Once sensitized to the GMTG, even wearing a protective glove while giving the acid perm, the hairdresser's hands can break out from just the trace amounts of the GMTG which penetrate through the glove material. After this and other hair treatments, many hairdressers will remove the gloves, insisting that they must "feel" the hair—another potential source of allergic contact. There are several other acronymic chemicals closely related to GMTG used in the acid perms which are only somewhat less potent as dermal sensitizers, but the particularly allergic or atopic hairdresser will often cross-react, so that substitution of another brand of acid perm is not an option for controling their problem.

There are usually lesser skin problems encountered with the bleaching treatment and hair dyeing, in part, because unlike shampooing, hairdressers find no hindrance in wearing gloves and they can see a benefit from wearing them. The hydrogen peroxide and ammonia bleaching mix used for making a brunette a lighter tone is a so-so skin irritant, but it can also cause a noncosmetic blanching of the hairdresser's hands and the hair dyes may also cause discoloration. When the bleaching power of the mixture is enhanced by the addition of ammonium or potassium persulfate to covert the brunette all the way to a blond, severely itching wheals, or urticaria, often results on the unprotected hands.

Whereas gentlemen may prefer blonds, it would appear from the use and choices of hair dyes that women repeatedly opt for change. A "temporary" color change chosen from well over a hundred dyes is produced by the rinses, which deposit an organic chemical film on the hair shaft and lasts as long as the next shampoo, wash, and rinse. Everyone in the salon understands that a "semipermanent" color change involves dyes of organic compounds complexed with chromophoric metals such as cobalt or chromium, or aromatic nitro or amino compounds. The coloring agent gets below the surface of the hair shaft and maintains the color through several shampoos. It is perfectly reasonable for cosmetologists to call "permanent" the most important dye treatment in which the color is maintained inside the hair shaft down to the roots for the six to eight weeks that it takes for a new growth of untreated hair to emerge. The permanent dye mixture consists of a color modifier and a colorless dye base which is oxidized usually with hydrogen peroxide just before the application. This forms the desired color dye which penetrates and deposits inside the hair shaft. The dye bases are mainly organic diamines and aminophenols, which include some of the more common and potent skin sensitizers. Most notably, *p*-phenylenediamine (PPD) produced a positive patch test response in 15 percent of European hairdressers and clients suspected of having a contact sensitization from cosmetic products.

The earlier use of "natural" hair dyes did not contain any known toxic hazard to the user, although lead combs dipped in vinegar which chemically produces lead acetate had been used in ancient Rome by men and women to darken their graying hair. Lead acetate is not used in the beauty salons today but continues to serve as the active agent in the most popular product used mostly by men for home treatment. Consistent with the new back to nature wave emphasizing natural ingredients in food, the use of the vegetable hair dyes of antiquity has been popularized, such as the auburn coloring derived from the henna plant, which still plays a cosmetic role in the Middle East. The active agent in henna, 2-hydroxy-1,4-napthaquinone, is reported in one well-known and authoritative text in occupational contact dermatitis to be a "common contact allergen" found in hair dyes, whereas an equally authoritative state-of-the-art literature review of occupational dermatosis in hairdressers states it is "not a sensitizer." Perhaps, only your hairdresser knows.

Other Work Health Concerns

There were more serious though less visible health concerns than dermatitis from the later modern-day use of hair dyes. In the mid-nineteenth century, a newborn synthetic chemical dye industry had produced a rainbow array of fast colors which were delightedly put into cosmetic applications. Many of these new hair dyes were aromatic hydrocarbons such as the aniline-base dyes derived from coal tars. The emerging occupational health professionals of the twentieth century became aware of the carcinogenic potency of some of these chemicals, having seen an unusually high incidence of tumors, notably of the bladder, liver, and skin, among the dye manufacturing workers. Some, such as beta-naphthyl amine, were judged to be so life-threatening to the workers that they were later effectively banned, and many of the related chemicals were demonstrated to produce tumors in animals by skin painting tests. Strangely, there was scant attention expressed by the health professionals about a cancer or serious health risk at the consumer end; that is, to the appliers and consumers of products containing these proven or suspect human carcinogens. In fact, it is unlikely that any awareness of a health risk from hair dyeing entered the minds of the hairdressers and the customers until well after the U.S. Food and Drug Administration Act of

1938 and subsequent amendments had established procedures requiring cosmetic manufacturers to prove the harmlessness of their products. More likely, serious attention by the general public and the cosmetologists to the issue was not raised until the much later television and popular press coverage in the 1970s—some may say, hype—of the chemical and environmental causes of cancer. Recently, a graduate student in toxicology reported that most members of her family were convinced that their grandmother, who had operated a home beauty salon in the basement, died from cancer resulting from many years of hair dyeing performed without gloves. An earlier generation had heard stories of some glamorous Hollywood actress, invariably a platinum blond, whose death from cancer was also, in its way, occupationally caused. Although rigorous FDA screening requirements and long-term experiences have probably reduced much of the cancer risk today, there has been a lingering suspicion that cosmetologists are inherently more vulnerable to not only cancer but other serious health effects from their exposures to chemicals, past and present. This association has been variably reinforced and questioned by studies, statistics, and surveys of cosmetologists and hairdressers reported in the scientific literature.

A first pass in the investigation of a possible life-threatening disease associated with cosmetologists might be to compare their standard relative mortality and morbidity with that of other occupations. This perhaps simplistically implies that if they die earlier or get sick more frequently than, say, accountants, carpenters, or stenotypists of similar age, sex, work tenure, and the like, it must have something to do with their unique exposures at work. A comparative breakdown of the *causes* of their deaths or illnesses might then suggest an occupational etiology for specific diseases and disorders such as brain tumors, spontaneous abortions, or depression. Very large populations of workers have to be compared to establish any meaningful trend and the reporting of much smaller groups can sometimes produce statistical anomalies which can send researchers off on the wrong track. What can be said then about the relative health risks of spending your life working in a beauty salon?

One fairly extensive occupational study of women in California involving almost 200,000 male and female deaths reported for 1979 through 1981 found that female cosmetologists were among the higher-risk occupations along with waitresses, certain health care workers, telephone operators, janitors, housekeepers, launderers, and dry cleaners. Contrary to the usual pattern, the males in these same occupations had a *lower* mortality risk. Apparently, the excess mortality rates for the female cosmetologists were not so compelling for the researchers to conclude that their work was responsible and tactfully retreated with the admonition for other researchers to conduct further study. Nonetheless, largely because of the cosmetologists' daily and extensive exposure to multiple chemicals, occupational health researchers have investigated the association of suspected systemic and reproductive health effects.

In order to evaluate the increased risk of developing an illness or adverse health effect from a particular job, it is necessary to compare statistically the observed rate of the workers at risk with the expected rate for the general population. Cancer was second only to heart disease as the leading cause of deaths in the United States in 1993, according to the National Center for Health Statistics in the U.S. Department of Health and Human Services. By the late 1980s, lung cancer had become the principal cause of the fatal forms for both men and women, whereas in the period 1958–1960, the death rate from breast cancer among women was more than five times greater than that for lung cancer and then gradually declined. The numbers never give the whole story. It is not that women were having fewer cases of breast cancer; in fact, the American Cancer Society had estimated that in 1994 there were 182,000 *new* cases of breast cancer, or more than two and a half times that for lung cancer. Earlier detection and more effective methods of treatment of breast cancer have been cited by the experts as having significantly reduced the fatality rate. The number of deaths from a lesser number of female lung cancer cases, however, was estimated to account for the highest number of cancer deaths, eclipsing that from breast cancer by thirteen thousand in 1994. During the same periods of comparison, the rate increase in lung cancer deaths and cases among women far exceeded that of the men, which is generally attributed to the greatly increased numbers and percentage of women smoking.

Although the investigators might well have predicted and expected to find an increased incidence of cancer, generally as well as for specific types, among the beauty shop workers, the results were less than confirmatory. In one large study of cancer patients in Japan, only breast cancer was cited as being elevated among the female cosmetologists, whereas no excess cancers of any kind were cited for male hairdressers, which could also mean that there are few, if any, male hairdressers in Japan. In a study in Finland which specifically addressed the cancer histories of female (3637) and male (168) hairdressers during 1970–1987, the cancer risks for both sexes were elevated in the first third of the observation period but, strangely, not thereafter. Although higher relative risks were reported for several gynecological types but, inexplicably, *not* breast cancer, only the risk for ovarian cancer was considered to be statistically significant. For the Finnish male hairdressers, lung and pancreatic cancer rates were excessive, but the small numbers in their cohort and apparent lack of corroboration from other studies qualified the risk. For whatever role geography and the uninterrupted work patterns of hairdressers may play in the etiology, the Nordic countries have reported several studies indicating higher risks for bladder cancer with no difference in sex. To add to the equivocal status of association, whereas elevated lung cancer risks were reported among female cosmetologists in Los Angeles, no correlation with their work or use of chemical products in the beauty shop could be established even taking into account their smoking status.

Brain cancers are relatively infrequent and difficult to treat successfully, but perhaps, because of their rarity, occupational health researchers have been intrigued with finding a possible occupational causation. The lay public is no less suspicious should they learn of a brain cancer case at work, but the report of more than one case in the same workplace or locality—which qualifies as a "cluster" of cases—practically constitutes in their minds proof of an association. Although it is generally agreed from the epidemiological studies that an occupational association with brain cancers has not been conclusively established, it has not deterred the quest. Thus, what started as a cluster case report of brain cancers in one rural town in Missouri showed no occupational association. When cascaded into an evaluation of brain cancer deaths in the entire state, the investigators reported significantly higher proportions for the individually listed but overlapping classifications of hairdressers, cosmetologists, and beauty shop workers. But so did the disparate occupations of motor vehicle manufacturers, managers and administrators, and elementary school teachers, but presumably not the junior and senior high faculty.

It would appear from the foregoing that the beauty care professionals may be at some increased risk of certain types of cancer with notable differences in the men and women. Occupational health professionals hope that this reflects the effects of past exposures and practices and that the future occupational cancer risk from the work will be reduced as the result of using safer products and work procedures. It is reasonable to assume that the manufacturers' own screening and compliance with FDA requirements for using only harmless ingredients in cosmetics have practically eliminated carcinogens in the cosmetic products. Exposures have been further reduced in that the beauty workers have become more attuned to the potential health hazards of their work and responsive to the need to use protective gloves and adequate ventilation. Of course, many will continue to smoke, so their elevated lung cancer risk may persist.

It was inevitable that occupational health researchers would investigate reproductive health and related effects in a predominantly female profession with such extensive chemical product contacts. A study of cosmetologists in North Carolina who were pregnant between 1983 and 1988 revealed that those who had worked full time during the first trimester had a 30 percent increased risk of spontaneous abortions compared to pregnant cosmetologists who did other full-time work in the same period. The increased risk was also associated with the weekly number of customers served and the degree of chemical exposures as indicated by the numbers of perms, hair dyes, and bleaches performed daily, the use of formaldehyde products, and nail treatments. There is always some question, however, regarding the findings in this and similar studies in which unverified data are self-reported by only those of the population who respond to a mail survey.

A study of almost fifteen thousand births in Venezuela strongly implicated occupational chemical exposures among seventy-six cases of neural tube defects

(NTD), representing the highest number of all the birth defects seen. Venezuelan women are well known for the fastidious attention given to their grooming and personal appearance, so the numbers of hairdressers in the population may be disproportionately high. Nonetheless, the report that 13.16 percent of all the mothers of NTD cases were hairdressers compared to only 1.32 percent among the mothers of the controls is strongly suggestive of an occupational association. The case for adverse birth effects from cosmetology is hardly settled. A Canadian study investigating 226 stillbirths and the chemical exposures of the mothers at work found that hairdressers had a significant *decreased* risk for stillbirth. Regardless or possibly because of the conflicting reports and the attention in the media, cosmetologists who have had spontaneous abortions, stillborns, children with birth defects, suffer from menstrual disorders, or have difficulty conceiving have come to suspect their chemical exposures at work.

Other health conditions which are not associated with chemical exposures at work have been reported disproportionately among cosmetologists; rather, they suggest the nature of the work or the nature of the worker. In what might imply a socio-economic stratification, it is widely believed that the upper class and the more prosperous white-collar workers are more prone to inflammatory bowel diseases, such as Crohn's disease and ulcerative colitis. In a study of over twelve thousand German workers who suffered sufficiently from a diagnosis of these conditions in 1982 to 1988 to warrant rehabilitation, low rates were predictably confirmed among low-paid blue-collar men working in construction, unskilled labor, and security, and low-paid women working in cleaning and maintenance or those without an occupation. High prevalence rates were unpredictably reported for men working as instrument makers, bakers, electricians, and technical assistants. The female occupations in the high prevalence groups include hairdressers, sales representatives, office workers, and health care. The investigators suggest that working inside with long and irregular shifts may be contributory to the colitis, whereas performing physical exercise in the freedom of the outdoors may be protective.

One long-suffering and skeptical hairdresser had another explanation.

"At times, the work can get pretty stressful for me. I'm sure that's why I got sick because I never had it before."

When asked why she didn't give up the work, she laughed, saying, "I love my work and wouldn't dream of doing anything else."

In an occupational mortality study covering 1979 to 1981 in California, cosmetologists were among female occupations having the highest death rates due to liver cirrhosis which, with the possible exception of bartending, is not usually associated with occupational exposure. Excessive drinking is the most suspect contributor to the disease, but whether the stress of the work causes someone to drink more or the nature of the work attracts people susceptible to cirrhosis bedevils any cause and effect conclusions.

Shared Health Problems

If customers have one subjective health complaint about the atmosphere in the shop, chances are it will have to do with the sometimes overwhelming odors.

"I feel sometimes like I can hardly catch my breath when they spray me," one inveterate female customer woman confessed.

Much of the redolence is, indeed, caused by the generous use of perfumed hair sprays, which help preserve the hairdresser's crowning achievement. The sprays are comprised of finely divided plastic polymers or lacquers dissolved in alcohol which are dispersed as an aerosol by a propellant gas. Even in a well-ventilated shop, because of their proximity to the frequent use of hair sprays throughout the shop, the hairdressers are repeatedly exposed to the airborne volatile chemicals. Some hairdressers report some annoyance or irritation principally from the alcohol vapors; others suspect that they have developed an asthmatic reaction to the spray or that a preexisting asthma condition has been exacerbated, and many just accept or ignore the room pollution. Occasionally, skin problems have been reported from their excessive use at home by consumers.

In response to a request from the owner of a super-size beauty salon for a survey regarding possible respiratory problems among twenty-five full- and part-time cosmetologists, NIOSH confirmed the airborne presence of ethyl alcohol and ammonia (from the alkaline perms), but failed to reveal any significant exposure concentrations of any contaminant based on the allowable workplace limits. Regardless, thirteen employees reported at least two symptoms of asthma, eight of whom ascribed their symptoms to the use of hair care products, principally the hair spray. The use of volatile products, principally hair sprays, in the beauty salon, may be a situation in which respiratory complaints may not be simply defined by compliance with the allowable exposure standards. NIOSH responded with the now standard industrial hygiene advice for dealing with indoor air complaints when the air sampling fails to explain the problem; simply, provide more fresh air.

The sprays may play an exacerbating role in a general health problem for cosmetologists that they share with workers who have close contact with the public, such as hospital and health care workers, dentists and dental technicians, fire fighters, police, and emergency squad personnel. Like habitues of the crowded New York or Tokyo subways, many of these people without benefit of scientific studies are certain that they suffer more colds and respiratory infections from their closely shared breathing spaces. Suspecting that hair sprays may have a drying and irritating effect on the nasal passages, a test on fifteen health volunteers in Sweden demonstrated that inhaling the hair spray significantly reduced the subjects' mucociliary transport mechanism for more than an hour after the exposure. This means that hairdressers and, to some extent, their clients are made even more vulnerable to infections from each other by being denied the normally protective mechanism of nasal secretions and clearance.

The clients may be subject to the same exposures as their cosmetologists but obviously to a much lesser degree and risk, recalling from Paracelsus that the dose makes the poison. Apart from the aforementioned annoyance of being blitzed with hair spray or choked by the blends of perfumes and tobacco smoke, the visits to the salon are often pleasurable and not usually regarded as posing any health and safety hazard to the customer. So said, every cosmetologist and many clients can recount some contradictory episodes.

One woman who had had regular and inviolable Saturday morning appointments for years without apparent incident was suddenly choking and gasping for breath within minutes of getting her hair dyed. A female police officer sitting under an adjacent hair dryer who was accustomed to responding to emergencies recognized symptoms of an asthmatic attack and quickly whisked the woman to the local hospital appropriately with a police escort. The victim claimed she had no prior history of asthma or allergy, but given the possible sensitizers among the multifarious chemical products and the vagaries of an allergic response even among the uninitiated, the improbable was inevitable. When the recovered victim returned to the shop the following weekend for her usual, she characteristically expressed irritation that she was taken to the hospital ". . . looking like such a mess."

The physical hazards to the hairdressers from self-inflicted cuts from scissors and burns from curling irons had been noted, but the customers are normally assumed to be safe. The same police woman and source of the previous incident learned otherwise when she went to the shop for just a hair trim and curling treatment before going on an extended trip to Mexico with her husband. Shortly after the hairdresser began to curl her tresses, her hair was almost set on fire caused by the inadvertent use of an overheated iron and to their mutual and near-tearful consternation, she had to leave with a new—and more closely cut—look.

Summary Thoughts

Any summary reflection on the health risks of the beauty care professionals ineluctably dwells on their inherent chronic skin problems and one must inevitably wonder why the most afflicted among them—a significant minority—tolerate their suffering and remain in the field. The previously cited statistical study of the work health histories with interviews of four hundred plus cosmetologists in the United States in 1982 gives some insight into an apparent dichotomy.

In the personal interviews, whether given during slow periods in the small-town shops in New Jersey or at breaks during the tumult of thousands attending a national meeting of the National Hairdressers and Cosmetologists Association in New York City, the appraisals of their work are invariably full of praise. Terms like “highly rewarding,” “creative and challenging,” and nondescriptively and simply, “the greatest” are the buzz words which precede the invariable conclusion, “I love it. There’s no other work I’d rather do.” These are the same people of whom fully half admit to having had dermatitis attributable to their work and half of those cases persist for weeks, months, or are continuous.

An apparent anomaly emerged from the statistical analysis of the data which plotted the cases of dermatitis as a function of tenure or years on the job, categorized as <5, 5–10, and >10 years. Normally, in industrial hygiene exposure studies one would expect to find the maximum health effects among the highest exposure group, which in this case implies those longest on the job. In this study, the occurrence of dermatitis was—perversely—inverse with the total time on the job. In fact, there was a significant drop in incidence among the longer-term veterans. At the lower end, a temporary high incidence of skin problems among the youngest practitioners might be expected because they often get the heavy-duty assignment with shampoos, they may not take the proper precautionary care, and, as some people believe, unlike the veterans, their tender skin has not yet been inured. It seems perfectly reasonable to conclude that the reason that the numbers of cases of dermatitis drop with tenure on the job is due to occupational dropouts. The cosmetologists with the most persistent and severe cases of dermatitis, who in the study were shown to account for 10–20 percent of their members, simply have to leave the profession.

What about the majority who continue to suffer occasional skin problems and justifiably have serious concerns about the long-term health effects from their chemical exposures? Rare among the work force today, they proudly remain as the willing assumers of the risks of their profession.

Chapter 2

The Fire Fighters

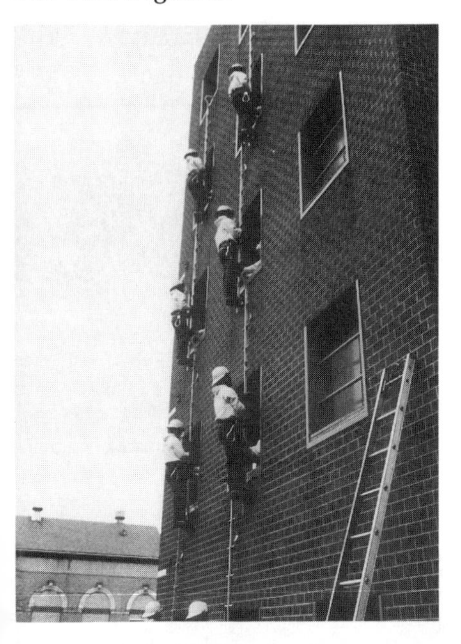

Left: Rookie firefighters in a training exercise at the Philadelphia Fire Academy are first gingerly introduced to ladder climbing and building entry, unencumbered with boots and heavy equipment.

Below: Fully-equipped with helmets, boots, heavy duty coveralls, and self-contained breathing apparatus (SCBA), which weigh up to 70 pounds, the trainees in a four-member crew practice raising a 35 foot ladder.

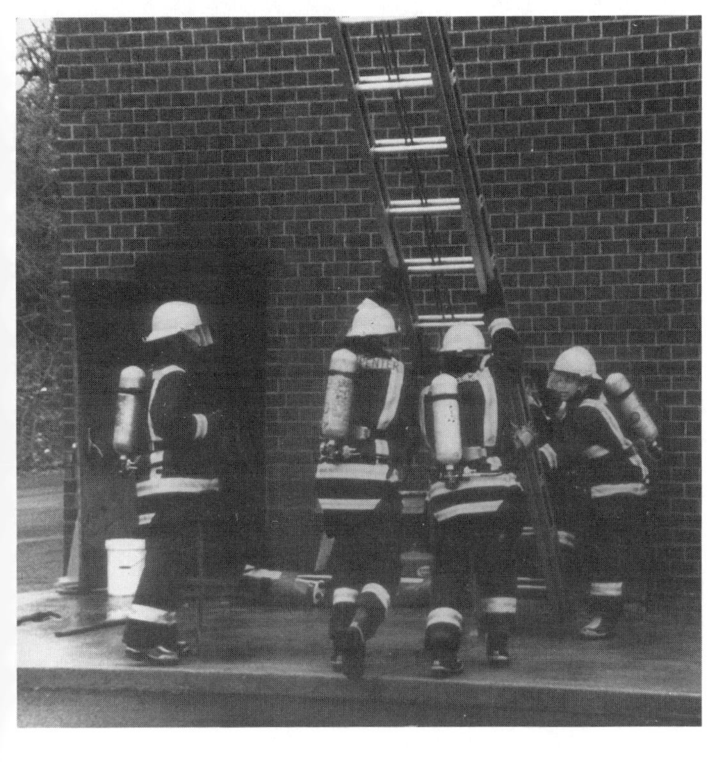

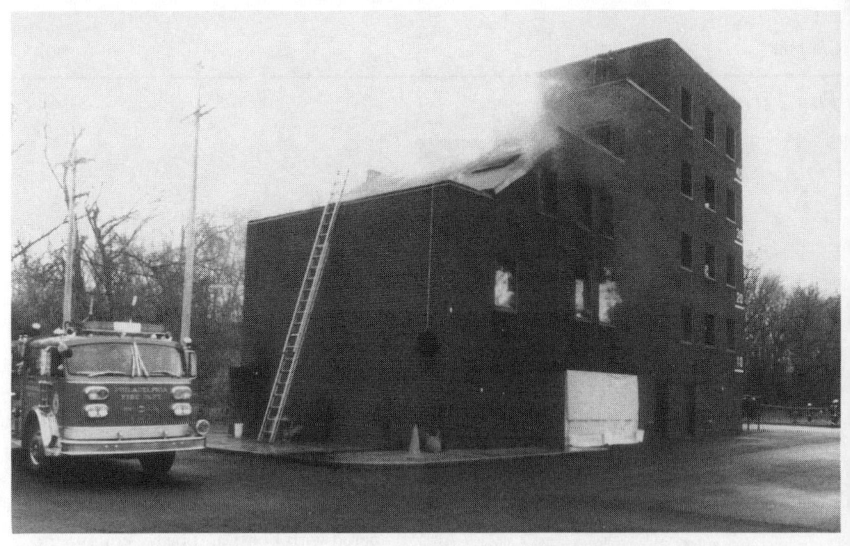

Fire conditions encountered in urban high rises and multiple dwellings are simulated in a training test facility at the Fire Academy.

No longer practicing, a city fire fighter directs a hand-held water hose toward the entrance of an enflamed city warehouse under the watchful eye of his lieutenant.

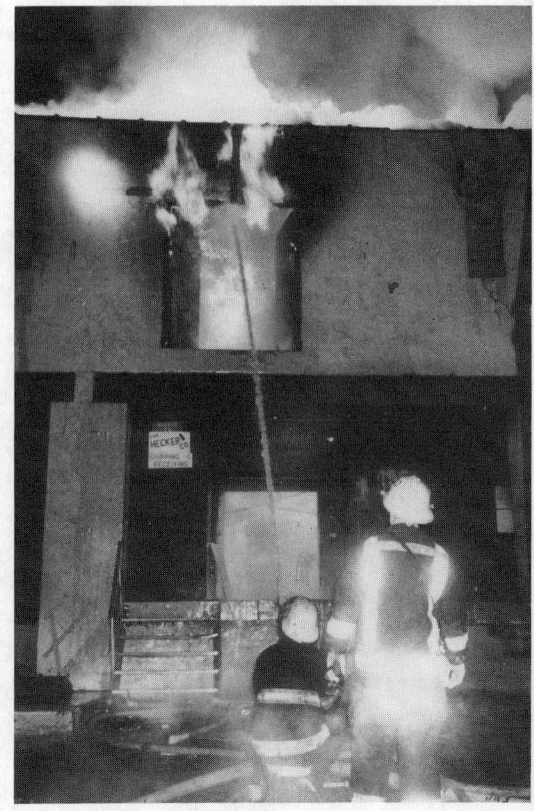

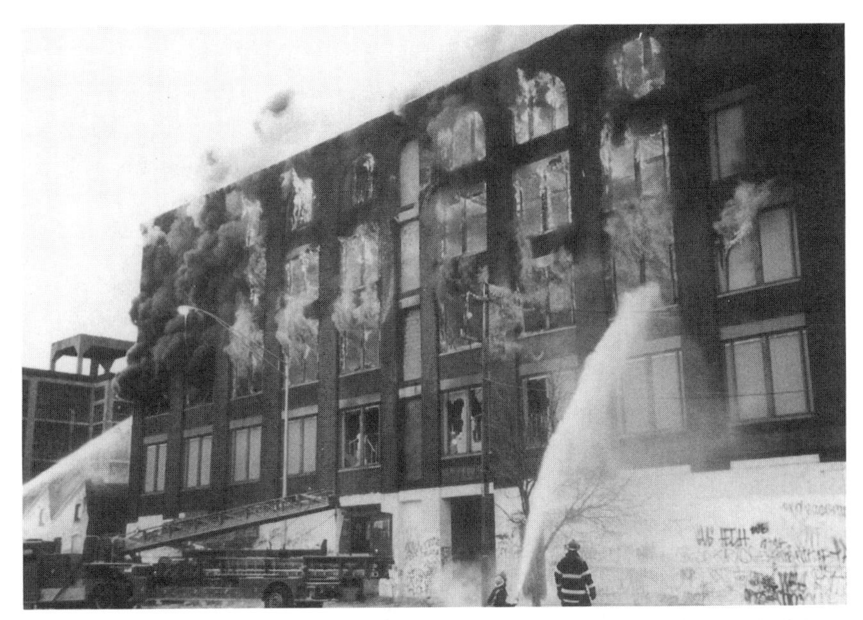

The members from four fire stations with approximately twenty pieces of major firefighting equipment were pressed into service in response to this four alarm fire at a storage warehouse in Philadelphia. At this advanced stage of the fire, the firefighters can only contain the spread of the conflagration from the outside with a barrage of water termed "surround and drown."

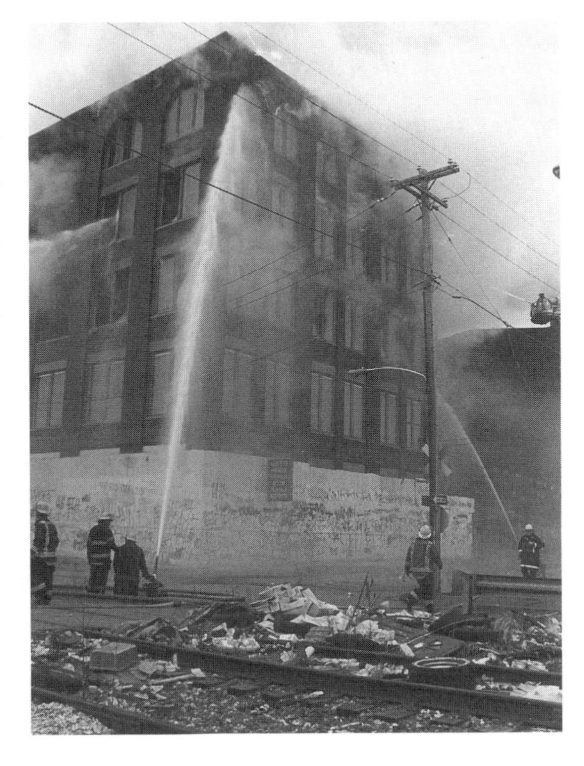

On an adjacent side of the same warehouse, water spray is delivered by a firefighter in an aerial lift (upper right.) Note the accumulation of trash and tires in the foreground, the ignition of which accounts for the most frequent type of fire call for most big city fire departments

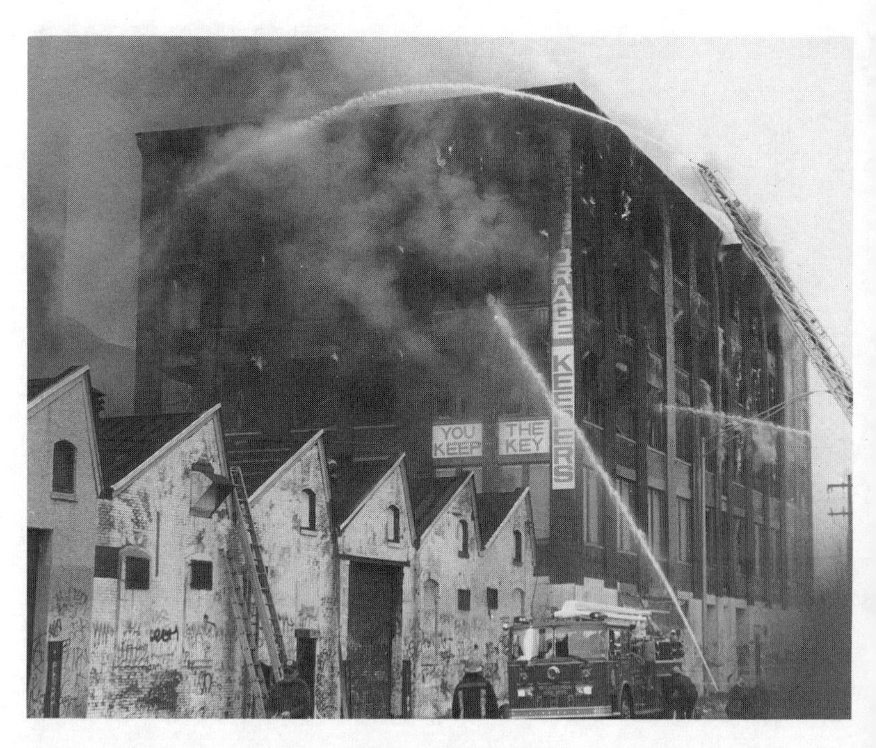

The near-empty warehouse fire was quickly brought under control as indicated by the reduction in flames and smoke.

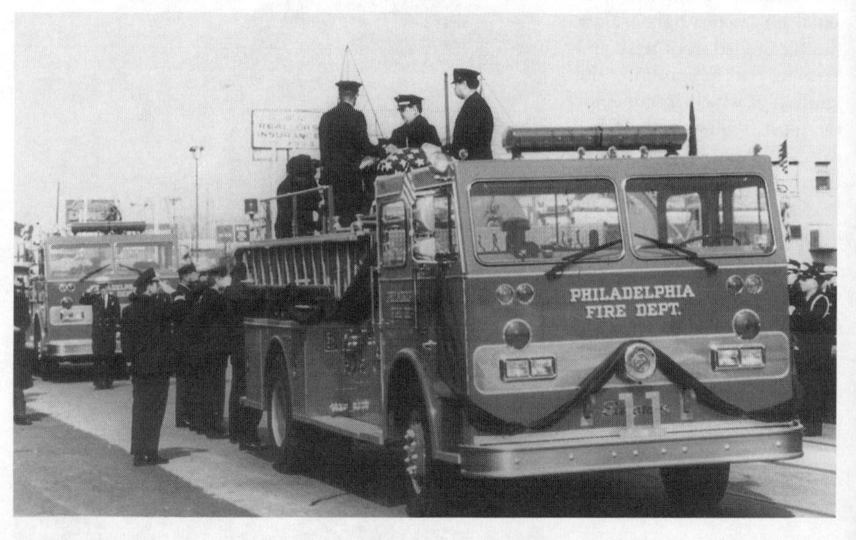

Virtually unique among the civilian work force, the deep professional bonding shared by fire fighters is no more dramatically demonstrated than at this funeral of a Philadelphia fire fighter killed in the line of duty. Members of fire departments from all over the state and country joined the victim's colleagues to pay their respects.

Credits: Photographs provided by Philadelphia Fire Department

Chapter 2

The Fire Fighters

The classic Jack London short story, *To Build A Fire,* depicts one man's lone battle to survive in the frigid Alaskan wilderness. A prospector, attempting to warm himself by making a fire en route to his base camp before dark, panics when his fingers have been immobilized by the seventy-five degrees below zero temperature and he is unable to strike a match. He desperately considers sacrificing his Alaskan husky companion for the animal's life-sustaining warm blood, but his paralyzed hands cannot release or hold his sheathed knife. That the animal is able to return to the base camp instinctively and survive whereas man succumbs to the forces of nature is vintage Jack London, but the tale also dramatically illustrates the primordial dependency of man on fire.

From the time that man learned to make and use fire, he also suffered from its afflictions. His possessions and housing often went up with the smoke from an accidental fire and sometimes in attempting to fight or flee from the flames, he would suffer from burns, choking, heat, and absolute panic. Small wonder that the torments from flame play a prominent role in Dante's descriptive tour of the circles of hell in the *Divina Comedia.* The home fires are also the original source of indoor and outdoor air pollution from human activities. It is not too farfetched to imagine some cave dweller having awakened with a bad headache—or just not awakening—due to carbon monoxide poisoning or lack of oxygen from a poorly ventilated fireplace.

Whether singed and choked by the experience of fighting a fire or not, it is difficult for most of us to believe that men and women would knowingly and willingly earn their livelihood by routinely facing such physical dangers and threats to their health. And yet that is exactly what career fire fighters do.

The Fire Fighters' Lot

There is probably no other job with a more consistently high incidence of injury, a higher line-of-duty death rate, and higher and regular exposures to toxic contaminants than fire fighters. Consequently, the occupational health sleuths have expended a lot of time and effort investigating their health and safety problems. There have been several doctoral dissertations and many research studies on the subject as evidenced by a recent literature search limited to the previous ten years which produced well over a hundred citations in the scientific journals. Hundreds of related articles and reports appear annually in the more popular fire-fighting and trade journals or are presented before the well-attended national meetings of professional and trade associations. There also are over a million volunteer fire fighters and firehouse groupies all across the United States who regularly share their fire-fighting experiences and information at weekly meetings. Judging by the popularity of such intensely dramatic and realistic films as *Backdraft* and *Towering Inferno* and the genre of books recounting the heroic exploits of actual fire fighters spawned by Dennis Smith's best selling *Report from Engine Co. 82*, even the general public has become more aware of the hazards of their job.

From their own formal training and experiences, fire fighters have a clear sense of the *health* risks from their work. This is certainly true with respect to the *acute* physical injuries—the burns, falls, cuts, fractures, and heat exhaustion—which they know more about than any researcher could tell them. To a similar degree, they are aware of the dangers from oxygen deprivation and inhaling smoke and carbon monoxide and, yet, when seen hacking their way into a burning building, they appear to be macho "smoke eaters" who are seemingly oblivious of any hazards to themselves. Their primary objective is to put out that fire as quickly and safely as possible and therein lies some of the conflict—virtually unique among occupational exposures—between assuming risks and avoiding personal injury. For example, there are some fires in buildings—the fire fighting manual and department policy may say, all—which require a fire fighter to wear respiratory protection. The breathing mask and air tank are heavy, restrictive to vision, and, if not essential, interfere with the ability to fight the fire. Whether there is the need or the time to don the mask—or whether to enter a room where the ceiling or floors may soon collapse—are judgment calls that often allow scant time to judge.

Notwithstanding the fire fighters' drive to extinguish the blaze in the face of many dangers, there is little question of their priorities in a residential fire; it is foremost to save lives, and that often preempts concern for their own personal risks. One revealing psychological study indicated that their highest-ranked occupational stressor was the report of children in a burning building. Such is the power of this life-saving commitment that psychological and emotional counseling are now considered essential to deal with the feelings of guilt and depression following a rescue attempt or fire call which failed to save a trapped resident—especially a child—or resulted in the death of a fellow fire fighter.

Industrial hygienists have concentrated on measuring and evaluating the sources and exposures during actual or simulated fire fighting with the practical goal of improving the protection for the firefighters. Do the respirators worn provide sufficient protection from the toxic levels of smoke and carbon monoxide that are likely to be encountered? Are there special health hazards in fighting a fire with new-age chemicals and products such as a transformer spilling over with polychlorinated biphenyls (PCBs), a warehouse filled with plastic sheets of polyvinyl chloride vinyl (PVC), or at a waste dump with a mountain of burning used rubber tires? There are also health concerns about the intense heat stress, hearing loss from the blare of the sirens, and even the biological hazards of giving mouth-to-mouth resuscitation during rescue operations.

The long-term health effects studies from the cumulative inhalation of smoke and toxic gases, the intense physical and emotional stresses of the work, and even, to some extent, their unusual work schedules and way of life in the firehouse are less evident. The fire fighters themselves intuit that they do not live as long as other workers and believe that they have more heart and breathing problems, but the information is largely anecdotal and limited to their acquaintances. However, it is a subject that they do not dwell on or care to discuss. Because of their inordinately high workplace hazards and the very special nature of their dedication and risk-taking, fire fighters are distinctive among the work force. This account of the health and safety hazards of being a fire fighter starts with the source of their raison d'être.

The Making and Nature of Fires

A fire is a self-sustaining chemical reaction involving the rapid oxidation of a fuel with oxygen, usually from the air, with the release of heat and light. For the reaction to occur, the fuel must be heated to its ignition temperature and be provided with sufficient oxygen. If these conditions are met, the combustion can be triggered by a source of ignition. More insidiously, if the temperature is sufficiently high, a fire can spontaneously erupt at the autoignition temperature of the fuel without a flame or spark. The most commonly used fuels are comprised mainly of carbon, such as coal, oil, and wood, but man learned to burn whatever was readily available and did the job. Eskimos have survived by burning the oil from whale and seal blubber and in many third world countries even today, dried animal dung serves as the principal fuel for heating and cooking to the detriment of local agricultural needs for fertilizer.

If the fuel burns completely, the oxygen is consumed producing predominantly carbon dioxide and water. Thus, a burning candle placed inside a sealed jar will soon consume the available oxygen and will be extinguished. In some open building fires, there is enough air sucked in by thermal drafts to support a fire, but in an enclosed building, the amount is often insufficient. Smoldering results in forming smoke and toxic gaseous products of incomplete combustion, most notably carbon monoxide. There are several insidious conditions at a fire scene that can create cataclysmic hazards for the fire fighters.

A fire inside a structure often starts slowly with smoldering furniture or a rug, as a high transfer of heat is required to cause most solid materials to be ignited and continue burning. The fire growth becomes exponential as the temperature rises. In the case of a smoldering structure, the heat produced in an enclosure gradually raises the temperature throughout the entire space to its autoignition temperature at which point, as long as there is sufficient oxygen present, an instantaneous fire, or *flashover* can engulf the area. In the case of an oxygen-deficient area, a fire fighter opening the front door or breaking into the building can unwittingly provide the necessary oxygen by the inward rush of air, or *backdraft* to cause an immediate conflagration. In both cases of flashback and backdraft, the instantaneous inferno that erupts makes escape or entry virtually impossible.

There is also a subset of unusual and often unknown dangers from fires involving hazardous materials—now familiarly called hazmats. These may involve fires of marked or unmarked chemical waste drums, radioactive materials, or cylinders of compressed explosive gases. In short, a fire fighter entering an enclosed burning structure with or without respiratory protection may be entering an occupational death chamber.

In the outside world, large-scale conflagrations such as from forest fires or in metropolitan areas of concentrated bombing attacks during warfare have sometimes created a colossal meteorological bellows that spreads the fire faster than it is humanly possibly to contain. The heated gases from such wide-base fires rise in a huge plume creating a chimneylike effect which sucks in air in a rapid whirling motion from the periphery at the base of the fire. This huge fanning of the fire literally produces a *fire storm*. In October 1871, what began as a local forest fire outside the small town of Peshtigo, Wisconsin, exponentially expanded into a fire storm which totally destroyed the town and caused the deaths of 1181 residents and fire fighters.

The Unmaking of Fire

Fire can be extinguished by controlling any one of the three critical factors necessary for combustion—fuel, heat, and oxygen. A fire can be contained by removing or shutting off the fuel from the flame, for example, by closing the valve of a gas line, or letting the burning fuel self-destruct in a safe area. A wastepaper basket which catches fire from a smoldering cigarette might be tossed out the window onto a snowy field, but the options for such actions are, at best, limited and often not well advised. Sometimes, as in fighting a forest fire, one section of the fire will be allowed to burn itself out while the fire-fighting efforts are directed toward containment and preventing further spreading. More practically, the fire fighter works on the other two factors: suffocating the fire by cutting off the essential oxygen or by cooling the fuel to a temperature that will not support combustion.

A blanket quickly thrown over a small fire or wrapped around a victim with burning clothing smothers the fire by restricting the replenishment of the oxygen. Because carbon dioxide gas is noncombustible and heavier than air, it, too, can displace the oxygen when it is released from a pressurized fire extinguisher over a fire. However, if the blanket of carbon dioxide gas is dissipated by air currents and the smoldering fuel is hot enough, the fire will reignite.

The alternative approach to oxygen exclusion is to reduce the temperature of the burning material to below its kindling temperature and the easiest and cheapest way to do this is to douse the fire with water. When applied to a burning or heated surface, the water rapidly absorbs the heat by its conversion into steam. The steam and excess water also provide some degree of cover over the burning surface, combining suffocation with cooling.

Fires of solid carbonaceous materials such as wood, paper, furniture, rubber, plastics, and textiles are termed Class A fires and are most often extinguished by water. To provide ongoing fire protection internally, many buildings and multiple residences are equipped with automatic water sprinkler systems on the ceilings which are activated by thermocouple sensors, smoke detectors, or, most commonly, low-melting metal links. Cities which have enacted ordinances requiring the installation of sprinkler systems in all high-rise buildings or multiple dwellings have seen a dramatic reduction in major fires and fire deaths.

Fires involving combustible liquids such as fuel oil and flammable gases like propane are classified as Class B fires. Water alone is generally not effective in putting out these fires and may actually cause the fire to spread. Small Class B fires can be extinguished with the carbon dioxide extinguisher or with the dry-chemical extinguishers. In certain buildings, ships, or storage areas where there may be large quantities of flammable liquids and gases, ongoing fire protection may be provided by the release of carbon dioxide gas from overhead piping analogous to the water sprinkler system. Because flooding the room with carbon dioxide will displace the oxygen in the breathing air to levels immediately hazardous to life, an audible alarm first gives the occupants sufficient time to evacuate the premises before the gas is released. In one case on a naval vessel, a failure in the alarm system tragically caused the suffocation deaths of crew members who were rapidly overcome by the anoxic conditions.

Fires which originate from live electrical power lines or equipment are classified as Class C fires in that they preclude the application of electrically conducting extinguishing agents like water and depend on electrically nonconducting agents such as carbon dioxide gas or dry-chemical powders. Otherwise fearless but savvy fire fighters admit to having qualms about facing live wires on the fire scene.

The rare Class D fire involves certain combustible metals such as magnesium, titanium, and sodium which require extinguishment with an agent which does not react with the metal such as specially formulated chemical powders.

Structure fires largely involve Class A materials and are routinely attacked with water delivered from high-pressure pumps at about two hundred gallons per minute (gpm) from hand-held hose lines. If the building is already ablaze, the firefighters will often "surround and drown" the fire from the outside utilizing larger semiportable or truck-mounted pumps delivering 1000 gpm or more. The largest metropolitan fire departments virtually have a water cannon with a maximum delivery of 10,000 gpm through mammoth four-and-a-half-inch hoses.

Although the high-powered water hose is the principal weapon for suppressing most fires, some innovative ways have been devised to fight unusually difficult and dangerous fires such as large gasoline or oil storage tanks adjacent to dozens of other tanks on a tank farm, which most fire fighters would be loath to approach. Through piping built in at the base, an aqueous foam solution is injected into the tank through an aspirating device to form a blanket of foam on the burning surface to exclude oxygen and, thereby, extinguish the fire.

Because combustion is a chemical reaction, it was inevitable that an attack based on chemistry would be developed. Combustion involves the formation of charged particles called "free radicals" which are highly reactive atoms or molecules which have at least one unshared electron in the outer orbit. These charged particles, in turn, activate other atoms or molecules in a chain reaction with such astounding speed that their half-lives, or time for half of their numbers to form and then disappear, is only 10^{-5} second, or a ten-millionth of a second. In combustion, the oppositely charged radicals of fuel and oxygen are attached and react instantaneously. It was discovered that special dry-chemical powders such as potassium hydrogen carbonate and ammonium dihydrogen phosphate will snuff out a fire by interrupting the chain-reaction process. These dry-chemical agents will extinguish Class A and B fires, and certain members, such as ammonium dihydrogen phosphate, also do not conduct electricity and are, therefore, termed "multipurpose" for extinguishing Class A, B, and C fires.

It was similarly discovered that the vapors of certain nonflammable halogenated hydrocarbons—identified by the trademark name of Halons—released into the fire zone could rapidly interrupt the free-radical formation and extinguish the fire at concentrations as low as 5 percent by volume in the atmosphere. Although breathing these vapors may cause cardiac effects like arrthymias in some individuals, the Halons have relatively low human toxicity at the suppression level. In a fire situation where neatness counts, the Halons are particularly attractive in that unlike water and dry-chemical sprays, they cause and leave no mess. Assuming that serious fire damage has been thwarted, computers, delicate electronic and laboratory instruments, computer records, and paper files would be spared the usual fire-fighting onslaught of water drenching or dry chemicals. Unfortunately, these halogenated hydrocarbons are believed to contribute to the destruction of the ozone layer in the stratosphere where their eventual fate as air pollutants would lead them. By an international agreement, they can no longer be manufactured and used for fire extinguishment, but this innovative chemical approach to fire fighting may lead to a more environmentally acceptable successor.

Fire-retardant chemicals, usually containing phosphorus or boron, have been developed which are incorporated in normally combustible materials such as textiles and plastics. It is believed that these key elements in the fire-retardant composition convert the smoldering material into a nonburning char that does what fire extinguishers are supposed to do: it provides an oxygen and heat cover. The retardant-treated material is not rendered noncombustible; rather, it is made more difficult to burn by increasing its kindling temperature. The wide use of fire retardants has unquestionably saved lives and cut down on the number of fire calls for the fire fighters, but there were some indications that in an intense fire, certain phosphorus-based fire retardants will emit unusually toxic thermal decomposition products.

The Emergence of Volunteer Fire Fighting

Benjamin Franklin wrote a paper on the accidental causes of fire and suggested means for their prevention which led to his organization of the Union Fire Company in Philadelphia in 1736 as the first volunteer fire-fighting company in the American colonies. The convivial thirty member company met monthly to exchange useful information about fire fighting and in short order, new applicants eager to join the popular company spawned the formation of other fire companies throughout the city enrolling most of the property owners. Franklin records in his autobiography that, "The small fines that have been paid by members for absence at the monthly meetings have been apply'd to the purchase of fire-engines, ladders, fire-hooks and other useful implements for each company, so that I question whether there is a city in the world better provided with the means of putting a stop to beginning conflagration; and in fact, since these institutions, the city has never lost more than one or two houses at a time, and the flames have often been extinguished before the house in which they began were half consumed."

In 1752, Franklin founded the first fire insurance company in Philadelphia and, subsequently, the various insurance companies would pay the volunteer fire company which responded to their client's fire. Consequently, each insurance companies had a distinctive wrought iron or lead marker about a foot high with the company symbol such as the four clasped hands for the Hand in Hand Company or an eagle or green tree. Sometimes, competing fire companies eager for the compensation fought each other before responding to the fire. A fire at an uninsured colonial row house was not, however, ignored as much for self-interest as a community service.

As long as Philadelphia and the other colonial cities remained as large towns relatively free from the urban congestion brought on by the later Industrial Revolution, Franklin's sanguine comments about fire-fighting protcction may have been justified. Nonetheless, Franklin anticipated the need to fireproof his own home specifying that, "None of the wooden work of one room communicate with the wooden work of any other room; and all floors, and even the steps of the stairs, are plastered close under the joints," adding that as he had observed in Paris, it would even be better if the stairways were stone, the floor tiled, and the roof covered with either tile or slate.

By the first half of the nineteenth century, the fire-fighting methods of bucket brigades, often dependent on nearby rivers and streams for their water supply, were already inadequate to protect the rapidly growing cities. In 1835, one massive fire in New York City destroyed an estimated five hundred buildings. Not only were the fire-fighting equipment and methods lacking, but there was also scant dedication and will from the fire fighters. In Philadelphia and other large cities, the wholly volunteer and independent fire companies evolved into highly polarized ethnic and political associations whose enmities severely compromised their members' fire-fighting missions. For the residents of a burning houses, there was little luck to the draw. In 1849, the Irish Catholic and Democratic Moyamensing Hose Company in Philadelphia joined up with the aptly named Killers gang to set four fires and ambush the rival Native American Shiffler Hose Company responding to the call.

The Tolls from Fire

Up until the second half of the nineteenth century, most cities in the United States continued to rely on the volunteer fire companies which were just beginning to be centralized. Salaried fire departments were instituted in the cities in the early 1870s, but the equipment, methods, and knowledge of fire fighting were once again woefully inadequate to contain the fire threats of the sprawling metropolises. Without a building and zoning code to help prevent fires, Chicago was virtually destroyed by its great fire in 1871 which caused 250 deaths and an estimated property loss of the then enormous sum of 196 million dollars.

By the mid-twentieth-century, the number of fires and the extent of fire damage in the cities was greatly reduced by the adoption of municipal building codes and insurance requirements which promoted the use of concrete, steel, and brick in lieu of wood in construction, building inspections for eliminating the potential for fires, and more sophisticated fire-fighting methods with automotive fire trucks and improved equipment and personal protection. On the debit side, the new age had to cope with fires from faulty electrical wiring, careless smokers, dilapidated and deserted housing, factories and warehouses in the urban centers, and the extensive use of plastics. Sometimes, intentional fires set for land clearing or for the open burning of trash resulted in desperate calls to fire companies. Less benevolently, the aerial incendiary bombing perfected during modern warfare produced the greatest man-man destruction by fire in history. Arson committed for insurance fraud, revenge, or malice, and the mindless torching of woodlands and property by pyromaniacs are simply more recent and malevolent contributions to man's toll of deaths, injuries, and huge property loss from intentional fires.

In terms of lives lost from fires, the most devastating events have been associated with the concentration of large numbers of people in an enclosed area. In what may have been the largest recorded loss of life under one roof, 1670 died in a theater fire in Canton, China in 1845. Theater fires in Vienna in 1881 and in Chicago in 1903 accounted for 850 and 602 fatalities, respectively. The crowded theaters were particularly vulnerable from the uninhibited smoking of the audience amidst so much combustible materials. The heavy cloth curtain often surrounded by flickering gas stage lights, in particular, drew the attention of the fire-wary. With the availability of asbestos textiles by the early twentieth century, many theaters installed fireproof asbestos curtains, often prominently bearing an identifying label, which became a familiar symbol to the patron anxiously awaiting the start of the show.

In more recent times, multiple deaths resulted from fires in night clubs, most notably the Boston Cocanut Grove fire in 1942 which claimed 491 lives. There was speculation that some of the victims succumbed to the inhalation of toxic decomposition products, principally oxides of nitrogen, from the highly flammable nitrocellulose decorations. A tabulation of the modern world's most notable fires includes such high-density locations and activities as nursing homes and hospitals, army barracks, circuses, churches, jails, schools, department stores, hotels, boarding houses, and even the London subway. In a one-of-a-kind event, fifty-three fans died in a fire at a soccer stadium in England in 1985.

With the exception of massive explosions and subsequent fires at munitions plants and storage areas, gas and oil pipelines, coal mines, and chemical plants, the human toll from industrial fires in modern times has usually been lower than in public buildings. This is mostly due to the much lower density of people at work and, in part, to greater anticipation, preparedness, and response to fires in the workplace. Most multiple deaths from workplace fires have been the result of virtually criminal violations of safety practices by company management such as having locked or no emergency exits, no sprinkler systems or fire detectors, or simply having no fire protection plans or employee education and training. For just such reasons, 25 employees died in a fire in a North Carolina chicken-processing plant in 1991, and 213 workers were trapped and died in possibly the highest human toll at a workplace fire in modern times in a toy factory in Bangkok, Thailand, in 1994.

Because knowledge of fire prevention and fire fighting is a standard requirement for employers with well-established fire hazards, OSHA has cited management for failure to have acted knowledgeably and responsibly in fire-related episodes where workers died or were put at unnecessary risk. Government agencies, no less than the private sector, are held accountable. An OSHA investigation of the 1994 forest fire near Glenwood Springs, California, in which an unprecedented fourteen fire fighters from federal agencies were trapped and died alleged that the respective managements were guilty of willful and serious violations demonstrating ". . . plain indifference to the safety and health of their employees." Specifically, OSHA faulted management for failing to provide the fire fighters with weather forecasts, the expected fire behavior, and the location of safety zones and escape routes that could have averted the tragedy.

That the numbers of fires and civilian deaths from building and forest fires have been drastically reduced in more recent times is variably attributable to the improved fire-fighting equipment and methods, the use of noncombustible and fire-retardant materials in construction, enforcement of the building codes, the widespread installation of smoke detectors and sprinkler systems, and the inspection of buildings for fire prevention. Preempting any complacency, the United States has consistently led the developed nations in the per capita numbers of property fires and dollar losses. Arguably, the critical key to the prevention and containment of damage and loss of life from fires to date has been the development of highly trained professional fire fighters and fire inspectors whose dedication to their work and each other is unparalleled among public service workers.

The Career Fire Fighters

Inasmuch as fires can break out in the cities, in the rural and wooded areas, at home, at work, on the roads and streets, at sea, and in the air, each locale requires its own organization of fire fighters to respond. There are many more volunteer and paid-on-call fire fighters in the suburbs, small towns and cities, and rural areas than there are paid career fire fighters. However, the greatest and most diverse fire-fighting challenges and tolls on the fire fighters are clearly in the larger cities. This is reflected in the distribution of the approximately 100,000 fire fighter injuries reported annually in the United States. Based on a 1992 National Fire Protection Association (NFPA) survey of fire departments, the average number of injuries and injuries per department requiring hospitalization for all types of duty rises disproportionately higher with the population of the community served (Table 1).

In 1992, the public fire departments in the United States responded to almost two million fires, or, on average, 1 every 3.74 minutes throughout the year with a property damage estimated by the National Fire Protection Association of $8.295 billion. There is a distinction between responding to an alarm and actually fighting a fire which requires an explanation to appreciate the varieties of challenges that the fire fighters in major cities face when the alarm of ear-shattering intensity goes off in the station house.

In 1993 and 1994, the Philadelphia Fire Department responded to approximately ninety thousand local alarms annually, or about one for every eighteen residents. Approximately two-thirds of these calls are classified as "first responder" or "emergency services." Perhaps fated by their past successes, it is to the local fire department that many local citizens immediately call for help in *any* emergency. This includes extricating the victims from vehicle accidents, diving under a river for a drowning child, safeguarding a neighborhood with downed live wires, retrieving the family cat from the upper branches of a tree, and responding to a medical emergency.

Fire fighters have traditionally been trained to give first aid, but recently, many in the large city departments have received advanced training to handle medical emergencies until relieved by the more professionally trained Emer-

Table 1. Fire Fighter Injuries per Department and Community Population Served (1992)

Community Population	Average Number of Fire Fighter Injuries	Average Number of Hospitalized Injuries
500,000 to 999,000	352.14	16.78
250,000 to 499,000	124.00	4.29
100,000 to 249,000	65.87	7.49
50,000 to 99,000	28.52	1.21
25,000 to 49,000	11.24	0.46
10,000 to 24,999	3.43	0.26
5,000 to 9,999	1.68	0.19
2,500 to 4,999	1.08	0.14
Less than 2,500	0.43	0.04

gency Medical Services (EMS) or, in some cases, to act in their stead. In New York City, partly in response to budgetary problems and partly because fire fighters routinely respond to an emergency in about four minutes, or half the time it takes the EMS personnel, there are plans to merge the two services. Some department members are resentful and complain they chose to be fire fighters to do just that; others, particularly the younger department members, welcome the challenge.

About 8 percent of the alarms in Philadelphia were "recalled" meaning that the services of the company called were not required in that there was no fire or it had already been put out. Fortunately, only 10 percent of the calls were intentional false alarms, down considerably after the street fire alarm boxes had been removed.

It is somewhat startling to learn that the remainder, or only one in six "fire" alarms, involved an actual fire and required the fire-fighting services of the station called. These fires are classified as structure or nonstructure and are broken down by the type and number of alarms in 1993 as shown in Table 2, derived from the City of Philadelphia Fire Department Perfomance Report.

City fire fighters respond to more than twice as many calls to put out a trash fire on the streets, in dumpsters, or in vacant lots than to structure fires and there are even slightly more calls to extinguish a burning vehicle than an occupied dwelling. The public commonly assumes that serious fire-fighting action is confined to the structure fires, which constitute only about 3.5 percent of all the alarms. Experienced firefighters have learned to expect the unexpected with *any* fire. On March 28, 1994, three New York City firefighters lost their lives responding to a trash fire.

False or true alarm, structure or nonstructure fire, medical emergency or fire call, when fire fighters with full protective gear leave the station to answer the call, their pulse rates and risks of serious injury or death shoot up in tandem.

Table 2. Classification of Fire Department Alarms in Philadelphia (1993)

Structure Fires	Alarms	Nonstructures	Alarms
Residential, single occupancy	1,561	Rubbish	6,933
Residence, multiple occupancy	589	Vehicle	3,535
Vacant	541	Brush or grass	1,327
Nonresidential assembly	224	Other	589
Mercantile	108		
Storage/special property	88		
Undetermined/unknown	77		
Manufacturing	3		
Total, structure	3,191	Total, nonstructure	12,384

Getting Hurt and Killed on the Job: The Numbers Game

Most fire fighters are either employees of local governmental agencies or unpaid volunteers and are not covered by OSHA; therefore, their employers are not required to record their occupational injuries and illnesses. As a further limit to comparisons with the national work force, fire fighters are not included in the U.S. Bureau of Labor Statistics (BLS) annual surveys of *lost-time* occupational injuries and illnesses which are based on a sampling of 250,000 establishments representing approximately 92 million workers (as of 1993) in private industry. The data we do have on fire fighters have largely been obtained from surveys of both career and volunteer fire departments by the NFPA and from a special program for that purpose administered by the United States Fire Administration (USFA) in conjunction with NIOSH and NFPA. Additional statistics have been amassed by the large city fire departments which characterize the distinctive hazards and non-fire-fighting activities of the municipal fire fighters.

As with most statistics, the numbers do not tell the whole story. Comparisons of relative hazards are difficult to make between fire fighters and all other workers, and between the volunteer and the career departments. For example, whereas the BLS survey of private industry only reports clearly defined lost-time injuries or illnesses (i.e., those serious enough to prevent the individual from performing usual duties at work), the report of a fire-fighter injury to the NFPA does not stipulate the degree of such injury, particularly with the volunteer departments. Then, the gross numbers of injuries and deaths reported do not mean much if we do not know the precise population they represent and their total time at risk; in other words, their incidence rates. For example, full-time fire fighters in a city spend a lot more time fighting fires than the rotating part-time volunteers in a suburban company who usually hold down full-time jobs elsewhere.

Finally, almost half of the NFPA reported injuries and deaths of fire fighters did not involve actual fireground activities. The president of one suburban volunter company with seventy-five active members could not recall a single serious injury of a volunteer fighting a fire and confessed that their most significant injuries involved road accidents from hot-rod respondents who never made it to the station. On reflection, he added that a former fire chief had died from a heart attack shortly after a fire call in which he had driven the fire truck but was not actually engaged in fighting the fire. Other injuries and deaths have been included in the NFPA report that happened during nonfire emergency responses and training. Although these events are clearly related to fire fighting, they do not represent the hazards of the actual fire fighting and have to be evaluated accordingly.

Whatever qualifications are made of the data, there is little doubt after reviewing the numbers and experiences that in ranking the dangerous trades, fire fighters are at the top of the ladder.

DEATHS

According to the Analysis Report on Fire Fatalities by the NFPA in 1994, the number of on-duty fire-fighter deaths has been on a generally downward trend from a high of 171 in 1978 to 78 in 1993. Slightly less than half of the fatalities (44.2 percent) in 1993 occurred on the fire ground, whereas most of the remaining non-fire-fighting deaths happened in accidents getting to or from the alarm (26.6 percent). Heart attacks have consistently been the leading cause of fire-fighter deaths which correlates with overexertion as being the largest single contributing factor to causing a fire-fighter's injury. About 40 percent of the heart attack fatalities in 1993 had a prior medical history of cardiac disease or predisposing medical conditions. Physical trauma including internal injuries and crushing accounted for a third of the deaths followed, in order, by burns, asphyxiation, electrocution, and—indicative of the recent wave in workplace fatalities—gunshot wounds. In previous years, there have been deaths from drowning, bleeding, stroke, and pulmonary embolism.

The NIOSH statisticians using the death certificates provided by the National Traumatic Occupational Fatalities surveillance system have calculated that during 1980–1989, the average annual occupational fatality rate from all causes for all *private industry* workers was 7.0 per 100,000 workers with a high of 31.91 per 100,000 for the top-ranked mining industry. By 1994, the average fatality rate had dropped to about 5 per 100,000, and because the annual number of fire-fighter deaths has dropped significantly during the same period, it is likely that their death rate has also decreased. Once again, it is difficult to make a rate comparison with other dangerous jobs, and between career and volunteer fire fighters without knowing precisely the populations from which the numbers are drawn and their at-risk time.

It would be rare for the largest city fire departments to experience no deaths of firefighters on the job in the course of a year. The tolls for individual fire departments are often high, highly variable, and episodic. In his book, *Report From Engine Co. 82*, Dennis Smith wrote that, on average, eight New York City firefighters out of a force of twelve thousand died annually in the years before 1972, an occupational death rate which is still more than double any other industry then or since. The use of an "average" to represent the expected number of firefighter deaths in a year even for a city as large as New York becomes meaningless when in one year, twelve fire fighters died there from a *single* fire. Similarly, Pittsburgh with about one-twentieth the population of New York and a fire department of slightly less than nine hundred full-time members suffered three deaths in one catastrophic fire alone in February 1995. Just about every career fire fighter with more than several years of tenure on the job knows personally of at least one brother—or now, sister—fire fighter who died on the job. This cannot be said across the board of any other civilian occupation.

Accidents and Physical Injuries

For many years, the BLS annual survey of workplace lost-time injuries have reported essentially the same distribution of the contributory conditions or manner in which the event occurred, as represented in Table 3 for the over two million cases reported in 1992.

If the public has a negative image about fire fighters, it might be based on their misconception that the fire fighters recklessly and unnecessarily destroy property as they charge into and through a heavily smoking building, smashing windows, ripping walls open, flattening doors, and chopping holes in the roof. This "knock-down" action is an essential part of the fire-fighting strategy for the purpose of venting the buildup of smoke and unburned gases and relieving the enormous pressure from the heated air and gases which would otherwise explode in flame with a backdraft. There are plenty of opportunities to fall or get hit by falling debris, plus all the special hazards of fighting the fire. With respect to the major contribution of overexertion to injuries, it takes a tremendous amount of physical energy for fire fighters just to climb stairs and ladders wearing full gear—helmet, jacket, hood, gloves, pants, and boots—which often weigh about fifty pounds and a respirator with a compressed air cylinder which typically adds another twenty pounds. They do so carrying fully charged hoses and tools into the building or carrying out adult victims on their backs with the added stress of intense heat, poor visibility, and an urgency that allows no rest for up to an hour of maximum exertion that might be required fighting a major fire. That most are able to do so frequently without collapsing attests to their generally good physical condition and endurance, but the overexertion puts them at greater risk of accidental injury from falling or getting cut by glass and, most critically, is the likely trigger for a heart attack waiting to happen.

Table 3. Contributory Conditions in Workplace Injuries, 1992

Contributory Condition	Percent of Total
1. Overexertion	28
2. Contact with objects and equipment	27
3. Falls and slips	18.5
4. Exposure to harmful substances	5
5. Repetitive motion	4
6. Transportation accidents	3
7. Assaults, violent acts by person	1
8. Fires, explosions	0.2

Source: U.S. Bureau of Labor Statistics.

Table 4. Nature of Workplace Injuries, 1992

Nature of Injury	Percent of Total
1. Sprains and strains	44
2. Bruises and contusions	10
3. Cuts and lacerations	7
4. Fractures	6
5. Multiple injuries	3
6. Heat burns	2
7. Carpal tunnel syndrome	1.4

Source: U.S. Bureau of Labor Statistics.

The BLS national surveys indicating the *nature* or type of injuries on the job have reported essentially the same ranking as in previous years except for the recent emergence of carpal tunnel syndrome (Table 4).

The breakdown of the 100,700 fire-fighter injuries from the 1979 NFPA survey reveals much that is similar with the BLS surveys of the private economy and yet distinctive for fire fighting (Table 5). Not surprisingly, the same top four injury categories account for approximately 67 percent, or two out of every three injuries, in both groups.

Fire fighters routinely suffer from all of these injuries with such frequency and intensity that in heavy-duty areas of major cities like the South Bronx in New York City, a physician is on duty at the firehouse during multiple-alarm fires. Burns, thermal stress, and smoke and toxic gas inhalation are especially and disproportionately associated with fire-fighting injuries.

Table 5. Nature of Fire-Fighter Injuries

Nature of Injury	Approximate Percent of Total
1. Sprain, strain, muscular pain	43.5
2. Bruise, wound, cut, bleeding	21.5
3. Smoke or gas inhalation	6.5
4. Eye irritation	6.0
5. Burns (thermal or chemical)	5.5
6. Thermal stress	3.5
7. Dislocation, fracture	3.0
8. Other respiratory distress	1.5
9. Heart attack or stroke	0.5

Source: NFPA 1989 Survey.

Burns

Heat burns account for slightly less than 2 percent of all the disabling injuries in the private sector, which excludes fire fighters, whereas the NFPA surveys of fire departments report that burns constituted almost 6 percent of all fire-fighter injuries. The disparity is even greater considering that the private sector tally by the BLS does not indicate whether the incident took place as the result of a fire. In fact, the burn centers and hospitals, which see the most serious cases, report that most of the occupational burns seen are caused by scalding, such as from hot grease spilled by a restaurant worker, the skin contact of a roofer with molten tar, or electrical burns by electricians.

Yet burns are arguably the most distinctive and severe injury from fighting a fire. Gloves, helmets, and breathing masks are often torn off during the frenzy of the battle, so that hands, face, and the ears, in particular, are frequently singed; embers drop into boots and the back of the neck. Surfaces including concrete floors become so intensely hot during a fire that knee burns result from kneeling and rubber boots are melted. Steam burns are common from the superheating of the water hosed into the building and even the lungs have been seared by the inhalation of superheated air, often with disabling or fatal consequences.

Fire fighters consistently and disproportionately incur more burns, and with more *serious* and often fatal outcomes, than any other job category based on the number of cases logged at the hospital burn centers. One such center in California noted in a study of 232 occupational burns over five years that in terms of severity, flame-related burns affected the highest average body surface area and specifically cited fire fighters among the most prevalent "occupational" cases.

Thermal Stress

The thermal stress category includes the health effects from exposure to extreme heat and cold, although with fire fighting we understandably concentrate on the former.

Harry Truman's admonition, "If you can't stand the heat, get out of the kitchen," is gratuitous advice to fire fighters. They not only *must* remain in the intense heat as an inherent part of the job but they cannot even exercise the option to rest in a cool spot available to most industry workers in hot jobs. Actually, Mr. Truman was referring to the inability of some people to make a decision under pressure, but that, of course, applies equally well to fire fighters. In most cases, excessive heat exposure will cause weakness, disorientation, and fainting; occasionally, the body temperature of a particularly susceptible individual will rise excessively due to a failure of the thermoregulatory mechanism to produce sweating and, if unattended immediately, he or she will often succumb from a fatal heat stroke.

Most healthy workers can function at a hot job without adverse health effects as long as their deep body temperatures are maintained below a maximum of about 38°C (100.4°F). Since hygienists cannot conveniently measure the worker's deep body temperature during work, the allowable limits or TLVs for heat stress incorporate surrogate environmental measurements and estimates of the total heat load on the worker's body that can be correlated with the *expected* physiological response. If these measurements indicate an excessive exposure, the hygienists can recommend rest periods during the hour, drinking more fluids, or cooling of the workplace to help prevent heat exhaustion. As indicated, all of these measures are largely academic considerations with respect to the control of heat stress during fire fighting. The use of relief fire-fighting teams in multiple alarm fires could reduce the individual heat stress load. However, the firefighters sometimes have a false sense of the heat stress because the airflow from their pressure-demand respirators has a cooling effect on the face. It should come as no surprise that thermal stress accounts for about 3.5 percent of all fire-fighter injuries, whereas it is relatively rare in the general work force.

Not all fire fighters have had serious problems with heat inside a burning structure. One veteran city fire fighter in Philadelphia reported that his singular experience with heat stress happened when as a probationary in full uniform, he had to perform all the outside gofer activities at a row house fire during an exceptionally hot August day. He collapsed from heat exhaustion and fell from a ladder while delivering a tool requested by a fire fighter, without ever having entered the burning building.

During severe winter weather, there are often chilling pictures in the newspapers and on television of fire fighters standing by water valves and pipes that are coated with ice and icicles formed from the flood of water and spray. Injuries from dry and wet cold exposures are less frequent than from heat stress because the fire fighters are protected with waterproof and warm clothing and gloves. However, the fire chief of a volunteer company reported that he almost lost the tips of three fingers from frostbite while supervising a difficult and lengthy fire during an unusually frigid and windy night. He confessed that in his zeal he simply forgot to wear gloves.

Smoke and Toxic Gas Inhalations

Acute Exposures

Industrial hygienists have become very adept at characterizing the expected range of airborne exposures for many job categories and operations based on having performed extensive industrial hygiene monitoring including lots of personal sampling. Fire fighting does not lend itself to that kind of analysis for a variety of reasons, starting with the practical difficulty of getting reliable personal samples under live fire-fighting conditions. Then, analogous to Tolstoy's description of unhappy families, each fire-fighting event is unhappy, unpredictable, and unrepeatable in its own way. Notwithstanding all the variables in the specific exposures, we have enough general information on the presence and concentrations of the main airborne contaminants during a fire to characterize the prospective health hazards. There is simply no other job in which exposures to excessive and lethal concentrations of smoke and toxic air contaminants are routinely and regularly faced as in fire fighting.

Fire fighters should—but do not always—wear operative self-contained breathing apparatus (SCBA) when they enter the fire ground. The smoke is a suspension in the air of a complex mixture of extremely tiny solid and liquid particles and toxic gases that form from the combustion of a carbon-containing fuel. It is acrid in smell, severely irritating to the eyes, and breathing it in heavy concentrations is choking, asphyxiating, and ultimately can be lethal. The lethality is underscored by the estimate that smoke inhalation is responsible for four out of five civilian fire deaths. In 1993, smoke and combustion gases accounted for about 5 percent of the firefighter deaths by asphyxiation and about 15 percent of the related injuries—namely, eye irritation, respiratory distress, and smoke and gas inhalation. Apart from the inhalation hazards, the smoke can be so dense and blinding that in tearing through the blackness of a heavily smoldering house, the fire fighters can easily get disoriented and sometimes by taking a strange turn, they have to find their way out of a closet.

Representative airborne measurements of individual combustion products in fires indicate why breathing the atmosphere without protection can be lethal. For example, carbon monoxide (CO) which is always present in fire atmospheres was found in several industrial hygiene studies of structural fires to be present in average concentrations up to 1450 ppm with a maximum of 27,000 ppm. A NIOSH survey of the CO exposure levels of fire fighters during the initial "knockdown" phase of fire fighting found that 10 percent of the personal samples exceeded 1500 ppm. For reference, a brief exposure to 1500 ppm of CO is considered to be immediately dangerous to life and health (IDLH). Using the CO levels alone to represent the hazards of breathing a smoky fire atmosphere understates the risk.

For one, the fire atmosphere will rapidly become deficient in oxygen and high in asphyxiating carbon dioxide, which is produced in huge quantities by the combustion. Second, the inhaled micron-sized smoke particles deposit in the respiratory tract and penetrate into the lungs, where they cause severe pulmonary distress and tissue damage while carrying other adsorbed toxic combustion gases. Finally, we would expect both independent and synergistic effects from these many other toxic components present. Some of these gases have been reported by researchers to occur at maximum concentrations in a fire well above the IDLH (Table 6).

Other combustion products reported at significantly toxic levels in fires include benzene, nitrogen dioxide, phosgene, sulfur dioxide, sulfuric acid, hydrogen fluoride, formaldehyde, and ammonia.

Chronic Exposures and Long-Term Health Effects

Fire fighters have expressed realistic and fatalistic perceptions of their immediate fate as conveyed in the sign in some firehouses announcing "This Could Be The Night." Perhaps, because long-term health effects from the job do not pose an immediate threat to their ability to continue doing what they love to do, these are not uppermost in their thoughts. However, many career fire fighters believe from personal observations and anecdotal reports that they do not live as long in retirement and more of them die from cancer and heart and lung disease than other people.

Physicians have been able to relate to some degree the effects of smoke inhalation immediately following a fire to changes in the fire-fighters' lung function tests. In studies on sixty fire fighters from Pittsburgh with normal preexposure lung function, twenty-two who later had symptoms were tested and found to have decreased lung function. A somewhat similar investigation of thirty-seven fire fighters in Buffalo, New York, responding to fourteen fire calls over a ten-day period pointedly showed significant lung function changes only in those fire fighters who did not wear their respiratory equipment. Another study of sixty-three forest fire fighters in the western United States, who do not regularly wear respiratory protection, revealed that there was universally a significant postseason loss of lung function and increase in airway responsiveness.

Apart from the acute respiratory and toxic effects from the inhalation of combustion products, there have been indications of delayed adverse health effects, particularly from chemical fires. Fourteen firefighters engaged in a transformer

Table 6. Maximum Reported Concentration and Source of Selected Toxic Combustion Products

Toxic Component	Burning Materials	IDLH (ppm)	Max. Concentration in Fires (ppm)
Acrolein	Wood, cotton	5	98
Hydrogen chloride	Polyvinyl chloride, chlorinated plastics	100	280
Hydrogen cyanide	Polyurethane, silk, wool	50	75

fire containing polychlorinated biphenyls (PCBs) showed neurophysiological and psychological effects, including significant impairment of memory more than six months later. Understandably, one of the admitted fears of generally fearless fire fighters is that of a fire involving "hazmats" (hazardous materials), particularly of unknown chemicals.

Occupational health researchers have investigated the suspected association of cancer and other chronic diseases in fire fighters that could result from their ongoing occupational exposures to carcinogenic combustion products such as the polycyclic aromatic hydrocarbons (PAHs) in soot and smoke and other chemicals. As is often the case with studies relating mortality experience to occupation, the answers depend on the choice of studies and the numbers of the cases and populations covered. So said, two independent long-term mortality studies of 7874 urban fighters in the United States and Canada agreed that firefighters actually live longer than the expectation for the general population. One explanation is that in order to be selected and remain a fire fighter, one has to be in good physical and mental condition, whereas the general population is, by comparison, less healthy. The U.S. study also found that their fire fighters had higher life expectancy compared with police officers who have similar physical qualifications but no occupational exposure to smoke. Both studies also concurred that the rates of heart disease and chronic respiratory diseases were also lower or about the same as expected, with the exception of a slightly higher incidence of emphysema among the U.S. group. Cancer was another story.

If *all* types of cancers are considered—meaning the nonmalignant and malignant forms—fire fighters experience no excess, but both the Americans and the Canadians report significantly higher incidence rates with malignant cancers. In particular, the incidence of lymphatic cancers and leukemia are well above normal, but there are anomalies. Canadian fire fighters are reported to die from *all* types of malignant tumors in greater proportions, with particularly high excesses with cancers of the kidney and urinary tract. Across the border, U.S. fire fighters are reported to experience a very low incidence of bladder and urinary tract, but unusually high numbers of brain and nervous system, tumors and cancer. Contrary to expectations for an occupation with regular exposures to smoke and airborne carcinogens *and* with a high percentage of cigarette smokers, the U.S. fire fighters do not show an excess incidence of lung cancer; the Canadian group, drawn from smaller numbers, experience an underwhelming excess. On balance, after a career as a fire fighter, there are very likely greater risks of dying from cancer.

Many other studies of the occupational exposures of fire fighters have been made, many of which might seem significant in any other job but are somewhat muted relative to the major hazards of the job. For example, the short but intense noise exposure from the sirens is largely believed to be responsible for some hearing loss seen among many fire fighters.

An Extended Family at Work

Because of their unusual work shifts and organization, career fire fighters are distinctive among workers—on land, at least—in that they work and, in a sense, live together. Furthermore, they share a loyalty and bonding in an extended family at work that is in sharp contrast to the increasing sense of isolation expressed by many contemporary workers. Their customary work shifts may be twenty-four hours followed by forty-eight hours off, or some variation involving one long shift with sleep-in time. In Philadelphia, it is two ten-hour day shifts followed by two fourteen-hour evening shifts with the next four days off. Due to their rotating work shifts, they forego a normal family life and social calendar, but as much for keeping busy as well as for extra income, most work at a flexible part-time job or operate a business in their time off.

Their organization in tightly knit squads (usually designated A, B, C, and D) which rotate as a unit throughout the week foments a bond of togetherness. They know in responding to an alarm that the life of each fire fighter is dependent on the utmost support and trust of their fellow fire fighters that transcends any differences in personality or race or sex. Their sense of identity with an empathy to all fire fighters extends outside their own fire house. Members of fire departments from over the country will attend the funeral of little-known fellow members they have never met who have died in the line of duty.

There are some unique aspects of life in the firehouse that have both positive and negative effects on their health and well-being. According to their own words, fire fighters are largely a contented and proud group. They have exceptionally low absenteeism, relatively few problems with alcoholism and drug abuse, tend to be family oriented, and enjoy generally good physical health as reflected in their vital statistics.

With heart attacks and stroke promoted by overexertion as the principal causes of on-duty deaths, preventive programs in many departments have been directed at maintaining desirable body weight, physical exercise, smoking cessation, and reducing stress. These goals are somewhat compromised by life in the firehouse. In a chore-sharing family-style life, enjoying high-calorie "hearty" meals prepared by their more culinary-gifted members may be no blessing. Rather, it frequently accounts for excess poundage, particularly among the more senior members, than can be compensated for by a sometime workout on the exercise units provided in each firehouse. When educational persuasion was unavailing in getting some members to reduce, one city fire department stipulated maximum weights for promotion with a grace period allowed for provisional appointees to meet the requirements.

The sight of an exhausted and sooty fire fighter drawing deeply on a cigarette after a battle in heavy smoke might appall the Lung Association and the American Cancer Society, but smoking-cessation programs have not made much headway. Possibly because of the inherent stress in anticipating and fighting a fire, it is estimated that about half of all city fire fighters seek relaxation in smoking, or more than twice the percentage of smokers in the adult population. A graduate industrial hygiene student aware of their dedication to their work undertook a program to convince a group of Philadelphia fire fighters to quit smoking by carefully explaining the adverse effects of the carbon monoxide in the inhaled cigarette smoke on their blood vessels and vital oxygen supply. Were they willing to stop smoking if it was demonstrated that it could contribute to a heart attack or, at least, seriously impair their ability to do their job? In a feat of instrumental black magic, she identified the smokers in the group by demonstrating that the residual CO in their breath samples alone—hours after their last smoke—caused a direct-reading CO instrument to rise to the top of the scale. They seemed impressed and some even said they would think about quitting.

A Career Not a Job

In 1993, there were 185,000 nominally full-time paid fire fighters and 18,000 fire inspectors, or fire marshals, and fire prevention professionals, according to the U.S. Bureau of Labor Statistics. There are severalfold that number of highly trained and well-equipped volunteer fire fighters to service the suburban developments and small towns without local public fire departments and those who respond part-time, as required, on board ships and aircraft, and in the military and in industry.

The applicant for the full-time career positions must meet rigorous physical requirements, pass a stiff written examination, sometimes with a screening interview, and then compete with other successful applicants for the limited openings. The larger governmental fire departments maintain their own training facilities which commonly provide as much as thirteen weeks of practical exercises and classroom lectures for the recruit, who remains on probation for six months. Supplementary training is ongoing for all fire fighters and many are sent to the National Fire Academy in Emmitsburg, Maryland, for either basic or specialized training. Courses and associate degrees in fire science are offered at hundreds of community and junior colleges and there are a few four-year degree college programs in fire protection and fire service management.

Most career fire fighters can retire at half-pay with twenty years of service, but many elect to stay on. A congressional proposal in 1995 to allow police and fire departments to force retirement at age 55 and older is strongly opposed by the rank and file even though most have retired by then. Unlike the fellow protective police services in which women have made significant inroads, the formerly designated occupation of fire*man* is still largely male dominated, with women accounting for less than 2 percent of total employed fire fighters.

Many senior veterans can recall childhood expressions of wanting to be a fireman—few young girls of that era considered the option—but the reasons for the eventual career choice are varied and less fanciful. For many, there were and still are practical reasons based on economics and security. When New York City and many of the large cities were largely settled by European immigrants, getting a job with the city government represented security and status, so a young Italian or Irish boy with limited education regarded a job as a fireman or a policeman as reaching the top of the heap. It then became traditional in many families of fire fighters for the sons to follow in their fathers' bootsteps, which to the outsider might seem to be a manifestation of hereditary madness. One fire captain of more than twenty-two years service in a midwestern city fire department admitted that he actually did chase fire engines as a kid and, although no one in his family had ever been a fire fighter, he never seriously considered any other work.

Many freely admit they get their "highs" from the excitement and challenge in putting out fires. How else does one explain the attraction of the many men and women otherwise employed as engineers, accountants, business people, dentists, teachers, students, and plumbers, among others, who staff the volunteer fire houses around the country? Part of the initial attraction may relate back to the mystique that fire created among primordial man, but it takes a very strong commitment for someone to accept facing death and danger so consistently at their work.

The fire fighters themselves explain it in words that are disarmingly heroic in their simplicity and honesty. In the final interview in Studs Terkel's book *Working*, a fire fighter reflecting on his career recounts tersely that, "I helped put out a fire. I helped save somebody. It shows something I did on this earth."

Index